Functional Bio-based Materials for Regenerative Medicine: From Bench to Bedside (Part 2)

Edited by

Mohd Fauzi Mh Busra

Centre for Tissue Engineering and Regenerative Medicine (CTERM)
Faculty of Medicine, Universiti Kebangsaan Malaysia, Jalan Yaacob Latif
Bandar Tun Razak, 56000 Cheras
Kuala Lumpur,
Malaysia

Daniel Law Jia Xian

Centre for Tissue Engineering and Regenerative Medicine (CTERM)
Faculty of Medicine, Universiti Kebangsaan Malaysia, 56000 Cheras
Kuala Lumpur,
Malaysia

Yogeswaran Lokanathan

Centre for Tissue Engineering and Regenerative Medicine (CTERM)
Faculty of Medicine, Universiti Kebangsaan Malaysia, Jalan

Yaacob Latif
Bandar Tun Razak, 56000 Cheras
Kuala Lumpur,
Malaysia

&

Ruszymah Haji Idrus

Centre for Tissue Engineering and Regenerative Medicine
(CTERM)
Faculty of Medicine Universiti Kebangsaan Malaysia Jalan
Yaacob Latif, Bandar Tun Razak, 56000 Cheras
Kuala Lumpur,
Malaysia

Functional Bio-based Materials for Regenerative Medicine: From Bench to Bedside (Part 2)

Editors: Mohd Fauzi Mh Busra, Daniel Law Jia Xian, Yogeswaran Lokanathan and

Ruszymah Haji Idrus

ISBN (Online): 978-981-5179-33-0

ISBN (Print): 978-981-5179-34-7

ISBN (Paperback): 978-981-5179-35-4

need for a court order if at any point you breach any terms of this License Agreement. In no event will any delay or failure by Bentham Science Publishers in enforcing your compliance with this License Agreement constitute a waiver of any of its rights.

3. You acknowledge that you have read this License Agreement, and agree to be bound by its terms and conditions. To the extent that any other terms and conditions presented on any website of Bentham Science Publishers conflict with, or are inconsistent with, the terms and conditions set out in this License Agreement, you acknowledge that the terms and conditions set out in this License Agreement shall prevail.

Bentham Science Publishers Pte. Ltd.
80 Robinson Road #02-00
Singapore 068898
Singapore
Email: subscriptions@benthamscience.net

BENTHAM SCIENCE

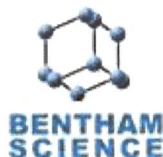

CONTENTS

PREFACE I

I would like to congratulate all the authors who took their valuable time to contribute to the book titled "FUNCTIONAL BIO-BASED MATERIALS FOR REGENERATIVE MEDICINE from Bench to Bedside". This book is a dedication to the founder of the Centre for Tissue Engineering and Regenerative Medicine (CTERM), University Kebangsaan Malaysia, Prof. Dato' Dr Ruszymah Hj. Idrus. It has been an honour to have been under her supervision and now expanding on our own across the continents through collaborating with talented, hardworking scientists in the tissue engineering and regenerative medicine field on various state-of-the-art technologies and biobased materials used for the tissue-engineered skin, bone, heart, respiratory tract and other vital organs.

In this marvellously insightful book, the authors offer some valuable strategies, technologies and artificial intelligence in the established technology covering tissue engineering as an essential field for various health applications to help not only scientists, researchers and healthcare providers but also the general public to remain updated with the current work happening worldwide.

Mohd Fauzi Mh Busra
Centre for Tissue Engineering and Regenerative Medicine (CTERM)
Faculty of Medicine, Universiti Kebangsaan Malaysia, Jalan Yaacob Latif
Bandar Tun Razak, 56000 Cheras
Kuala Lumpur,
Malaysia

Daniel Law Jia Xian
Centre for Tissue Engineering and Regenerative Medicine (CTERM)
Faculty of Medicine, Universiti Kebangsaan Malaysia, 56000 Cheras
Kuala Lumpur,
Malaysia

Yogeswaran Lokanathan
Centre for Tissue Engineering and Regenerative Medicine (CTERM)
Faculty of Medicine, Universiti Kebangsaan Malaysia, Jalan Yaacob Latif
Bandar Tun Razak, 56000 Cheras
Kuala Lumpur,
Malaysia

&

Ruszymah Haji Idrus
Centre for Tissue Engineering and Regenerative Medicine (CTERM)
Faculty of Medicine Universiti Kebangsaan Malaysia Jalan
Yaacob Latif, Bandar Tun Razak, 56000 Cheras
Kuala Lumpur,
Malaysia

PREFACE II

The regenerative medicine is currently an established technology, covering tissue engineering as a significant field in various health applications. Traditionally, tissue engineering is a combination of cells, biomaterials, and biomolecules to replace or repair damaged tissues. The current advanced technology in the tissue engineering field focuses on the functionalisation of invented bio-based materials. It includes the development of a hybrid or composite biomatrix together with cells-secreted products and related active compounds for better performance in enhancing the rapid therapeutic mechanism. The mode of action for the invented product depends on its formulation or a three-dimensional design of the biomatrix.

This book provides detailed information on the latest advancements in bio-based materials treatment strategy for various tissue applications, encompassing skin, bone, heart, respiratory tract and other vital organs. This is followed by future perspectives on the new emerging treatment in the field of tissue engineering and regenerative medicine.

Mohd Fauzi Mh Busra
Centre for Tissue Engineering and Regenerative Medicine (CTERM)
Faculty of Medicine, Universiti Kebangsaan Malaysia, Jalan Yaacob Latif
Bandar Tun Razak, 56000 Cheras
Kuala Lumpur,
Malaysia

Daniel Law Jia Xian
Centre for Tissue Engineering and Regenerative Medicine (CTERM)
Faculty of Medicine, Universiti Kebangsaan Malaysia, 56000 Cheras
Kuala Lumpur,
Malaysia

Yogeswaran Lokanathan
Centre for Tissue Engineering and Regenerative Medicine (CTERM)
Faculty of Medicine, Universiti Kebangsaan Malaysia, Jalan Yaacob Latif
Bandar Tun Razak, 56000 Cheras
Kuala Lumpur,
Malaysia

&

Ruszymah Haji Idrus
Centre for Tissue Engineering and Regenerative Medicine (CTERM)
Faculty of Medicine Universiti Kebangsaan Malaysia Jalan
Yaacob Latif, Bandar Tun Razak, 56000 Cheras
Kuala Lumpur,
Malaysia

List of Contributors

Abdul Manaf Abdullah	School of Mechanical Engineering, College of Engineering, Universiti Teknologi Mara, 40450 Shah Alam, Selangor, Malaysia
Asma Abdullah Nurul	School of Health Sciences, Universiti Sains Malaysia, 16150 Kubang Kerian, Kelantan, Malaysia
Anton Kusumo Widagdo	Indramayu Indramayu Bhayangkara Hospital, Indonesian National Police, Jawa Barat, Indonesia
Ahmad Syaify	Department of Periodontology, Faculty of Dentistry, Universitas Gadjah Mada, Yogyakarta, Indonesia
Antonella Motta	Biotech Research Center, Department of Industrial Engineering, University of Trento, Mattarello (TN), Italy
Akib Jabed	Department of Materials Science and Engineering, Rajshahi University of Engineering and Technology (RUET), Rajshahi, Bangladesh
Bakiah Shaharuddin	Regenerative Medicine Cluster, Advanced Medical and Dental Institute, Universiti Sains Malaysia, Bertam, Kepala Batas, Pulau Pinang, Malaysia
Dasmawati Mohamad	School of Dental Sciences, Health Campus, Universiti Sains Malaysia, 16150 Kubang Kerian, Kelantan, Malaysia
Fan Ying Zhen	School of Health Sciences, Universiti Sains Malaysia, Kubang Kerian, Kelantan, Malaysia
Francesca Agostinacchio	University of Trento, Department of Industrial Engineering, via Sommarive 9, Trento (TN), Italy and BIOtech Research Center – Center for Biomedical Technologies, via delle Regole 101, Mattarello (TN), Italy
Genieve Ee Chia Yeo	Centre for Tissue Engineering and Regenerative Medicine, Faculty of Medicine, Universiti Kebangsaan Malaysia, Cheras, Kuala Lumpur, Malaysia
Hasan Subhi Azeez	School of Dental Sciences, Universiti Sains Malaysia, Kubang Kerian, Kelantan, Malaysia
Heng J. Wei	Centre for Tissue Engineering and Regenerative Medicine, Faculty of Medicine, Universiti Kebangsaan Malaysia, Cheras, Kuala Lumpur, Malaysia
Ishak Ahmad	Department of Chemical Sciences, Faculty of Science and Technology, Universiti Kebangsaan Malaysia (UKM), Bangi Selangor, Malaysia
Jia Xian Law	Centre for Tissue Engineering and Regenerative Medicine, Faculty of Medicine, Universiti Kebangsaan Malaysia, Cheras, Kuala Lumpur, Malaysia
Jun W. Heng	Centre for Tissue Engineering and Regenerative Medicine, Faculty of Medicine, Universiti Kebangsaan Malaysia, 56000, Cheras, Kuala Lumpur, Malaysia
Kok-Lun Pang	Department of Pharmacology, Faculty of Medicine, Universiti Kebangsaan Malaysia, Cheras, Kuala Lumpur, Malaysia
Kok-Yong Chin	Department of Pharmacology, Faculty of Medicine, Universiti Kebangsaan Malaysia, Cheras, Kuala Lumpur, Malaysia
Lim Wei Lee	Centre for Tissue Engineering and Regenerative Medicine, Faculty of Medicine, Universiti Kebangsaan Malaysia, Cheras, Kuala Lumpur, Malaysia

Marzuki Omar	School of Dental Sciences, Health Campus, Universiti Sains Malaysia, 16150 Kubang Kerian, Kelantan, Malaysia
Min Hwei Ng	Centre for Tissue Engineering and Regenerative Medicine, Faculty of Medicine, Universiti Kebangsaan Malaysia, Cheras, Kuala Lumpur, Malaysia
Mohd Nor Ridzuan Abd Mutalib	School of Health Sciences, Universiti Sains Malaysia, Kubang Kerian, Kelantan, Malaysia
Mohamed Salih	Regenerative Medicine Cluster, Advanced Medical and Dental Institute, Universiti Sains Malaysia, Bertam, Kepala Batas, Pulau Pinang, Malaysia
Mohd Reusmaazran bin Yusof	Material Technology Group, Agensi Nuclear Malaysia, Bangi, Selangor, Malaysia
Maliha Rahman	Department of Materials Science and Engineering, Rajshahi University of Engineering and Technology (RUET), Rajshahi, Bangladesh
Md Enamul Hoque	Department of Biomedical Engineering, Military Institute of Science and Technology (MIST), Dhaka, Bangladesh
Mohamad Fikeri Ishak	Centre for Tissue Engineering and Regenerative Medicine, Faculty of Medicine, Universiti Kebangsaan Malaysia, Cheras, Kuala Lumpur, Malaysia
Norazlina Mohamed	Department of Pharmacology, Faculty of Medicine, Universiti Kebangsaan Malaysia, Cheras, Kuala Lumpur, Malaysia
Nur Atiqah Haron	Centre for Tissue Engineering and Regenerative Medicine, Faculty of Medicine, Universiti Kebangsaan Malaysia, Cheras, Kuala Lumpur, Malaysia
Nadiah Sulaiman	Centre for Tissue Engineering and Regenerative Medicine, Faculty of Medicine, Universiti Kebangsaan Malaysia, Cheras, Kuala Lumpur, Malaysia
Osa Amila Hafiyyah	Department of Periodontology, Faculty of Dentistry, Universitas Gadjah Mada, Yogyakarta, Indonesia
Renatha Jiffrin	Bio Inspired Device and Tissue Engineering Research Group, School of Biomedical Engineering and Health Science, Faculty of Engineering, Universiti Teknologi Malaysia, Skudai, Johor, Malaysia
Rohaina C. Man	Department of Pathology, Faculty of Medicine, Universiti Kebangsaan Malaysia, Cheras, Kuala Lumpur, Malaysia
Retno Ardhani	Department of Dental Biomedical Sciences, , Indonesia, Faculty of Dentistry, Universitas Gadjah, Yogyakarta, Indonesia Centre for Tissue Engineering and Regenerative Medicine, Faculty of Medicine, Universiti Kebangsaan Malaysia, Cheras, Kuala Lumpur, Malaysia
Saiful Izwan Abd. Razak	Bio Inspired Device and Tissue Engineering Research Group, School of Biomedical Engineering and Health Science, Faculty of Engineering, Universiti Teknologi Malaysia, Skudai, Johor, Malaysia
Sophia Ogechi Ekeuku	Department of Pharmacology, Faculty of Medicine, Universiti Kebangsaan Malaysia, Cheras, Kuala Lumpur, Malaysia
Tamrin Nuge	Department of Mechanical, Materials and Manufacturing Engineering, Faculty of Science and Engineering, University of Nottingham Ningbo China, 199 Taikang East Road, Ningbo315100, China

Ubashini Vijakumaran Centre for Tissue Engineering and Regenerative Medicine, Faculty of Medicine, Universiti Kebangsaan Malaysia, Cheras, Kuala Lumpur, Malaysia

Wan Hafizi Wan Ishak Department of Chemical Sciences, Faculty of Science and Technology, Universiti Kebangsaan Malaysia (UKM), Bangi Selangor, Malaysia

Wan Kartini binti Wan Abdul Khodir Department of Chemistry, Kulliyyah of Science, International Islamic University Malaysia Kuantan Campus, Bandar Indera Mahkota, Kuantan, Pahang, Malaysia
SYNTOF, Kulliyyah of Science, International Islamic University Malaysia Kuantan Campus, Bandar Indera Mahkota, Kuantan, Pahang, Malaysia

Xiaoling Liu Advanced Polymer Composite Group, Faculty of Science and Engineering, University of Nottingham Ningbo China, 199 Taikang East Road, Ningbo315100, China

Yogeswaran Lokanathan Centre for Tissue Engineering and Regenerative Medicine (CTERM), Faculty of Medicine, Universiti Kebangsaan Malaysia, Jalan Yaacob Latif Bandar Tun Razak, 56000 Cheras, Kuala Lumpur, Malaysia

Zahra Rashidbenam Centre for Tissue Engineering and Regenerative Medicine, Faculty of Medicine, Universiti Kebangsaan Malaysia, Cheras, Kuala Lumpur, Malaysia

CHAPTER 1

Recent Advancement on Polyamide Composites as an Alloplastic Alternative in 3D Printing for Craniofacial Reconstruction

Abdul Manaf Abdullah[1], Marzuki Omar[2] and Dasmawati Mohamad[2,*]

[1] *School of Mechanical Engineering, College of Engineering, Universiti Teknologi Mara, 40450 Shah Alam, Selangor, Malaysia*

[2] *School of Dental Sciences, Health Campus, Universiti Sains Malaysia, 16150 Kubang Kerian, Kelantan, Malaysia*

Abstract: Polymer-based biomaterials are a material of choice for many surgeons due to their availability and durability. Many types are available on the market, but the search for improved properties to cater to technology demands, such as 3D printing, continues. Polyamide, to be used as an alternative in craniofacial reconstruction, has been a subject of interest recently. This chapter explores the physical and mechanical properties of polyamide composites fabricated *via* injection moulding and 3D printing techniques along with their biocompatibility. With promising physical, mechanical, and biocompatibility properties, polyamide composites are expected to emerge as an alternative biomaterial for craniofacial reconstruction soon.

Keywords: 3D printing, Craniofacial reconstruction, Polyamide composites.

INTRODUCTION OF BIOMATERIALS

Biomaterials are natural or synthetic materials used for implantation in the human body. They are designed to be able to adapt and function in a biological environment. A biomaterial should possess adequate mechanical characteristics, have a surface texture that supports adhesion, and be biocompatible and reproducible [1].

Biomaterials for implantation purposes can be divided into natural and synthetic materials. The classifications of biomaterials are shown in Fig. (**1**). Natural implant materials consist of autograft, allograft, and xenograft. Grafts, such as the cornea, skin, nerve, muscle, *etc.*, depend on donor availability, which limits their

---

* **Corresponding author Dasmawati Mohamad:** School of Dental Sciences, Health Campus, Universiti Sains Malaysia, 16150 Kubang Kerian, Kelantan, Malaysia; E-mail: dasmawati@usm.my

Mohd Fauzi Mh Busra, Daniel Law Jia Xian, Yogeswaran Lokanathan and Ruszymah Haji Idrus (Eds.)

application Despite providing similar mechanical properties and being compatible with the receiver, pre-treatment, such as preservation and sterilisation, are a serious issue that needs to be considered to prevent complications [2].

Synthetic biomaterials or alloplastics are classified as metallic, polymeric, ceramic, and composite materials. In craniofacial reconstruction, metallic materials are widely used due to their high strength and ability to maintain shape. Polymeric materials are becoming popular due to their desirable properties, composition, and easy processing. However, their flexibility and lack of mechanical properties limit their application. Polymers can be divided into two categories, namely resorbable and non-resorbable. Resorbable polymers are mainly made from natural sources, such as cellulose, chitosan, collagen, and starch. Sometimes, extracted starch and cellulose are blended with synthetic polymers to make them resorbable. Non-resorbable polymers are made from long repetitions of hydrogen and carbon atom chains that produce strong molecule bonds.

Meanwhile, ceramics are well-known for their biocompatibility, brittleness, and difficult fabrication that limits their manipulation. Ceramics are classified into three different groups, namely bioinert, bioactive, and bioresorbable [3]. A mixture of the aforementioned materials and composites appears to be a likely prospect to enter the biomaterials field, as they possess the blended properties of those materials - even though the processing method needs to be addressed.

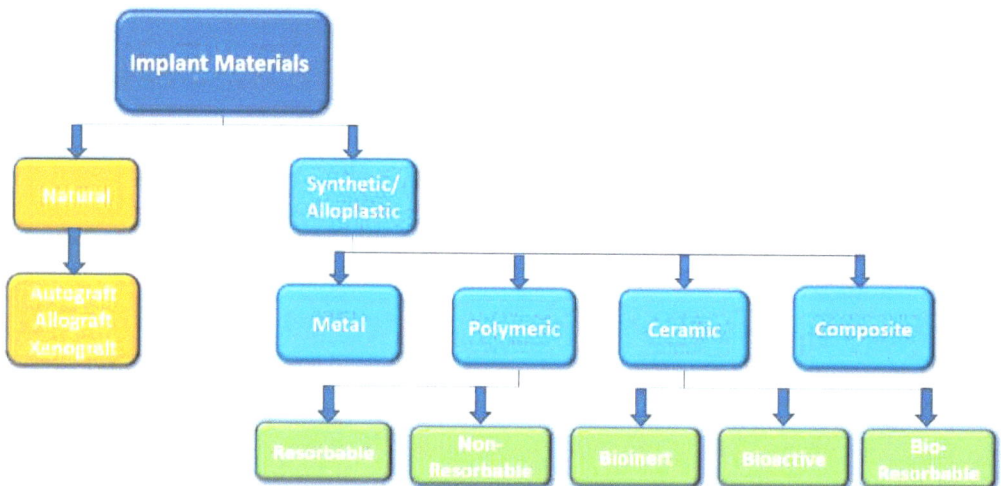

Fig. (1). Classification of biomaterials.

POLYMERIC MATERIALS

Polymeric materials, such as polymethyl methacrylate (PMMA) are the most common material for craniofacial bone reconstruction (4). They have excellent properties, such as biocompatibility, biological inertness, and rigidity, and are widely used to repair craniofacial anomalies. PMMA usually comes with a packaging set of powder and liquid. The powder component contains PMMA polymer and benzoyl peroxide (BPO), whereas the liquid consists of methyl methacrylate (MMA) monomer, N, N-Dimethyl-p-toluidine (DMPT), which acts as activator and hydroquinone to stabilise the liquid monomer. DMPT initially decomposes the BPO. Free radical molecules result from the decomposition during the polymerisation process. Mixing these two components, as instructed by the supplier, will result in polymerisation. Although PMMA offers ease of handling, its brittleness, shrinkage, and heat release, due to exothermic reaction during polymerisation, may damage surrounding tissue. Furthermore, the temperature inside PMMA, with the adjacent tissue exposed, may reach a maximum of 50°C. Therefore, preoperative implant preparation is highly recommended [5].

Porous polyethylene (PE) is widely used by surgeons as it is well tolerated by surrounding tissue, and the porous structure allows for fibrovascular ingrowth that promotes biological fixation. However, PE available on the market, such as Medpor, comes in a standard shape. Therefore, needs to be trimmed and moulded manually prior to the implant placement, thus increasing the operating time [6].

The polymeric material that is currently getting attention from surgeons and researchers is polyether ether ketone (PEEK). PEEK possesses excellent mechanical properties that are said to be comparable with cortical bone [7]. However, this material lacks osteointegration properties, which leads to various complications, such as infection and implant loss [8]. Furthermore, the melting point of PEEK is around 343°C, which can therefore only be processed by a high-end polymer processing machine equipped with high heating capabilities, such as selective laser sintering (SLS). Though exclusive and expensive in nature, the introduction of PEEK as a patient-specific implant (PSI), processed *via* current additive manufacturing (AM) techniques, has helped patients with craniofacial anomalies to regain their regular cosmesis [9]. PSI is designed to fit each patient or is customised by utilising the patient's CT scan data.

POLYAMIDE

Polyamide (PA), also known as nylon, consists of repeating units of amide –CO-NH– linkages. PA is formed by the polycondensation of a diacid with a diamine or by ring-opening polymerisation of lactams with 6, 11, or 12 carbon atoms. PA generally exhibits good mechanical properties and chemical resistance. Most importantly, PA is biocompatible and can be easily contoured and sutured. PA also enhances the growth of fibrous tissue and has been successfully used as an orbital floor implant. Moreover, it has been used to produce skull model pre-surgical planning and young surgeon training [10]. The hygroscopic factor makes PA not durable, so certain materials need to be incorporated to tailor the properties.

Extensive research has been carried out to tailor the property incorporation of bioactive materials to simultaneously create a new value-added material. For example, PA 6,6 has been incorporated with 65wt% of nano-hydroxyapatite (n-HA) to show remarkable moulded tensile properties, with a tensile strength of 87 MPa [11]. This newly blended material has proved biocompatible, showing a non-cytotoxic effect when cultured with mesenchymal stem cells (MSCs) [12]. The material was successfully implanted in a patient in China to construct the condylar *via*SLS (Li *et al.*, 2011), thus indicating its potential as an alternative implantation material. However, evaluation with more patients and a longer follow-up is necessary.

Polyamide 12 (PA 12) is another type of polyamide that is gaining attention for its easy processing. It possesses a low melting temperature and high flowability. PA 12 can be prepared from lauryl lactam [13] and aminolauric acid [14]. PA 12 is the current material of choice for selective laser sintering (SLS) due to its relatively lower cost than PEEK. High flowability properties make it appropriate for the SLS process. Although prominent in the SLS segment, SLS-graded PA 12 is never applied to other processing methods. Current manufacturers of PA 12 include 3D Systems and EOS, which supply PA 12 using the commercial names Duraform® and PA2200, respectively [15]. Production of Duraform® and PA2200 is dedicated to their SLS machine. Investigation of the tensile properties of specimens produced by these materials revealed that specimens using PA2200 produced higher tensile properties than specimens of Duraform® [16]. Since the introduction of polyamide 6,6 (PA 6,6) by Carothers in 1934, various types of polyamides have been developed and commercialised. Details of currently available PA, their properties, and repeating units of molecular structure are summarised in Table **1**. The polar molecular (-CO- NH-) structure in the polyamide chain incidentally mimics the structure of collagen [17], an essential factor that promotes osteoblast. Therefore, this collagen mimicked structure could be manipulated by introducing PA as a potential biomaterial for craniofacial reconstruction.

Table 1. Aliphatic polyamides and their monomers.

Polyamide	Monomer(s)	Molecular Structure
Polyamide 6	Caprolactam	
Polyamide 6,6	Hexamethylene Diamine/Adipic Acid	
Polyamide 12	Lauralactam	

PROPERTIES OF PA AND COMPOSITES

This section discusses the physical, mechanical, and biocompatibility properties of PA and composites. The presence of filler mainly affects these properties. The incorporation of ceramic fillers may attribute to higher strength. Most importantly, the non-radiopaque nature of polymers can be improved to be radiopaque, which is essential in the radiological assessment of the implant position. However, the effect of the processing method is an area that can be explored to understand the behaviour of PA. Injection moulding (IM) is the most common polymer processing technique. However, the current progression in polymer 3D printing and its composites is an exciting prospect to be focused on. The melting point is a crucial factor that needs to be considered when selecting PA for processing. The PA with the lowest melting point is constantly a subject of interest regarding the machine's capability and processing window.

Physical Properties

Quantification of biomaterial physical properties is deemed important as it determines the biological performance of the materials. The surface of the material will first encounter the biological host before the surrounding cells interact and attach to the respective surface. A rough surface was observed to provide a better environment for the early response of cells [18]. Furthermore, surface modification, performed by Zareidoost *et al.* [19], resulted in a strong correlation between a rough surface and the biological response of the employed cells. However, the surface roughness of PA 12 composites at different filler loadings fabricated *via*IM and 3D printing techniques are shown in Fig. (**2**).

The utilisation of filler is desirable to reduce the shrinkage that occurs during the polymer processing cooling stage. However, composites with a combination of high filler loading and micro filler often result in a rougher surface; therefore, low filler loading and nano-filled composites are preferred. The effect of a combination of both micro and nano-fillers on the physical properties of PA 12 composites prepared *via*injection moulding and 3D printing techniques showed that the surface roughness of PA 12 composites was not significantly affected by the increment of filler loading [20, 21].

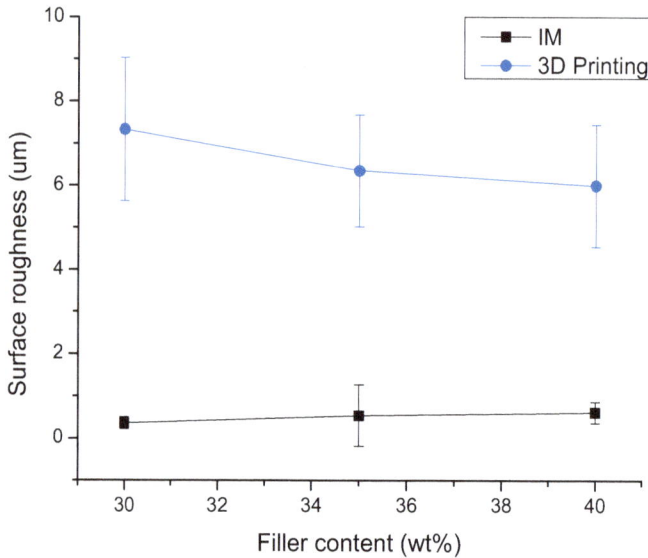

Fig. (2). Surface roughness of PA composites at different filler loadings and processing techniques.

A combination of 15 wt% of micro-beta tricalcium phosphate (β-TCP) and 15 wt% nano zirconia filler significantly reduced the roughness of the injection moulded specimens. On the contrary, rough surfaces were observed in a 3D-printed specimen at a similar filler loading [20]. A similar composition does not necessarily resemble physical properties when different processing techniques are employed. During the moulding process, polymer composites are injected at high speed so that the composites can flow and fill the hot cavity in a short time frame, which results in a smooth and compact surface. However, 3D printing is a rather time-consuming process, where a semi-molten polymer is deposited onto a build plate, layer by layer. The process continues until the desired build is complete, which typically results in a rough surface.

The surface roughness of 3D printed specimens is highly dependent on printing orientation (Fig. **3**). and layer thickness [22]. Alteration of these factors could affect printing duration, where more time is needed to print a specimen in a y-z orientation coupled with a low layer setting. For example, a nozzle size of 0.4 mm can be set to extrude a single layer ranging from 0.1 to 0.4 mm.

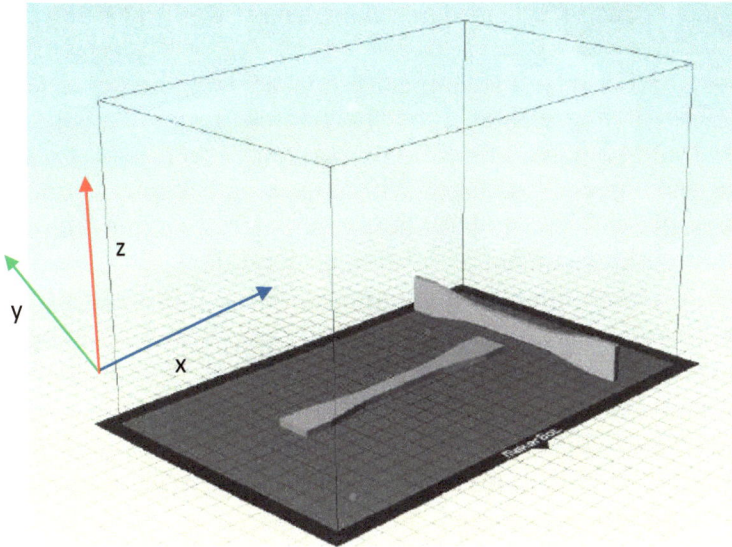

Fig. (3). Various orientations of specimens.

A specimen printed in an x-z orientation generally results in a higher surface roughness than a part printed in a y-z orientation see Fig. (**4**). However, the printing duration is considerably shorter in that orientation; therefore, the balance between surface quality and time needs to be considered prior to starting the 3D printing process.

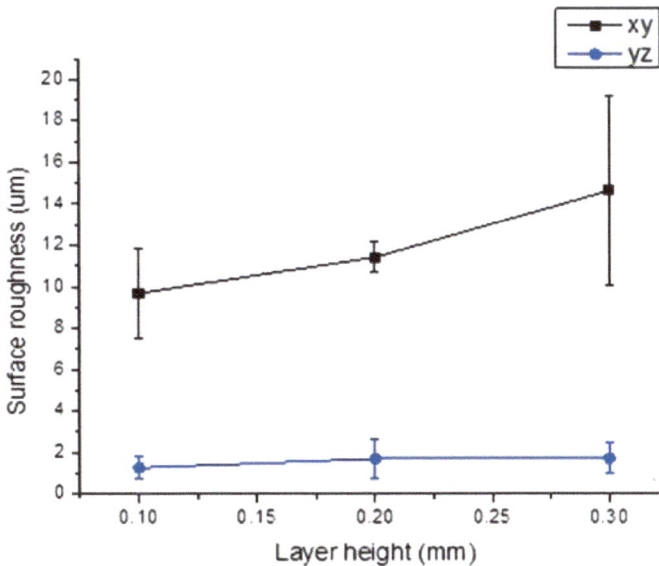

Fig. (4). Effect of layer thickness and printing orientation on surface quality.

MECHANICAL PROPERTIES

Besides physical properties, mechanical properties are another area of interest in the development of composites. The mechanical properties of the developed biomaterials should be equal to the anatomical part that aims to be reconstructed. For instance, biomaterial implants with higher mechanical properties than a natural bone will lead to implant failure as stress cannot be homogenously distributed to the adjacent bone, resulting in implant loosening [23]. Several factors influence the mechanical properties of bone. Ethnicity difference where Asian men are found to possess denser cortical than Caucasian men, although they are smaller in bone size and trabecular area [24]. Furthermore, sexual dimorphism also contributes to apparent differences in the microstructure of both compact and cancellous bones during puberty [25]. Meanwhile, age is an undeniable factor that contributes to the mechanical properties of bone. It is a fact that physical activity results in greater bone strength compared to calcium intake, as observed in rat models [26].

The general tensile properties of PA and its melting point, together with craniofacial bone tensile properties as a comparison, are displayed in (Table **2**). PA 6,6 exhibited the highest melting point due to the presence of more hydrogen bonds in every repeating unit.

Table 2. General properties of polyamides and craniofacial bone.

-	Melting Point (°C)	Tensile Strength (MPa)	Tensile Modulus (GPa)
PA 6	220	72.5	2.35
PA 11	187	78.4	2.84
PA 12	178	49.0	1.29
PA 6,6	260	78.4	2.80
PA 6,10	213	58.8	1.96
PA 6,12	210	60.8	1.96
Craniofacial Bone	-	35-283	0.5-7.0

The mechanical properties (maximum value) of PA 12 composites fabricated *via*injection moulding and 3D printing techniques are displayed in Table **3**. In general, 3D printing techniques result in lower mechanical properties (except impact strength) compared to the injection moulded part. These results are not alarming due to the nature of the processing itself. As mentioned previously, injection moulding produces compact parts, while 3D printing results in an apparent porous structure due to layer arrangement during the printing process. Nevertheless, a 3D-printed impact specimen exhibited a higher value of 16.95

kJ/m^2, which could be linked to its ability to absorb impact during testing due to its porous nature. Therefore, specific properties should be taken into consideration when designing a new biomaterial for certain applications.

Table 3. Mechanical properties of experimental PA 12 composites

Properties	Test Method	Injection Moulded (Maximum value)	3D Printed (Maximum value)
Tensile strength (MPa)	ASTM D638	36.60	24.25
Tensile modulus (MPa)	ASTM D638	1286.80	994.71
Flexural strength (MPa)	ASTM D790	61.75	30.03
Flexural modulus (MPa)	ASTM D790	1692.0	631.14
Impact strength (kJ/m^2)	ASTM D256	10.49	16.95

Fig. (**5**) shows the behaviour of injection moulded, and 3D printed PA 12 composites after being subjected to tensile testing. The injection moulded part is quite strong and flexible, as it can elongate more than 60% of its original length. Meanwhile, the 3D-printed part is only able to resist up to 15% expansion before catastrophic failure. While this is the result of using particulate filler, a future study could be designed to optimise the current setting of the 3D printer and consider a fibrous filler for reinforcement purposes.

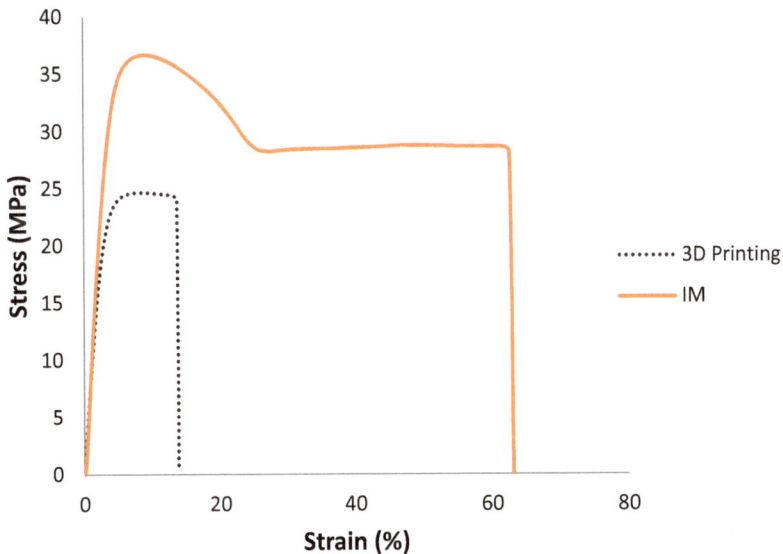

Fig. (5). Stress-strain graph of polyamide 12 composites fabricated *via* injection moulding and 3D printing techniques.

BIOCOMPATIBILITY PROPERTIES

The development of biomaterials involves various stages that need to be accomplished prior to a clinical trial. One of the tests that need to be conducted is in vitro cytotoxicity [27]. The complete polymerisation process generally produces a non-toxic polymer. In most cases, the presence of residual monomer or other solvents induces a cytotoxic effect on the respective cells. The residual monomer could cause irritation, inflammation, and allergic reactions [28]. Studies have shown [29, 30] that PA has good biocompatibility because it is chemically similar to collagen proteins and therefore possesses excellent stability in human body fluids.

The cytotoxicity properties of PA 12 and its composites are illustrated in Fig. (6). Significant enhancement in cell viability of the composites was observed compared to unfilled PA 12 at high concentrations, indicating the presence of filler might have contributed to the phenomena. It is well documented that β-TCP alone induces cell proliferation [31]. Meanwhile, a more recent study indicated that zirconia possesses a positive effect on the cell, and the elements β-TCP and Zirconia, present in the composites, increased the viability of the cells [32].

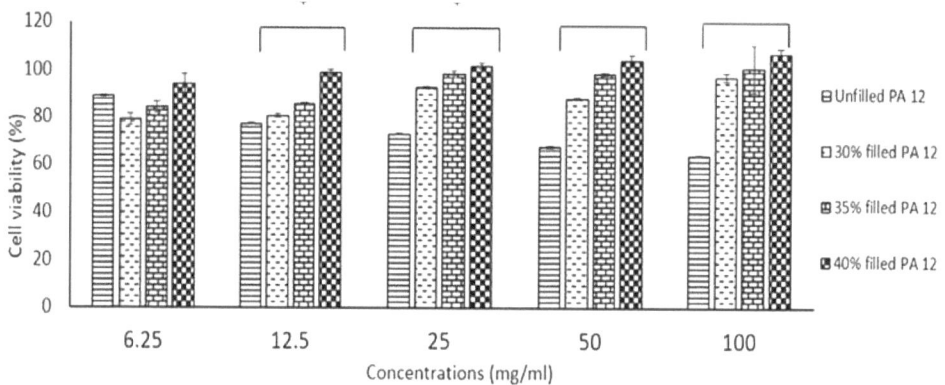

Fig. (6). Cytotoxicity properties of PA 12 and its composites, adapted from Abdullah *et al.* [33], reproduced with permission from Elsevier.

Meanwhile, the attachment of cells on the 3D printed PA 12 composites, namely 3D orbital polyamide customised composite (3D-OPACC), compared to commercial materials, is shown in Fig. (7). 3D-OPACC is a PA 12 composite-based material, which contains both zirconia and β-TCP. More cells were observed on the experimental 3D-OPACC printed surface compared to other polyethylene materials (Medpor & Synpor). The synergistic effect between the rough surface and the presence of calcium phosphate-based materials probably contributed to a better cell attachment compared to others.

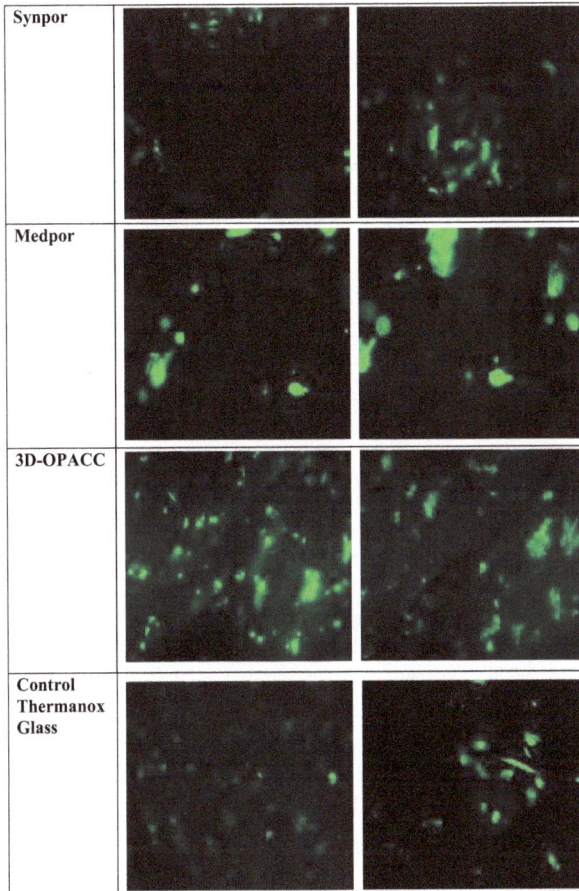

Fig. (7). Live and dead staining of osteoblast cell attachment on different materials, adapted from Sheng *et al.* [34].

CONCLUSION

The advancement of polyamide composites for craniofacial reconstruction was explored. Polyamide composites discussed in this chapter were fabricated *via*two different techniques, injection moulding, and 3D printing, and the physical and mechanical properties were assessed and compared. The surface profiles of 3D printed parts were rougher than injection moulded parts, which were preferred for cell attachment. Nevertheless, lower mechanical properties were seen compared to injection moulded parts. The melting temperature of polyamide is far lower than currently available polymeric materials for PSI, such as PEEK. Therefore, polyamide can easily fit a filament-based 3D printer. However, greater attention needs to be paid during processing, as tangling tends to occur during extrusion and shrinkage during the 3D printing processes. With the enhancement in cell viability attributed to the presence of fillers, polyamide composite can potentially be used as an alloplastic alternative in non-load-bearing areas, such as craniofacial parts. Further research should be carried out to enhance the mechanical properties of 3D printed parts *via* optimisation of filler loading and printing parameters. Furthermore, *in vivo* assessment should be proposed to further explore the performance of polyamide to meet the regulations stated by the Medical Device Act.

ACKNOWLEDGEMENTS

This study was made possible by funding from a Research University Grant (1001/PPSG/8012241) and a Fundamental Research Grant Scheme from the Ministry of Education (FRGS/1/2021/SKK0/USM/02/13).

REFERENCES

[1]   Ramakrishna S, Mayer J, Wintermantel E, Leong KW. Biomedical applications of polymer-composite materials: a review. Compos Sci Technol 2001; 61(9): 1189-224.
[http://dx.doi.org/10.1016/S0266-3538(00)00241-4]

[2]   Ali SHR, Almaatoq MM, Mohamed ASA. Classifications, surface characterization and standardization of nanobiomaterials. IACSIT Int J Eng Technol 2013; 2(3): 187-99.
[http://dx.doi.org/10.14419/ijet.v2i3.1005]

[3]   Thamaraiselvi TV, Rajeswari S. Biological evaluation of bioceramic materials - A review Trends Biomaterial and Artificial Organs 2004; 18(1): 9-17.

[4]   Chiarini L, Figurelli S, Pollastri G, *et al.* Cranioplasty using acrylic material: a new technical procedure. J Craniomaxillofac Surg 2004; 32(1): 5-9.
[http://dx.doi.org/10.1016/j.jcms.2003.08.005] [PMID: 14729042]

[5]   Golz T, Graham CR, Busch LC, Wulf J, Winder RJ. Temperature elevation during simulated polymethylmethacrylate (PMMA) cranioplasty in a cadaver model. J Clin Neurosci 2010; 17(5): 617-22.
[http://dx.doi.org/10.1016/j.jocn.2009.09.005] [PMID: 20189395]

[6]   Sevin K, Askar I, Saray A, Yormuk E. Exposure of high-density porous polyethylene (Medpor®) used for contour restoration and treatment. Br J Oral Maxillofac Surg 2000; 38(1): 44-9.
[http://dx.doi.org/10.1054/bjom.1998.0038] [PMID: 10783447]

[7]   Shah AM, Jung H, Skirboll S. Materials used in cranioplasty: a history and analysis. Neurosurg Focus 2014; 36(4): E19.
[http://dx.doi.org/10.3171/2014.2.FOCUS13561] [PMID: 24684331]

[8]   Khonsari RH, Berthier P, Rouillon T, Perrin JP, Corre P. Severe infectious complications after PEEK-derived implant placement: Report of three cases. J Oral Maxillofac Surg Med Pathol 2014; 26(4): 477-82.
[http://dx.doi.org/10.1016/j.ajoms.2013.04.006]

[9]   Lethaus B, Poort ter Laak M, Laeven P, *et al.* A treatment algorithm for patients with large skull bone defects and first results. J Craniomaxillofac Surg 2011; 39(6): 435-40.
[http://dx.doi.org/10.1016/j.jcms.2010.10.003] [PMID: 21055960]

[10] Wanibuchi M, Ohtaki M, Fukushima T, Friedman AH, Houkin K. Skull base training and education using an artificial skull model created by selective laser sintering. Acta Neurochir (Wien) 2010; 152(6): 1055-60.
[http://dx.doi.org/10.1007/s00701-010-0624-7] [PMID: 20401499]

[11]   Wei Jie , Li Yubao . Tissue engineering scaffold material of nano-apatite crystals and polyamide composite. Eur Polym J 2004; 40(3): 509-15.
[http://dx.doi.org/10.1016/j.eurpolymj.2003.10.028]

[12]   Wang H, Li Y, Zuo Y, Li J, Ma S, Cheng L. Biocompatibility and osteogenesis of biomimetic nano-hydroxyapatite/polyamide composite scaffolds for bone tissue engineering. Biomaterials 2007; 28(22): 3338-48.
[http://dx.doi.org/10.1016/j.biomaterials.2007.04.014] [PMID: 17481726]

[13]   Kim I, White JL. Anionic copolymerization of lauryl lactam and polycaprolactone for the production of a poly(ester amide) triblock copolymer. J Appl Polym Sci 2003; 90(14): 3797-805.
[http://dx.doi.org/10.1002/app.12980]

[14]   McKeen L. Polyamides (Nylons). In: McKeen L, Ed. The effect of temperatureand other factors on plastics and elastomers: William Andrew. 2014; pp. 243-378.

[15]   Goodridge RD, Tuck CJ, Hague RJM. Laser sintering of polyamides and other polymers. Prog Mater Sci 2012; 57(2): 229-67.
[http://dx.doi.org/10.1016/j.pmatsci.2011.04.001]

[16]   Zarringhalam H, Hopkinson N, Kamperman NF, de Vlieger JJ. Effects of processing on microstructure and properties of SLS Nylon 12. Mater Sci Eng A 2006; 435-436: 172-80.
[http://dx.doi.org/10.1016/j.msea.2006.07.084]

[17]   Li J, Hsu Y, Luo E, Khadka A, Hu J. Computer-aided design and manufacturing and rapid prototyped nanoscale hydroxyapatite/polyamide (n-HA/PA) construction for condylar defect caused by mandibular angle ostectomy. Aesthetic Plast Surg 2011; 35(4): 636-40.
[http://dx.doi.org/10.1007/s00266-010-9602-y] [PMID: 20972567]

[18]   Yamashita D, MacHigashira M, Miyamoto M, *et al.* Effect of surface roughness on initial responses of osteoblast-like cells on two types of zirconia. Dent Mater J 2009; 28(4): 461-70.
[http://dx.doi.org/10.4012/dmj.28.461] [PMID: 19721284]

[19]   Zareidoost A, Yousefpour M, Ghaseme B, Amanzadeh A. The relationship of surface roughness and cell response of chemical surface modification of titanium. J Mater Sci Mater Med 2012; 23(6): 1479-88.
[http://dx.doi.org/10.1007/s10856-012-4611-9] [PMID: 22460230]

[20]   Abdullah AM, Tuan Rahim TNA, Mohamad D, Akil HM, Rajion ZA. Mechanical and physical properties of highly ZrO2 /β-TCP filled polyamide 12 prepared *via* fused deposition modelling (FDM) 3D printer for potential craniofacial reconstruction application. Mater Lett 2017; 189: 307-9.
[http://dx.doi.org/10.1016/j.matlet.2016.11.052]

[21]   Abdullah AM, Mohamad D, Rahim TNAT, Akil HM, Rajion ZA. Enhancement of thermal, mechanical and physical properties of polyamide 12 composites *via* hybridization of ceramics for bone replacement. Mater Sci Eng C 2019; 99: 719-25.
[http://dx.doi.org/10.1016/j.msec.2019.02.007] [PMID: 30889745]

[22]   Abdullah AM, Mohamad D, Tuan Rahim TNA, Md Akil H, Ahmad Rajion Z. 3D printer's parameter optimization for potential patient specific implant fabrication. J Teknol 2015; 76(7): 75-9.
[http://dx.doi.org/10.11113/jt.v76.5718]

[23]   Niinomi M, Nakai M. Titanium-based biomaterials for preventing stress shielding between implant devices and bone. Int J Biomater 2011; 2011: 1-10.
[http://dx.doi.org/10.1155/2011/836587] [PMID: 21765831]

[24]   Kepley AL, Nishiyama KK, Zhou B, *et al.* Differences in bone quality and strength between Asian and Caucasian young men. Osteoporos Int 2017; 28(2): 549-58.
[http://dx.doi.org/10.1007/s00198-016-3762-9] [PMID: 27638138]

[25]   Cheuk KY, Wang XF, Wang J, *et al.* Sexual Dimorphism in Cortical and Trabecular Bone Microstructure Appears During Puberty in Chinese Children. J Bone Miner Res 2018; 33(11): 1948-

55.
[http://dx.doi.org/10.1002/jbmr.3551] [PMID: 30001459]

[26]   Welch JM, Turner CH, Devareddy L, Arjmandi BH, Weaver CM. High impact exercise is more beneficial than dietary calcium for building bone strength in the growing rat skeleton. Bone 2008; 42(4): 660-8.
[http://dx.doi.org/10.1016/j.bone.2007.12.220] [PMID: 18291744]

[27]   ISO 10993-5. Biological evaluation of medical devices Part 5: Tests for in vitro cytotoxicity. United Kingdom: International Organization for Standardization; 2009.
[http://dx.doi.org/10.1016/j.bone.2007.12.220] [PMID: 18291744]

[28]   Ivković N, Božović D, Ristić S, Mirjanić V, Janković O. The residual monomer in dental acrylic resin and its adverse effect. Contemp Mater 2013; 4(1): IV-1.
[http://dx.doi.org/10.7251/COMEN1301084I]

[29]   Makhlouf ASH, Khalil A. Fabrication of durable high performance hybrid nanofiber scaffolds for bone tissue regeneration using a novel, simple in situ deposition approach of polyvinyl alcohol on electrospun nylon 6 nanofibers. Mater Lett 2015; 147.

[30]   Winnacker M. Polyamides and their functionalization: recent concepts for their applications as biomaterials. Biomater Sci 2017; 5(7): 1230-5.
[http://dx.doi.org/10.1039/C7BM00160F] [PMID: 28561076]

[31]   Neamat A, Gawish A, Gamal-Eldeen AM. β-Tricalcium phosphate promotes cell proliferation, osteogenesis and bone regeneration in intrabony defects in dogs. Arch Oral Biol 2009; 54(12): 1083-90.
[http://dx.doi.org/10.1016/j.archoralbio.2009.09.003] [PMID: 19828137]

[32]   Criseida Ruiz-Aguilara, Alcántara-Quintanab LE, Aguilar-Reyesc EA, Olivares-Pintoa U. Fabrication, characterization, and in vitro evaluation of β-TCP/ZrO2-phosphate-based bioactive glass scaffolds for bone repair. Boletín de la Sociedad Española de Cerámica y Vidrio. 2020;Article in press 1-12.

[33]   Abdullah AM, Rahim TNAT, Hamad WNFW, Mohamad D, Akil HM, Rajion ZA. Mechanical and cytotoxicity properties of hybrid ceramics filled polyamide 12 filament feedstock for craniofacial bone reconstruction *via* fused deposition modelling. Dent Mater 2018; 34(11): e309-16.
[http://dx.doi.org/10.1016/j.dental.2018.09.006] [PMID: 30268678]

[34]   Sheng SB, Abdullah AM, Omar M, Mohamad D. Cytotoxicity and Cell Adherence Evaluation of 3D Orbital Polyamide Composite Customised Implant. Malaysian Journal of Microscopy 2020; 16(1): 17-27.

CHAPTER 2

Advances and Issues in Biomaterials for Coronary Stenting

Tamrin Nuge[1], Xiaoling Liu[2], Yogeswaran Lokanathan[3] and **Md Enamul Hoque[4,*]**

[1] *Department of Mechanical, Materials and Manufacturing Engineering, Faculty of Science and Engineering, University of Nottingham Ningbo China, 199 Taikang East Road, Ningbo315100, China*

[2] *Advanced Polymer Composite Group, Faculty of Science and Engineering, University of Nottingham Ningbo China, 199 Taikang East Road, Ningbo315100, China*

[3] *Center for Tissue Engineering and Regenerative Medicine (CTERM), Faculty of Medicine, Jalan Yaa'cob Latiff, 56000 Cheras Kuala Lumpur, Malaysia*

[4] *Department of Biomedical Engineering, Military Institute of Science and Technology (MIST), Dhaka, Bangladesh*

Abstract: Polymer-based biomaterials are a material of choice for many surgeons due to their availability and durability. Many types are available on the market, but the search for improved properties and to cater to technology demands, such as 3D Printing, continues. Polyamide, used as an alternative in craniofacial reconstruction, has become a subject of interest recently. This chapter explores the physical and mechanical properties of polyamide composites fabricated via injection moulding and 3D printing techniques, along with their biocompatibility. With promising physical, mechanical, and biocompatibility properties, polyamide composites are expected to emerge as an alternative biomaterial for craniofacial reconstruction soon.

Keywords: 3D printing, Patient-specific implant, Polyamide composite.

IN VIVO USE OF STENT BIOMATERIALS

Tissue engineering and regenerative medicine are evolving interdisciplinary and multidisciplinary research areas that encompass living cells and material engineering knowledge to engineer biological substitutes as body implants. The general strategies adopted in tissue engineering rely on a construct of biomaterial scaffolds, cells, and bioactive molecules to orchestrate tissue formation and regeneration within the host environment. The strategies can be explained using

---

* **Corresponding author Md Enamul Hoque:** Department of Biomedical Engineering, Military Institute of Science and Technology (MIST), Dhaka Bangladesh; E-mail: enamul1973@gmail.com

an illustration, as shown in Fig. (**1**). The core knowledge in cell-biomaterial construct can be classified into three areas *viz.* [2]; (i). Cell technology (ii). Scaffolds design and construct technology (iii). Novel approach for an *in-vivo* implant.

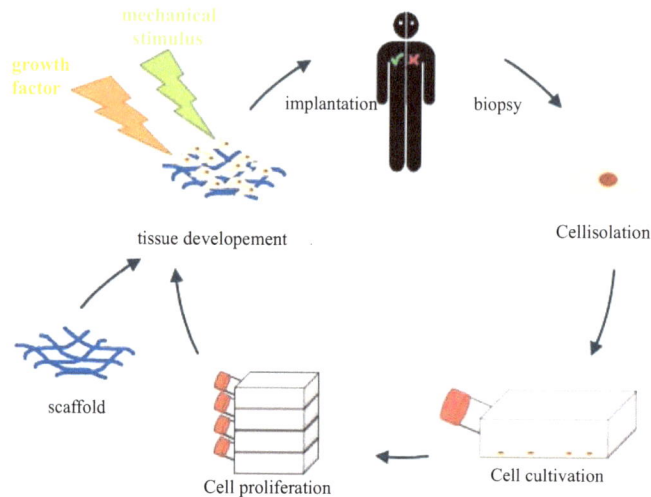

Fig. (**1**). General strategies adopted in tissue engineering and biomaterials as an implant [3].

CARDIOVASCULAR IMPLANTS

Cardiovascular implants can be categorised as permanent internal, temporary internal, and temporary external implants. The biocompatibility of cardiovascular implants highly depends on the implant location and the duration of the implants that come in contact with blood (permanent (>30 days), prolonged (Between 24 h to 30 days), and temporary (less than 24 h). Regardless of the contact duration, blood compatibility will be assessed for all blood-contacting implants. Cardiovascular implants include biocompatible biomaterials such as polymers, metallic alloys, and biological materials (Fig. **2**).

Metallic biomaterials such as titanium alloys, cobalt-chromium, and stainless steel have been used widely as stent-endovascular and stent-graft in cardiovascular implants for more than a century due to their strength and biocompatibility. The metallic stents support endothelial revascularisation and maintain patency after vessel damage. A breakthrough in bioresorbable metallic stents was reported in 2013 with zinc exploitation and its alloy with a slow degradation rate (0.02 mm/y) and it did not induce an inflammatory response. The design of metallic products with excellent biocompatibility and inherent mechanical and surface properties makes the metallic stent a preferential choice over their polymeric counterparts (Table **1**). To enhance the cardiovascular stenting biocompatibility, inorganic coatings such as iridium oxide coating, carbon coating, and oxide layer were examined but failed to exhibit conclusive and compelling performance over the stent lifetime [5]. The coating had caused neointimal proliferation and restenosis. Unfortunately, the adverse effect of corrosion-resistant stents' remains a significant concern for stent thrombosis.

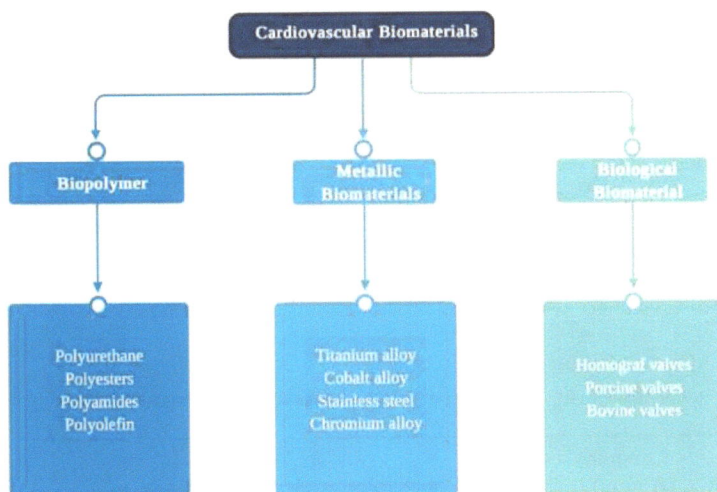

Fig. (2). Classification of cardiovascular stenting biomaterial [4].

Table 1. Commercial metallic biomaterial for the coronary stent. Data is available from the company website.

Stent Name	Manufacturer/Country	Material	Properties
BX velocity®	Johnson& Johnson, USA	Stainless steel 316L	Thickness – 140 µm Yield Strength- 340 MPa
Express®	Boston Scientific, USA	Stainless steel 316L	Thickness – 132 µm Yield Strength- 340 MPa
Driver®	Medtronic, USA	Cobalt-Chromium alloy	Thickness – 91 Yield Strength – 415
Vision™	Abbott, USA	Cobalt-Chromium	Thickness – 81 Yield Strength – 510

Stents are generally graded into three categories based on their mode of use and function: (i) Bare-metal stents (BMS), (ii) Drug-eluting stents (DES), and (iii) Bioabsorbable stents. The introduction of the drug-eluting stent has dramatically reduced restenosis rates and the need for repeat revascularisation compared to the BMS and bioabsorbable stents. The DES commonly consists of an antiproliferative drug, polymeric materials for drug delivery, and a metallic platform (Fig. **3**).

A new generation of DES bifurcation stents has been developed to address the issue associated with bifurcation lesions, distortion of the main vessel, and failure to contain the side branch ostium. The new generation DES has considerably reduced restenosis by approximately 80%. Table **2** describes the commercially available second-generation DES in the market.

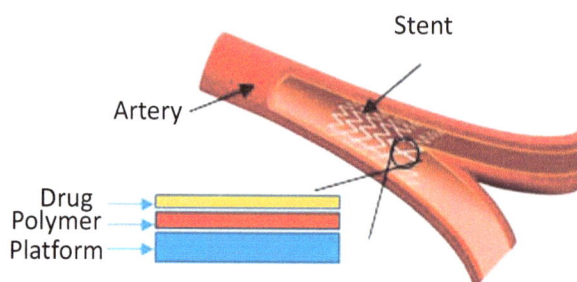

Fig. (3). Drug-eluting coronary stent (DES).

Table 2. Second-generation drug-eluting stent (DES). Data available from the company website

DES	Company /Country	Compositions	Properties
Axxess Plus™	Devax Inc, USA	Self-expanding nickel-titanium alloy	Struts covered with bio-resorbable polymer loaded with Biolimus A9.
TAXUS Petal™	Boston Scientific, USA	Platinum–chromium platform	Coated with poly(styrene-b-isobutylen--b-styrene) which elutes Paclitaxel.
Nile Pax™	Minvasys, France	Chromium–cobalt	Coated with polymer-free abluminal paclitaxel for better drug delivery to the arterial wall and to avoid long-term lack of endothelisation.
STENTYS™	Stentys, France	Self-expanding nitinol (Nickel-Titanium)	It is coated with polysulfone and polyvinylpyrrolidone loaded with paclitaxel.
ENDEAVOR®	Medtronic, USA	Chromium-cobalt	Coated with phosphorylcholine, which elutes zotarolimus.
RESOLUTE Onyx ™	Medtronic, USA	Chromium-cobalt	Coated with Bio links loaded with zotarolimus.
XIENCE Sierra	Abbott, USA	Chromium-cobalt	Coated with poly-butyl methacrylate and PVDF-HFP and loaded with everolimus-eluting drug.
PROMUS Premier ™	Boston Scientific, USA	Chromium-cobalt	Coated with polyn-butyl methacrylate and PVDF-HFP and loaded with everolimus-eluting drug.
ELUNIR ®	Medinol, USA	Chromium-cobalt	Coated with Carbosil and PBMA. Loaded with ridaforolimus eluting drug.

(Table 2) cont.....

DES	Company /Country	Compositions	Properties
SYNERGY ™	Boston Scientific, USA	Platinum-chromium	Eluting everolimus over abluminal bioresorbable polymer coating.

A fully bioresorbable polymeric stent was developed to overcome the limitation of current metallic DES *viz.* late in-stent restenosis and permanent cage vessel. Hence, the idea of using a bioresorbable polymer is an attractive strategy as it provides necessary temporary support to the vessel and degrades in due time, allowing the vessel to heal. To date, the bioresorbable polymeric stent has advanced significantly relative to their more desirable metallic counterparts. Several bioresorbable polymeric stents have already received a green light for market approval in Europe or are still under clinical trials. Polymers such as a polycaprolactone (PCL), poly-DL-lactic acid (PDLLA), and polycarbonate (PCB) have been explored as potential materials for the bioresorbable stent. Some materials offered higher strength and stiffness, such as polyglycolide, poor processing, and low ductility, which have hindered its application in the polymeric stent. Table **3** depicts the FDA-approved bioresorbable polymeric stent.

Table 3. FDA-approved bioresorbable polymeric stent. Adapted from (Gunatillake & Adhikari, 2003).

Polymer	Modulus (GPa)	Strength (MPa)	Elongation at break (%)	Degradation (month)
Polylactic acid	4	65	2-6	18-30
Poly-DL-lactic acid	3.5	40	1-2	3-4
Poly-L-lactic acid	2-4	60-70	2-6	More than 24
Polycaprolactone	0.34	23	More than 4000	24-36
Polylactide-co-glycolide	3.3-3.5	65	2-6	12-18

The advancement of new-generation polymeric stents still encounters many challenges, especially with insufficient controllable degradation time and mechanical properties. Other than poor control in the degradation time, concerns about toxicity always hindered their employability as implants in the human body. The toxicity from implant degradation is always associated with the release of polymer degradation products and by-products in a local acidic environment at the implant site. The tiny particles from the polymer degradation could trigger an inflammatory response, especially when captured in a confined space. Hence, polymeric stent materials that inhibit the inflammatory reaction and offer mechanical support at an appropriate time are highly desired. To date, many studies have been carried out to synthesise novel bio-based materials by employing non-harmful natural polymers such as palm oils and soybean oil *via* solvent-free polymerisation techniques to reduce the toxicity resulting from the solvent impurity and formation of residual monomers during degradation.

Natural polymers are mostly the main components in the extracellular matrix (ECM), a macromolecular network present within cells compared with synthetic polymers. This makes the natural polymer mostly biocompatible with a less inflammatory response, hence providing a conducive environment for cell proliferation [6]. Attempts have been made to use natural polymer implants for bioresorbable stents. The natural polymer-based scaffold properties are expected to closely resemble those of the ECM macromolecular network that offers mechanical stability and structural integrity to tissue and organ [7]. The inherent capacity for cell binding is exerted by the presence of the following molecular sequences: Polypeptide base - carrying specific protein structural motifs such as RGD (arginine/Glycine/aspartic acid) and polysaccharides base – numerous hydroxyl groups that provide multiple sites for the attachment of side groups [8]. Bueno *et al.*, 2009 [9] implanted stents covered with cellulose in the rabbit artery model and found that the stents coated with cellulose exhibited no adverse effect with no acute or late vessel occlusion caused by stent thrombosis.

Similarly, excellent hemocompatibility and biocompatibility were also observed on the stent covered with type 1 collagen implanted in small diameter vessels in rabbits [10]. A biodegradable stent fabricated from chitosan was reported to exhibit drug elution delivery consistently to the vascular wall without any noticeable damage to the membrane [11]. Nevertheless, further *in vivo* analyses are required to prove the concept before clinical application. Fig. (**4**) depicts the stent covered with a chitosan membrane.

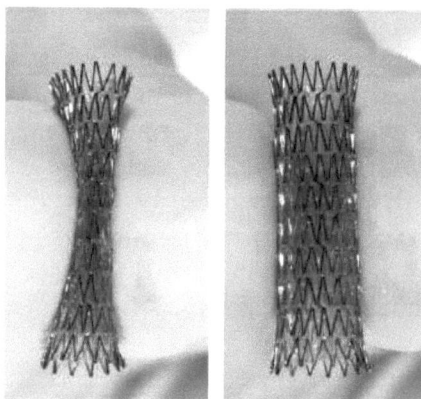

Fig. (4). Chitosan membrane-covered stent exhibits the membrane's ability to withstand the metallic stent's mechanical deformation [11]. Copyright © 2005 Wiley & Sons, Inc. Reprinted by permission of John Wiley & Sons.

Advancement in additive manufacturing has opened a new avenue in stent cardiovascular for potential drug delivery to the placement site. Park *et al.*, 2015 [12] successfully fabricated a helical biodegradable and biocompatible polycaprolactone stent *via* a 3D rapid prototyping technique coated with sirolimus mixed with poly-(*lactide-co-glycolide*) (PLGA) and polyethylene glycol for controllable drug release. The *in-vivo* study into the porcine femoral artery exhibited no complications and was found to reduce neointimal hyperplasia. The limitation of 3D scaffold construction especially related to unfavourable host response and necrosis at the implantation site has inspired the polymer research community to explore the possibility of fabricating scaffold-free engineered tissue constructs. Norotte *et al.*, 2009 [13] successfully fabricated fully biological tubular grafts by bioprinting technology. Despite the advances, poor cell infiltration surrounding vessel construction could lead to cell ischemia. Hence, creating a construct containing a complex hierarchical macro to a micro-vascular tree *in vitro* is highly desirable to escalate the cells' infiltration and migration. Besides, cell maturation is also pivotal in attaining the necessary mechanical properties for implantation. Fig. (**5**) shows the development of bioprinted tubes for the fabrication of uniform and sturdy engineered constructs.

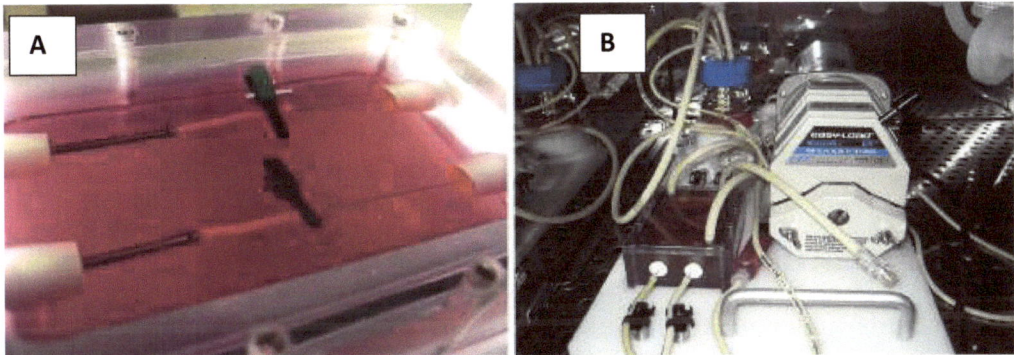

Fig. (5). Maturation bioprinted tubes composed of porcine aortic smooth muscle cells (A) in a perfusion bioreactor (B) [13] Copyright © 2010 Elsevier Ltd. Reprinted by permission of Elsevier Ltd.

ISSUES IN BIOMATERIALS FOR CORONARY STENTING

Immunosuppression-free implants and an inexhaustible source of organs are the goal standard in regenerative medicines. The current advances in regenerative therapies offered bioengineered organs fabricated from patients' cells and biomaterials to produce organ-on-demand genesis. Undesired host responses such as chronic and acute inflammation triggered by foreign bodies always limit the biomedical implant's functionality and longevity (Fig. **6**). Numerous studies have been undertaken to reduce the host response, which is regarded as implant biocompatibility [14]. The cascade of host responses on the implants involves blood-biomaterial interaction, protein-material surface contact, blood coagulation, and complement fixation cascade have been systematically investigated. Designing materials with instructive properties is highly desirable to inhibit extensive chronic inflammation and scar tissue formation. These responses depend on several aspects, such as the injury magnitude during the trauma and surgery, the nature of biomaterials used as implants, and their interaction with the tissue or organs. The following section outlines the main concerns associated with the host response resulting from stent implantation.

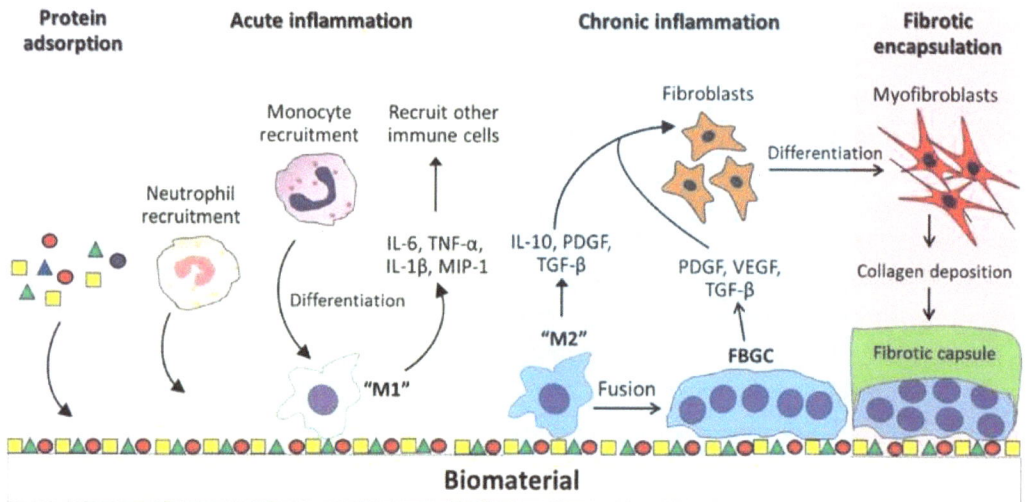

Fig. (6). Biomaterials interaction on host cellular. Adapted [15]. Copyright © 1999-2021 John Wiley & Sons, Inc. Reprinted by permission of John Wiley & Sons, Inc.

OCCLUSIVE THROMBOSIS INDUCED BY STENT IMPLANT

Biomaterials' functional failure is always associated with insufficient hemocompatibility at the implant site, triggering adverse reactions, such as thrombus formation and occlusion in the blood vessels. In interventional cardiology, the most feared complication related to percutaneous coronary interventions is stent thrombosis which almost 60-80% of patients were at risk of mortality or myocardial infarction. In their study, Madhavan *et al.*, 2020 [16] presented more than 25 000 pooled individual present data (IPD) related to stent thrombosis after coronary stent implantation. It was also found that the risk of stent thrombosis is common to all metallic stents. However, the complications related to stent implantation had reduced with BMS evolution to DES 1 AND DES 2. Several mechanisms have been purported to explain stent thrombosis, including stent under-expansion, malapposition, uncovered struts, device fracture, and neo-atherosclerosis. Stent thrombosis could be diagnosed by a significant increase in bio-humoral and systemic cellular markers during inflammation [17].

Stent Under-Expansion

Stent under-expansion is a well-known risk factor for stent thrombosis, with an almost 25% incidence rate related to it [18]. The incidence frequently associates with technique or operator-related factors and lesion calcification (Fig. **7**). In-stent under-expansion, shockwave coronary intravascular lithotripsy (IVL) has been employed to treat stent under-expansion over a 0.014" coronary guidewire with a rapid exchange intravascular lithotripsy balloon catheter into the stented segment. The shockwave is generated to pass through non-reflective tissue but is reflected and amplified within calcific tissues. The IVL shockwave disrupted both superficial and deep calcium, limiting stent expansion without damage to non-calcified tissue [19]. IVL is considered a novel and practical approach to mitigating chronically under-expanded stents by disrupting calcified plaque without destroying the stent. Hence, the approach could avoid additional stent implantation and provides a solution to lower the subsequent risk of stent thrombosis and restenosis. Fig. (**8**) illustrates the IVL equipment for treating the stent under-expansion.

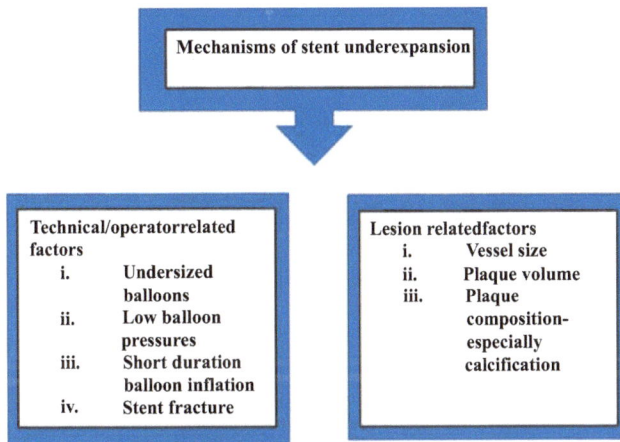

Fig. (7). Mechanism of stent under-expansion.

Malapposition Stent Thrombosis

Stent malapposition is the post-procedure due to the absence of contact of strut with the vessel wall and major causes of coronary thrombosis due to strut exposure and local flow disturbance. European expert consensus recently defined the stent malapposition as a lesion with a length of more than 1 mm and depth of more than 400 μm and suggested that malapposed struts should be fixed when anatomically feasible [21]. The stent malapposition could be reliably detected using optical coherence tomography (OCT) (Fig. **9**). OCT is the most precise and sensitive to evaluate stent malapposition due to its high spatial resolution and imaging quality. With OCT, metallic struts exhibit highly reflective surfaces that cast shadows on the underlying vessel wall [22]. A study by Hong *et al.*, 2020 [23] reported that in OCT follow-up on 390 DES-treated lesions, 45% exhibited significant stent malapposition on the OCT. Fortunately, with earlier intervention, the stent malapposition reduced to 34% after three months of intervention.

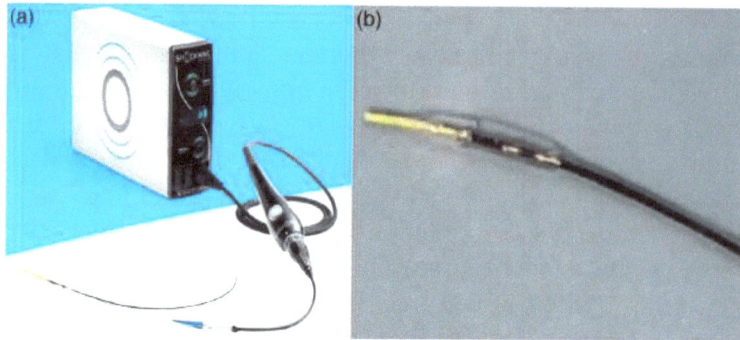

Fig. (8). coronary intravascular lithotripsy (IVL) equipment (a). Shockwave generating console (b). Lithotripsy balloon catheter – high energy shockwave generating pulse transducers [20]. Copyright © 1999-2021 John Wiley & Sons, Inc. Reprinted by permission of John Wiley & Sons, Inc.

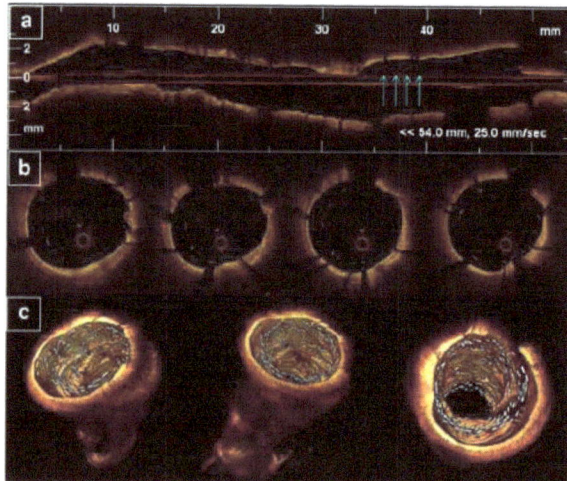

Fig. (9). Optical coherence tomography in a different way of visualisation. (a). 2D longitudinal display (b). 2D cross-sectional views (c). 3D rendered [24]. Copyright © 2021 Springer Nature. It is reprinted with the permission of Springer Nature.

Stent Fracture

Metal stents implant at the peripheral vessel and pulmonary arteries is always associated with stent fracture incidence. Almost 1 to 2% of patients turned up during 8 to 10 months of follow-up have been diagnosed with stent fractures [25]. The stent fracture can be associated with various clinical implications such as stent thrombosis, myocardial infarction, and unstable angina. Mechanical fatigue and excessive movement/pressure are the essential contributions to stent implant failure. The stent placement at the high curves and twisted arteries is vulnerable to fracture, especially longer stent size, due to the strong forces exerted by the vessel's motion during cardiac diastole and systole. Moreover, over-expansion of the stent could weaken its struts, rendering it susceptible to fracture [26].

In most cases, the vessel movement's struts fracture would propagate from the highly rigid area resulting from the metal overlapping, which acted as a fulcrum for metal deformation. The struts fracture would induce local inflammation and destruction of the stent architecture. The debris may have principate acutely and accumulate; thus, it may later risk patients for stent thrombosis. Fig. (**10**) shows the failure of stent implants following DES implantation.

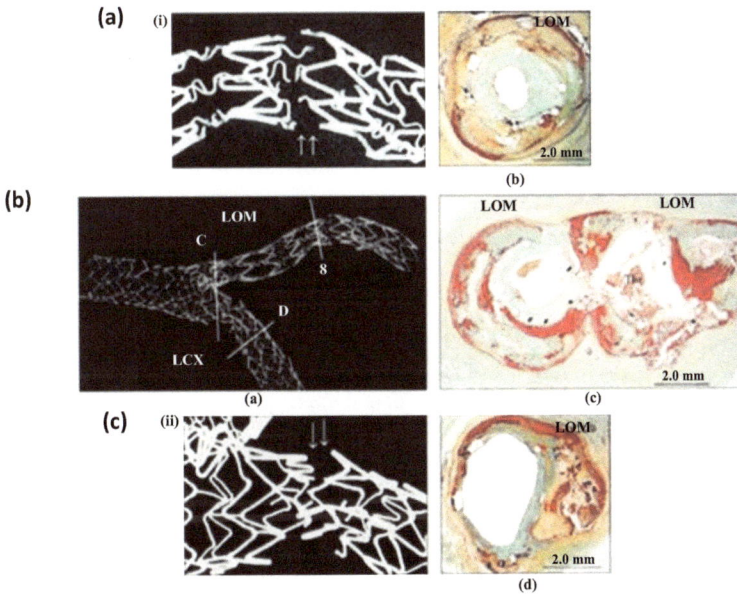

Fig. (10). Stent fracture in a left circumflex artery that leads to stent thrombosis to the patient. The failure occurred 172 days after coronary stent implantation (a). Fracture at the bifurcation site (Histology image shows the thrombosis location) (b). The fracture incidence of a stent with sirolimus-eluting grade (c). The fracture pattern at the stented segment [27]. Copyright © 2009 American College of Cardiology Foundation. It was reprinted with permission of Elsevier Ltd.

ACUTE AND CHRONIC INFLAMMATION STENTING

Foreign body reaction to the implanted stent occurred as early as 15 minutes after the procedure. The reaction involves the incipient period, phase progression, and phase resolution. The cascade was initiated with macrophages (M1) and giant cells to the stenting materials' surface. The stent's coronary endothelium injury has also triggered the overexpression of ligands arrays and potent chemoattractant molecules such as interleukin (IL), tumour necrosis factor, and leukocytes at the injury site. While stent-induced mechanical injury to the vessel is inevitable, the local acute inflammation reaction is directly related to individual susceptibility. In certain patients, a high incidence of restenosis is reported with the patient with the higher release of IL6 in the acute inflammation after a stent implant (Fig. **11**). Genetic factors play a significant role in modulating inflammatory response to stent implantation.

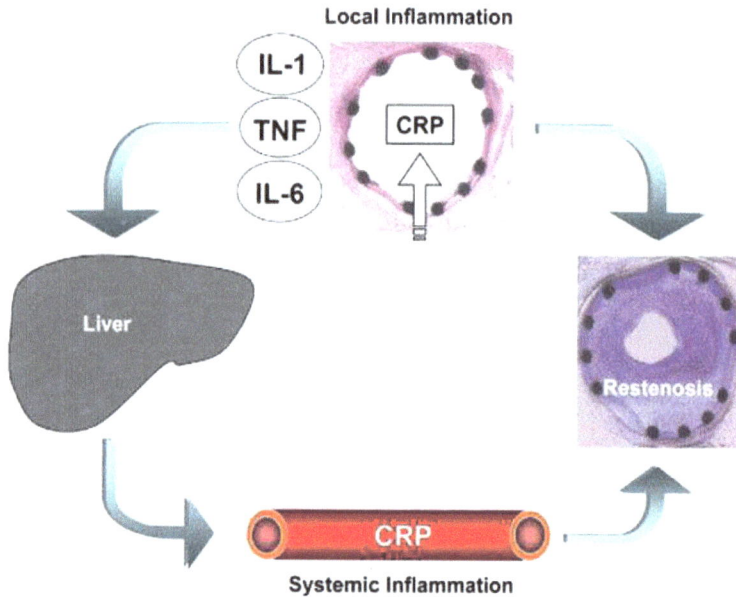

Fig. (11). Local and systemic inflammatory response to stent implantation [28].

Within four weeks after stent implantation, the acute inflammation is superseded by chronic inflammatory cells and propagating smooth muscle cells. The patients expressing a high affinity of cellular activation are at a high prevalence of restenosis and cardiovascular events. Other than restenosis, a high cellular activation level after implantation may consequent in endothelial dysfunction and ischemia. Nevertheless, both incidence related to the inflammatory event is not well studied. Other than genetic factors, the stent insertion technique could also contribute to the prolonged expression of the cells' bioactive cellular. More profound arterial injury during the stenting procedure has caused macrophages' prolonged and high-level appearance within site. Besides severe injury and trauma on the arterial wall, the macrophages' higher expression could also be inherent by the permanent radial strain, metallic residual from the struts, and endothelial dysfunction. The chronic inflammatory and proliferative reaction is not limited to the vessel wall but extends from the injured vessel throughout the surrounding tissues, including the adjacent myocardium. Various drugs have been developed to cater to the inflammatory reactions resulting from stent implantation complications and increase local resistance to cell proliferation and apoptosis. Table **4** depicts the commercially available synergistic therapeutic approach in controlling local and systemic inflammation.

Table 4. Complementary synergistic therapeutic approach in controlling stenting inflammation reaction.

Class	Drugs	Action
Antiplatelet drugs	Aspirin Clopidogrel Triclopidine	Anti-inflammatory response by decreasing the expression of the transmembrane protein and CD40 ligand.
Statin	3-hydroxy-3-methylglutaryl co-enzyme A	Reduces platelet aggregation Leukocyte adhesion Monocyte activation Reduces plasma level of C-reactive protein.
Corticosteroid	Glucocorticoids	Anti-inflammatory agents. Inhibits the inflammatory process and influence platelet function, smooth muscle proliferation, and collagen synthesis.

CHALLENGES AND FUTURE PERSPECTIVES

The significant challenges for coronary stenting are numerous, including biocompatibility, materials selection, geometry, and manufacturing processes. There is a great need to develop new methods for assessing the ability of biodegradable stents to provide not only acute support but also a reliable structure for an appropriate time. In all these properties, the material and manufacturing process play an essential role in manufacturing bioresorbable polymeric stenting with desirable mechanics while maintaining its integrity and controllable degradation within an appropriate time.

ACKNOWLEDGEMENTS

This research was supported by the Fundamental Research Grant Scheme (FRGS) grant number FRGS/1/2020/SKK0/UKM/02/7 provided by the Ministry of Higher Education (MOHE), Malaysia.

REFERENCES

[1]　Hoque ME. 2019.https://doi.org/https://doi.org/10.1016/B978-0-12-816771-7.00005-3

[2]　Devices PS. Tissue Eng 2000; 18: 18-20.

[3]   Nuge T, Liu Z, Liu X, *et al.* Recent Advances in Scaffolding from Natural-Based Polymers for Volumetric Muscle Injury. Molecules 2021; 26(3): 699.
[http://dx.doi.org/10.3390/molecules26030699] [PMID: 33572728]

[4]   Jaganathan SK, Supriyanto E, Murugesan S, Balaji A, Asokan MK. Biomaterials in cardiovascular research: applications and clinical implications. BioMed Res Int 2014; 2014: 1-11.
[http://dx.doi.org/10.1155/2014/459465] [PMID: 24895577]

[5]   Bowen PK, Shearier ER, Zhao S, *et al.* Biodegradable Metals for Cardiovascular Stents: from Clinical Concerns to Recent Zn-Alloys. Adv Healthc Mater 2016; 5(10): 1121-40.
[http://dx.doi.org/10.1002/adhm.201501019] [PMID: 27094868]

[6]   Nuge T, Tshai KY, Lim SS, Nordin N, Hoque ME. Characterization and optimization of the mechanical properties of electrospun gelatin nanofibrous scaffolds. World J Eng 2020; 17(1): 12-20.
[http://dx.doi.org/10.1108/WJE-04-2019-0119]

[7]   Hoque M. Gelatin Based Scaffolds for Tissue Engineering – a Review. Polymer Research Journal 2014; 9(1): 15-32.

[8]   Nuge T, Tshai K Y, Lim S S, Nordin N, Hoque M E. (2017). Preparation and characterization of CU-, FE-, AG-, ZN- and NI- doped gelatin nanofibers for possible applications in antibacterial nanomedicine. Journal of Engineering Science and Technology, 12(Special Issue 1).

[9]   Bueno RRL, Tanguay J-FC, Brito FS Jr, *et al.* Evaluation of the efficacy and safety of a stent covered with biosynthetic cellulose in a rabbit iliac artery model. J Invasive Cardiol 2009; 21(8): 392-6.http://europepmc.org/abstract/MED/19652252
[PMID: 19652252]

[10]   Fujiwara NH, Kallmes DF, Li ST, Lin HB, Hagspiel KD. Type 1 collagen as an endovascular stent-graft material for small-diameter vessels: a biocompatibility study. J Vasc Interv Radiol 2005; 16(9): 1229-36.
[http://dx.doi.org/10.1097/01.RVI.0000171690.21149.8F] [PMID: 16151064]

[11]   Thierry B, Merhi Y, Silver J, Tabrizian M. Biodegradable membrane-covered stent from chitosan-based polymers. J Biomed Mater Res A 2005; 75A(3): 556-66.
[http://dx.doi.org/10.1002/jbm.a.30450] [PMID: 16094632]

[12]   Park SA, Lee SJ, Lim KS, *et al. In vivo* evaluation and characterization of a bio-absorbable drug-coated stent fabricated using a 3D-printing system. Mater Lett 2015; 141: 355-8.
[http://dx.doi.org/10.1016/j.matlet.2014.11.119]

[13]   Norotte C, Marga FS, Niklason LE, Forgacs G. Scaffold-free vascular tissue engineering using bioprinting. Biomaterials 2009; 30(30): 5910-7.
[http://dx.doi.org/10.1016/j.biomaterials.2009.06.034] [PMID: 19664819]

[14]   Nuge, T., Liu, X., Tshai, K. Y., Lim, S. S., Nordin, N., Hoque, M. E., & liu, Z. (2021b). Accelerated wound closure – Systematic evaluation of cellulose acetate effects on biologically active molecules release from amniotic fluid stem cells (AFSCs). Biotechnology and Applied Biochemistry, n/a(n/a).
[http://dx.doi.org/10.1002/bab.2162]

[15]   Zhou G, Groth T. Host Responses to Biomaterials and Anti-Inflammatory Design-a Brief Review. Macromol Biosci 2018; 18(8): 1800112.
[http://dx.doi.org/10.1002/mabi.201800112] [PMID: 29920937]

[16]   Madhavan MV, Kirtane AJ, Redfors B, *et al.* Stent-Related Adverse Events >1 Year After Percutaneous Coronary Intervention. J Am Coll Cardiol 2020; 75(6): 590-604.
[http://dx.doi.org/10.1016/j.jacc.2019.11.058] [PMID: 32057373]

[17]   Del Pace S, Boddi M, Rasoini R, *et al.* Acute infection–inflammation and coronary stent thrombosis: an observational study. Intern Emerg Med 2010; 5(2): 121-6.
[http://dx.doi.org/10.1007/s11739-010-0350-4] [PMID: 20169424]

[18]   Taherioun M, Namazi MH, Safi M, *et al*. Stent underexpansion in angiographic guided percutaneous coronary intervention, despite adjunctive balloon post-dilatation, in drug eluting stent era. ARYA Atheroscler 2014; 10(1): 13-7.https://pubmed.ncbi.nlm.nih.gov/24963308
[PMID: 24963308]

[19]   Yaginuma K, Werner GS. Resolving chronic stent under-expansion in calcified lesions by intravascular lithoplasty. J Cardiol Cases 2021; 23(3): 136-9.
[http://dx.doi.org/10.1016/j.jccase.2020.10.018] [PMID: 33717380]

[20]   Yeoh J, Cottens D, Cosgrove C, *et al*. Management of stent underexpansion using intravascular lithotripsy—Defining the utility of a novel device. Catheter Cardiovasc Interv 2021; 97(1): 22-9.
[http://dx.doi.org/10.1002/ccd.28715] [PMID: 31912981]

[21]   Lee SY, Im E, Hong SJ, *et al*. Severe Acute Stent Malapposition After Drug-Eluting Stent Implantation: Effects on Long-Term Clinical Outcomes. J Am Heart Assoc 2019; 8(13): e012800-0.
[http://dx.doi.org/10.1161/JAHA.119.012800] [PMID: 31237187]

[22]   García-Blas S, Jiménez-Valero S, Bonanad C, Sanchis J, Bodi V. OCT in the evaluation of late stent pathology: restenosis, neoatherosclerosis and late malapposition. 2019.
[http://dx.doi.org/10.1088/2053-2563/ab01fach1]

[23]   Hong SJ, Park KH, Ahn CM, *et al*. Severe acute stent malapposition follow-up: 3-month and 12-month serial quantitative analyses by optical coherence tomography. Int J Cardiol 2020; 299: 81-6.
[http://dx.doi.org/10.1016/j.ijcard.2019.06.075] [PMID: 31279662]

[24]   Chamié D, Prabhu D, Wang Z, *et al*. Three-Dimensional Fourier-Domain Optical Coherence Tomography Imaging: Advantages and Future Development. Curr Cardiovasc Imaging Rep 2012; 5(4): 221-30.
[http://dx.doi.org/10.1007/s12410-012-9145-5]

[25]   Alqahtani A, suwaidi JA, Mohsen MK. Stent fracture: How frequently is it recognized? Heart Views 2013; 14(2): 72-81.
[http://dx.doi.org/10.4103/1995-705X.115501] [PMID: 23983912]

[26]   Al Mamary A, Dariol G, Napodano M. Late stent fracture – A potential role of left ventricular dilatation. J Saudi Heart Assoc 2014; 26(3): 162-5.
[http://dx.doi.org/10.1016/j.jsha.2014.02.001] [PMID: 24954989]

[27]   Nakazawa G, Finn AV, Vorpahl M, *et al*. Incidence and predictors of drug-eluting stent fracture in human coronary artery a pathologic analysis. J Am Coll Cardiol 2009; 54(21): 1924-31.
[http://dx.doi.org/10.1016/j.jacc.2009.05.075] [PMID: 19909872]

[28]   Gaspardone A, Versaci F. Coronary stenting and inflammation. Am J Cardiol 2005; 96(12) (Suppl. 1): 65-70.
[http://dx.doi.org/10.1016/j.amjcard.2005.09.064] [PMID: 16399095]

CHAPTER 3

Cell Sheet Technology for Tendon and Ligament Tissue Engineering

Lim Wei Lee¹, Zahra Rashidbenam¹, Genieve Ee Chia Yeo¹, Min Hwei Ng¹ and Jia Xian Law¹,*

¹ *Centre for Tissue Engineering and Regenerative Medicine, Faculty of Medicine, Universiti Kebangsaan Malaysia, Cheras, Kuala Lumpur, 56000, Malaysia*

Abstract: Tendon and ligament injuries are very common and affect many people worldwide. Tendon and ligament injuries may cause serious morbidity to the patients as these tissues play a very important role in body mobility. Cell sheet technology is one of the new tissue engineering approaches introduced to promote tendon and ligament repair. Cell sheets for tendon and ligament repair are commonly prepared using mesenchymal stem cells and tendon/ligament-derived stem cells. Due to their poor mechanical properties, cell sheets are used to wrap around the ligated tendon/ligament, the graft, and the engineered tendon/ligament to hasten tissue regeneration. To date, the application of cell sheet technology in tendon and ligament repair is still at an early stage. However, results from the preclinical studies are promising. Generally, cell sheets were found to hasten tendon and ligament healing, promote graft integration at the tendon-bone interface, and improve the mechanical strength of the healed tissues. More studies, especially the randomised clinical trials, are needed in the future to validate the efficacy of cell sheets in tendon and ligament repair.

Keywords: Cell sheet, Ligament, Mesenchymal stem cell, Tendon, Tissue engineering.

INTRODUCTION

Tendon and ligament injuries are very common. In the United States, tendon and ligament injuries constitute 50% of the 33 million musculoskeletal injuries reported annually [1]. As both tendon and ligament are important connective tissues that connect muscles to bones and bones to bones, respectively, tendon and ligament injuries can lead to serious morbidity and drastically reduce the patients' quality of life. The injured tendon and ligaments will cause pain and significantly

---
* **Corresponding author Jia Xian Law:** Centre for Tissue Engineering and Regenerative Medicine Faculty of Medicine, 12th Floor, Clinical Block, Universiti Kebangsaan Malaysia Medical Centre, Jalan Yaacob Latif, Bandar Tun Razak, Cheras, Kuala Lumpur, Malaysia; E-mail: lawjx@ppukm.ukm.edu.my

reduce the flexibility and range of motion of the affected joints. Additionally, the management of tendon and ligament injuries is also a huge financial burden to the healthcare system.

The most common cause of tendon and ligament injuries is traumatic injuries that involve the application of a sudden external force or impact to the tissues. Tendon and ligament injuries can happen in many forms, most commonly involving tears or ruptures of the connective tissues [2]. In addition, ageing can lead to tendon and ligament tissue degeneration, and the overuse of joints can lead to repetitive injuries that subsequently cause chronic tendon and ligament injuries [3, 4].

Treatment of tendon and ligament injuries can be divided into nonsurgical and surgical methods [5]. One of the surgical techniques is to replace the beyond-repair tendon and ligament with autograft and allograft. More recently, advancement in regenerative medicine and tissue engineering research has led to the development of stem cell therapy to stimulate tissue regeneration, as well as engineered tendons and ligaments as a substitute for damaged tissues [6].

Cell sheet technology is one of the new tissue engineering approaches introduced by Yamato and Okano [7]. This technology is utilised to fabricate a cell sheet that can be used to wrap around the injured tendon and ligament to facilitate tissue regeneration. In addition, cell sheet technology also has been used in the blood vessels, cardiac, cornea, skin, bladder, and urethral tissue engineering. This technique involves the secretion of extracellular matrix (ECM) by the cultured cells, which in turn entraps the cells. When the technology was first introduced, temperature-responsive polymers were used to detach the cell sheet undamaged from the culture dish [8, 9]. The cells were detached as a sheet as this technique could preserve the cell-cell and cell-ECM connections. Nowadays, more techniques such as electro-responsive systems, pH-responsive systems, photo-responsive system, magnetic systems and mechanical systems have been developed and used for the fabrication of cell sheets [9, 10].

Cell sheets for tendon and ligament injuries can be fabricated using many cell types, including mesenchymal stem cells (MSCs), tendon-derived stem cells, and periosteal progenitor cells [11]. MSCs can be harvested from various tissue sources, *e.g.*, bone marrow, umbilical cord, cord blood, and adipose tissue [12 - 14]. MSCs have been widely tested preclinically and clinically for the treatment of tendon and ligament injuries [15]. The use of MSCs is advocated as they do not only secrete paracrine factors that facilitate tissue regeneration. Furthermore, they also produce cytokines that attenuate tissue inflammation [16, 17]. The tendon-derived stem cells are used as they are the native cells of the tendon tissue, while the periosteal progenitor cells are beneficial in promoting the repair of tendon and ligament at the tendon-bone junction and ligament-bone junction, respectively [18, 19].

The application of cell sheet technology can bypass the limitation of cell injection, whereby the cells can be implanted precisely in the intended area. Furthermore, the cells are retained at the transplantation site as they are entrapped within the self-secreted matrix. Additionally, the close proximity of the transplanted cell sheet and injured tissue facilitates the integration of transplanted cells into the host tissue [20]. All these beneficial effects are expected to accelerate tissue regeneration.

In this chapter, we discuss the use of cell sheet technology to facilitate tendon and ligament repair. Focuses are given to the different cell sheet fabrication techniques and the application of cell sheet technology in tendon and ligament regeneration.

TENDON AND LIGAMENT

Structure, Function, and Biomechanical Properties

Tendon is a connective tissue that is responsible for the transfer of force from the muscle to bone, whereas the ligament connects and transmits the force between 2 bones. These tissues are known to sustain stress and force during movement, and the stress and force can increase drastically during intense physical activities such as exercise [21]. Tendon is a tissue with relatively few cells, with tenoblasts and tenocytes constituting 90-95% of the cells found in the tissue [22]. These cells are responsible for the secretion of tendon ECM. Tendon mainly consists of collagen (predominantly collagen type I) with a small quantity of proteoglycans, glycosaminoglycans, glycoproteins, and elastin [23, 24]. The most prominent proteoglycan in the tendon is decorin.

Nonetheless, hyaluronan, fibromodulin, lumican, and biglycan also can be found [25, 26]. The collagen fibrils in the tendon are highly organised and aligned. This orientation is crucial for the mechanical extension of the tendon [27].

Tendon plays an important role in preventing muscle damage by absorbing shock and withstanding tension. Tendon is extended when force is applied and can recoil to the original state once the force is removed. Extension of the tissue beyond the limit will lead to tendon tears or ruptures [28]. Fig. (**1**) shows the structure and strain-stress curve of tendon tissue.

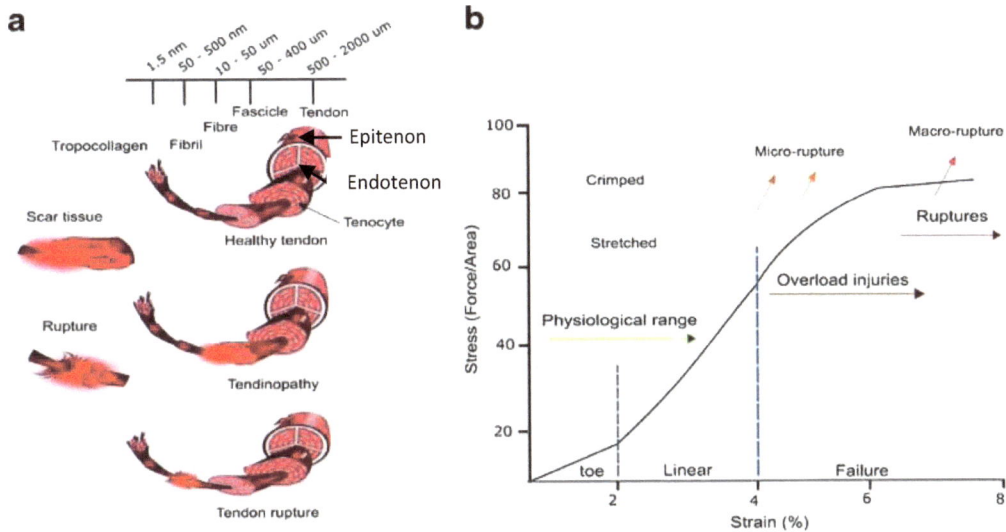

Fig. (1).   Structure and strain-stress curve of tendon tissue. (a) Structure of tendon. Starting with tropocollagen as the smallest unit to a collagen fibril, collagen fibre, subfascicle, and the largest fascicle that forms the endotenon. The endotenon is covered by the epitenon. Tenocytes represent the majority of the resident cells in tendons. Tendinopathy is characterised by disorientated collagen fibres, whereas tendon rupture is indicated by the breaking of collagen fibres. (b) The strain-stress curve of tendon tissue. The collagen fibres in the tendon retain the crimped structure in strains below 2% and become stretched when the strains increase up to 4%. Strains beyond 4% will cause micro-rupture of the collagen fibres, and the tissue will be ruptured once the strains exceed 8%. (reproduced with permission from reference [28])

The ligament is pliable, but unlike the tendon, it is not elastic. Ligaments and tendons share a lot of similarities in terms of their composition, structure, and mechanical property. Both tissues consist predominantly of water (approximately 55-70%), with slightly higher water content in the tendon. Similar to the tendon, collagen (mainly collagen type I and some collagen type III) is the most abundant ECM of the ligament. The fibroblasts that reside in the ligament and are responsible for ECM production are called ligamentoblasts when it is still immature and ligamentocytes when it becomes mature [24].

TENDON AND LIGAMENT INJURIES AND REPAIRS

Tendon and ligament injuries represent the most common musculoskeletal injuries [29]. Tendons and ligaments can be found all over the body. Nonetheless, most tendon and ligament injuries happen in the knee, ankle, hip, shoulder, elbow, and wrist [30]. The Achilles tendon, anterior crucial ligament, and rotator cuff tendons are the most commonly injured tendon and ligaments [31]. As these tissues play a very important role in joint motion and stability, injury to these tissues can lead to serious complications and significantly restrict the body movement.

Tendon and ligament injuries can be categorised into 2 types, *i.e.*, acute injuries caused by traumatic injury to the previously healthy tissue and chronic injuries due to tissue degeneration [32]. The prevalence of tendon and ligament injuries is higher among older adults and those who are exposed to tissue overuse and weight-bearing activities, such as athletes. As the population ages and more and more people getting involved in sport activities, the incidence of tendon and ligament injuries also increases. Other intrinsic factors that increase the prevalence of tendon and ligament injuries are gender, genetic and systemic diseases such as rheumatoid arthritis. Environment and occupation are the extrinsic factors that increase the risk of tendon and ligament injuries [33].

Upon injury, tendon repair occurs*via* intrinsic and extrinsic mechanisms. The intrinsic pathway, which involves the proliferation and migration of the fibroblasts residing in the endotenon and epitenon, is believed to be the main mechanism of healing. The extrinsic pathway involves the migration of inflammatory cells and fibroblasts from the surrounding tissues [34, 35]. The regeneration of an injured tendon and ligament is slow due to the low cellularity, vascularity, and metabolic nature of these tissues. Thus, the regeneration of damaged tendons and ligaments can take up to several months. Additionally, the repair process cannot fully restore the structure and functionality of the tissues, resulting in the formation of regenerated tissue with poorer mechanical strength and functionality [2]. Patients with poor tendon and ligament function will suffer from reduced motility, and the regenerated tissues are also more prone to recurrent injury.

Prompt treatment is crucial in the management of tendon and ligament injuries to confine the damage, to expedite the healing, and to restore the original structural and functional characteristics of the tissue. Treatment of tendon and ligament injuries can be categorised as surgical and non-surgical approaches. The non-surgical approaches include rest, bracing, biophysical stimulation (*e.g.*, cryotherapy, laser therapy, physical therapy, and ultrasound), growth factor therapy (single or multiple growth factors), biologic therapy (*e.g.*, platelet-rich plasma) and pharmacological therapy (*e.g.*, non-steroidal anti-inflammatory drugs (NSAIDs) and corticosteroid) [6, 36]. Generally, the goal of non-surgical therapies is to control pain and reduce inflammation but not to address the underlying cause of the disease.

Even though many therapies are available to treat tendon and ligament injuries, the repair often results in a tissue that is weaker and is more prone to injury [28]. In fact, the recurrent rate of tendon and ligament injuries is quite high [37]. The recurrence of tendon and ligament injuries is very common among athletes that are exposed to the repetitive use of the tissues. Many athletes suffer deterioration in their performance and are forced to end their careers prematurely due to tendon and ligament injuries. Thus, developing a new and more effective therapy for tendon and ligament injuries is very important as the currently available therapies are limited by suboptimal healing, long rehabilitation time, and high recurrent rate [38]. Cell sheet technology is one of the new techniques that has been introduced in the field of regenerative medicine and tissue engineering to tackle this issue. Cell sheets are often used in combination with a graft or a scaffold to stimulate tendon and ligament healing as well as to cover the ligated tissues to expedite the regeneration process.

CELL SHEET TECHNOLOGY

Principle of Cell Sheet Technology

Cell sheet technology is a scaffold-free approach to produce cell patches and engineered tissues for transplantation. Basically, this technology allows the detachment of cells in culture as a sheet as it does not or only cause little damage to the cell-cell and cell-matrix connections. This technology is compatible with many types of cells and has been utilised to produce many types of tissue, including urethral [39], cardiac patch [40], bone [10], cartilage [10], tendon [41], ligament [42], skin [43] and corneal [44].

Cell sheet technology involves the expansion of cells in culture until confluence. Upon confluence, the cells will adhere to each other. At the same time, the cells also secrete ECM, which also helps to link them together. Typically, proteolytic enzymes such as trypsin and trypsin-EDTA are used to detach the cells from the culture surface. However, trypsin will destroy the cell adhesion molecules and the ECM. Thus, the cells will detach from culture surface individually as single cells. To detach the cells as a single confluence layer, specific techniques are needed to loosen the bonding between the cells and the culture surface without affecting the cell-to-cell adhesion (Fig. **2**). illustrates the cell sheet technology, and (Fig. **3**). shows the techniques used to detach cell sheets from the culture surface.

When it was first introduced, Yamato and Okano used the temperature-responsive polymer poly(N-isopropyl acrylamide) (PIPAAm) to detach the cell sheet from the culture surface [46, 47]. In brief, the authors thinly coated culture dishes with the polymer and grew the cells on top of the polymer. The polymer supported cell attachment and proliferation at 37°C. However, PIPAAm changed from relatively hydrophobic (resembling surface characteristics of commercially available culture dishes) to becoming hydrophilic at a temperature below 32°C. The changes in surface hydrophilicity resulted in the spontaneous detachment of cells without the use of trypsin. Thus, a mere temperature change is sufficient to detach the cells as a sheet when using PIPAAm. The detached cell sheets can be stacked to form a 3-

dimensional (3D) tissue construct and be used for *in vitro* testing, for transplantation to promote tissue regeneration and so on.

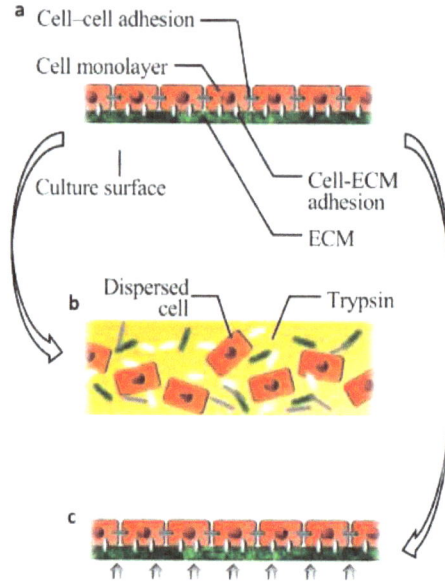

Fig. (2). Illustration of cell sheet technology. (a) Cells are cultured to confluence in a culture dish. (b) Cell detachment using proteolytic enzymes such as trypsin and trypsin-EDTA will destroy the extracellular matrix and cell adhesion proteins. Thus, the cells will detach as a single cell and become dispersed. (c) Selective loss of the adhesion between the cells and culture surface is required to detach the confluence cells as a cell sheet. (Reproduced with permission from reference [45]).

Afterwards, many types of PIPAAm derivatives and co-polymers have been developed and used for cell sheet fabrication. These PIPAAm derivatives and co-polymers include poly(N-isopropylacrylamide-co-glycidylmethacrylate) [48], poly(N-vinylcaprolactam-co-N-iso-propylacrylamide) [49], poly(N-isopropylacryl amide-co-diethyleneglycol methacrylate) [50] and poly(N-isopropylacryl amide-co-butyl methacrylate) [51]. PIPAAm can be deposited on the surface of tissue culture dishes using several techniques, including electron beam irradiation, plasma irradiation, UV irradiation with a photoinitiator, and visible light irradiation with a photoinitiator. Additionally, atom transfer radical polymerisation (ATRP) and reversible addition-fragmentation chain transfer (RAFT) can be used to create a PIPAAm-brush surface [52]. The biggest challenge of using PIPAAm is the relatively long detachment time, whereby it will take approximately 40-60 minutes for the cell sheet to detach. Another issue with PIPAAm is the cell sheet shrinkage after detachment. However, this problem can be tackled using polymer support to prevent shrinkage [53].

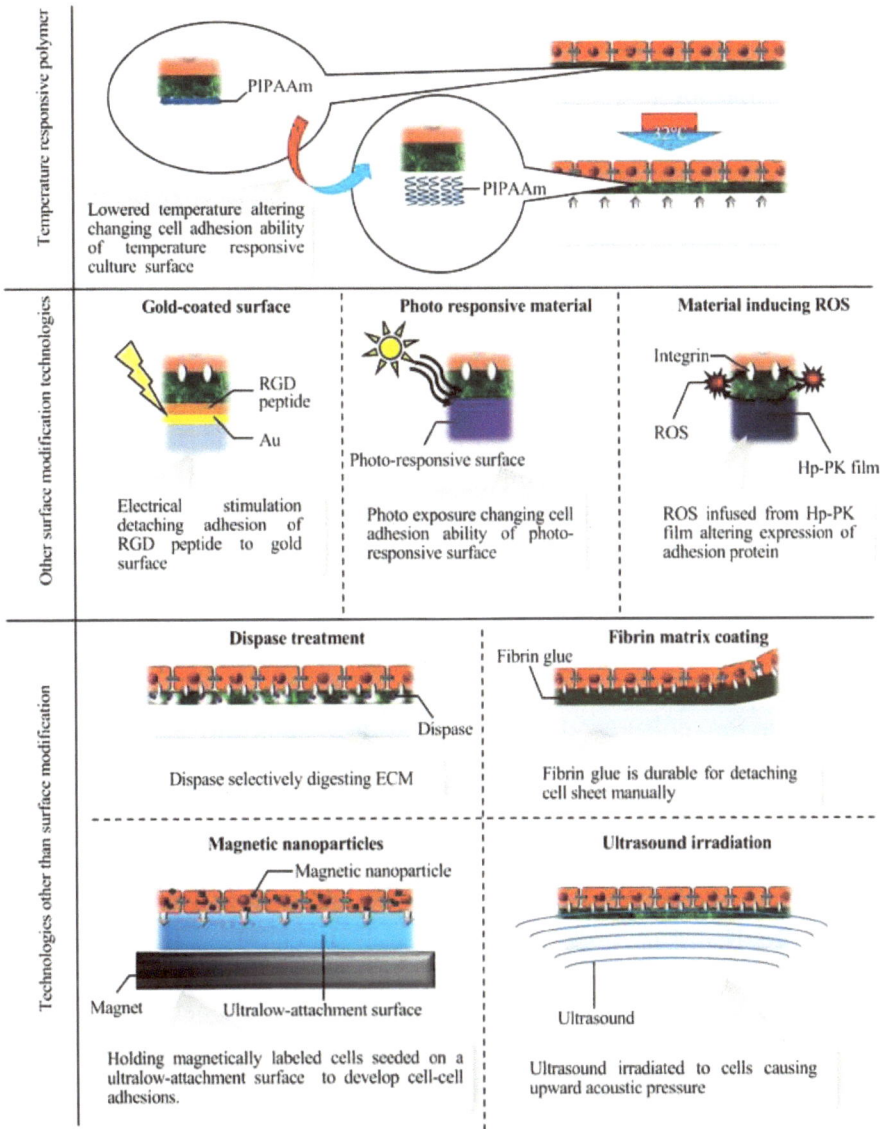

Fig. (3). Techniques to detach the confluence cells as a cell sheet. Conventionally, the temperature-responsive polymer is used to detach the cell sheet. Afterwards, other surface modification techniques, such as gold-coated surfaces, photo-responsive material, and material-inducing reactive oxygen species, have been developed. In addition, Dispase treatment, fibrin matrix coating, magnetic nanoparticles, and ultrasound irradiation also can disrupt the adhesion between the cells and the culture surface. (Reproduced with permission from reference [45])

The gold-coated surface is another method used to prepare acell sheet. In this technique, cell sheet is detached using specific electrochemical reactions [54]. A zwitterionic oligopeptide is used to create a gold-thiolate bond on the gold surface and the other terminal of the oligopeptide contains a domain that supports integrin-mediated cell adhesion. In this case, the cells are not in direct contact with the gold surface. Upon confluence, the cell sheets can be detached from the surface by applying an electrical stimulus that cleaves the gold-thiolate bond, followed by desorption of the oligopeptide layer. The entire process takes round 5-10 minutes, which is much faster compared to the PIPAAm approach [55, 56]. The direct transplantation of the cell sheets detached from the gold-coated surface has been done successfully. This approach can also be used to prepare tailor-made cell sheets using customised 3D molds [53].

Next is the use of photo-responsive materials to detach the cells. Light has the advantage of high spatiotemporal resolution, and using low-intensity biocompatible light to disrupt the attachment between the cells, and the culture surface is not harmful. It will not interfere with other cellular processes [57]. Many light-responsive systems have been used to detach the cell sheets. Generally, these methods can be divided into 2 mechanisms. The first is using light to interrupt the attachment between the cell and the culture surface. The second is disrupting the interaction between the adhesion protein and culture surface [45]. In the first method, light exposure will modify the electrical charge or wettability of the light-responsive materials, subsequently interrupting the cell attachment on the culture surface. Many biocompatible materials have been reported to change their wettability or electrical change through exposure to different types of light. These materials include metal oxides (e.g., zinc oxide (ZnO) and titanium dioxide (TiO_2) and azobenzene that are modifiable by ultraviolet (UV) light [58]. TiO_2 nanodot films with Arg-Gly-Asp (RGD) peptide immobilisation have been used to detach mouse calvaria-derived preosteoblasts (MC3T3-E1) cell sheets [59]. In addition, cell sheets also can be detached from the culture surface*via* the photothermal method. For example, the near-infrared (NIR) photothermal effect of poly(3,4-ethylene dioxythiophene) (PEDOT) allows the detachment of cell sheets from the collagen layer on top of the PEDOT layer [60]. NIR irradiation will cause local heating that induces the dissociation of collagens and release of the cell sheet. Only a few minutes of NIR irradiation is required to detach the cell sheets [61]. A unique advantage of the PEDOT method is the reusability of the PEDOT surface, as the NIR irradiation does not cause photo breakage and photodegradation [62].

Previously, studies have found that reactive oxygen species (ROS) influence cell attachment, and elevation in intracellular ROS will lead to cell detachment [63]. Afterwards, the rise in extracellular ROS also has been found to cause cell detachment by damaging the cell membrane, decreasing the number of integrin-related adhesion molecules, and interrupting the cell-ECM interaction [64, 65].

Thus, materials inducing ROS production have been utilised to detach as cell sheets. In a recent study, the authors seeded various types of cells on the hematoporphyrin-polyketone film and the cells were detached in a sheet *via* irradiation with a green light-emitting diode (510 nm) [66]. Different types of cells can be detached without damage by controlling the irradiation power and time. The cell detachment is caused by the protein structural changes induced by the ROS produced upon green light irradiation.

Changes in pH also can be used to detach the cell sheet even though this application is hampered by the limited range of pH (6.8-7.4) that allow normal cell function. Cells have been reported to detach as a sheet by lowering the environmental and local pH. In the study, the authors fabricated the pH-responsive surface by stacking cationic poly(allylamine hydrochloride) layers and anionic poly(styrene sulfonate) layers on a conductive indium tin oxide surface [67]. The cell sheet detached within 10 to 20 minutes upon trigger with a current density of 30 μA/cm^2. It is postulated that the cells detached because of the drop in the local pH. Thus, in the subsequent experiments, the authors decreased the environmental pH and found that the cell sheet only detached at pH 4.0 (within 2 to 3 minutes), while no changes in cell adhesion were observed at pH 5.0 to 7.4. Even though the cells were exposed to low pH, the recovered human placenta-derived MSCs are viable and capable of differentiating into adipogenic and osteogenic lineages.

Dispase is a protease that selectively digests the ECM to detach the cell sheets from the culture surface [68]. Dispase is a milder enzyme that causes less damage to the cells compared to trypsin. Dispase has been widely used to detach the epidermal cell sheet for transplantation [69]. However, the usage of Dispase will disrupt the ECM protein, which is important for the survival of transplanted cell sheets. In fact, a study has found that the survival rate of the cell sheets detached with temperature-responsive polymer is higher compared to the cell sheets detached with Dispase [70]. Apart from Dispase, collagenase also has been used to detach oral mucosal epithelial cell sheets [71].

Cells can also be seeded on top of the fibrin-coated surface and detach as a cell sheet using forceps [72]. This is a relatively simple technique, and the cell sheets are relatively easier to handle due to the presence of the fibrin glue layer. However, in another study, the rat cardiomyocytes secreted protease that digested the fibrin glue [73]. Thus, the cell sheets are easier to detach and are in direct contact with other cells, allowing the transfer of electrical signals that permit synchronous beating of the multilayered cell sheets.

Magnetic systems can also be used to regulate cell attachment and detachment. The magnetically labelled cells are attracted to attach to the ultralow attachment culture surface when exposed to the magnet. When the cell sheet is formed, the magnet will be removed, and the cell sheet will detach from the surface. Generally, the magnetic nanoparticles used to label the cells have excellent biocompatibility and are compatible with many types of cells. More importantly, the cells retained their therapeutic potential [74, 75].

Cell sheets can be detached from the culture surface using ultrasonic vibration. The advantage of this technique is that it does not involve changes in temperature and pH as well as addition of chemicals that may influence cell functionality. Thus, excellent biocompatibility can be expected. Furthermore, it is also not technically complicated. This technique can be used to detach cells from normal culture dishes at a relatively low cost [76]. Lastly, it is also possible to detach intact cell sheets from the culture dish mechanically using a cell scrapper. However, the usage of cell scrappers might cause mechanical damage to the cell sheets.

Cell Sheet for Tendon and Ligament Repair

Cell sheet technology is not ideal for fabricating tendon and ligament substitutes as it is fragile and lack of mechanical strength. Mechanical strength is important for tendon and ligament substitutes because these tissues must sustain high mechanical loading to allow joint motility. However, the cell sheets can be used to wrap around the sutured tendon/ligament, the tendon/ligament graft, and the engineered tendon/ligament to stimulate and enhance tissue regeneration. To the best of our knowledge, a cell sheet has yet to be used clinically to enhance tendon and ligament repair. Nonetheless, the preliminary results from the animal studies have shown very promising results.

The cells delivered *via* cell sheet technology can migrate and recellularise the injured tendon and ligament as well as secrete paracrine factors that stimulate the native cells to proliferate and regenerate. Tendon/ligament stem cells and MSCs have been utilised to prepare cell sheets for tendon and ligament repair. It remains ambiguous about which cell type is more effective in tendon and ligament repair, as positive results have been reported with both types of cells. In the future, a comparison between the different types of cells should be conducted.

Harada *et al.* used cell sheets prepared from human rotator cuff-derived cells to repair rotator cuff injury in a rat model [77]. The results showed that the cell sheets promoted tendon regeneration and angiogenesis as well as increased the mechanical strength of the repaired tendon. In another study, Mifune *et al.* prepared a human anterior cruciate ligament (ACL)-derived CD34+ cell sheet and tested it in a rat model of ACL reconstruction [78]. The authors found that the cell sheets promoted the maturation of the tendon graft, stimulated blood vessel formation, enhanced healing at tendon-bone junction (higher angiogenesis and osteogenesis), supported proprioceptive recovery, and enhanced the mechanical strength of the healed tendon graft. In another study, Lui *et al.* wrapped the tendon graft with a tendon-derived stem cell (TDSC) sheet and used it to treat a rat model of ACL reconstruction [18]. Results showed that the TDSC cell sheet enhanced tendon repair improved the mechanical properties of the graft, and gave rise to better graft osteointegration. Chang *et al.* reported that wrapping the tendon graft with a periosteal progenitor cell sheet enhanced the tendon-bone junction healing in a rabbit model of extra-articular tendon-bone healing as indicated by the better fibrocartilage formation at the tendon-bone junction at week 4 and the presence of matured fibrocartilage at the tendon-bone junction at week 8 [19].

Liu *et al.* reinforced the engineered tendon-fibrocartilage-bone composite with bone marrow-derived MSC (BM-MSC) cell sheet and used it to promote rotator cuff healing in a canine model [79]. After 6 weeks, cell sheets were found to enhance tendon repair, increase the mechanical strength of healed tendon, and promote graft integration at the tendon-bone interface. Maruyama *et al.* implanted the rat BM-MSC cell sheet in a rat model of Achilles tendon injury. They found that it enhanced the mechanical strength of the tendon tissue at day 5 and day 6 post-transplantation compared to the animals that received sutures alone [80]. The faster improvement in mechanical strength suggested that the patients might be able to start the rehabilitation earlier. Zhao *et al.* combined the poly(lactide-c--glycolide) (PLGA) scaffold with basic fibroblast growth factor (bFGF) and BM-MSC cell sheet to treat Achilles tendon injury in rats and found that the cell sheet promoted tendon repair [81]. A synergistic effect was seen when both bFGF and cell sheet were incorporated into the PLGA scaffold. In a recent study, Zhou *et al.* examined the potential of the book-shaped acellular tendon scaffold (ATS) augmented with a BM-MSC cell sheet in promoting the healing of bone-tendon interface injury [82]. The authors reported positive results whereby the more prominent regeneration and higher mechanical strength were recorded in the injured bone-tendon interface treated with ATS + cell sheet. In addition, they also found macrophage polarisation towards the M2 phenotype, which resolves inflammation.

CHALLENGES IN USING CELL SHEETS FOR TENDON AND LIGAMENT REPAIR

The biggest challenge of applying cell sheet technology for tendon and ligament repair is the poor mechanical property of the cell sheets. Thus, a cell sheet is used together with scaffolds for tendon and ligament repair. Additionally, it is difficult to prepare a cell sheet with complicated structure and morphology, albeit newer cell sheet fabrication techniques have shown the possibility of producing patterned cell sheets. Stacking of the cell sheets often leads to cell apoptosis. This is because gaseous and nutrient transportation as well as the waste removal*via* diffusion is not sufficient to meet the metabolic demand of the cells residing in the centre of the 3-dimensional multi-layered cell sheet. This shortcoming limited the number of cell sheets that could be stacked together. Furthermore, even though the cell sheets contain ECM proteins, the components of the cell sheet ECM proteins and native tissue ECM proteins are different. Conditioning of the culture cells might be useful for the modulation of the cell sheet ECM protein. Additionally, application of mechanical stimulus might also stimulate the cells to secrete more ECM protein to attain a thicker cell sheet.

Table 1. Cell sheets used to support tendon and ligament repair.

Reference	Cells used to Prepare Cell Sheet	Animal Model	Grouping	Key Outcomes
Harada *et al.* [77]	Human rotator cuff-derived cells	Rats with infraspinatus tendons resected bilaterally at the enthesis	1. Transosseous technique 2. Transosseous method + cell sheet	1. Faster tendon regeneration with better mechanical strength 2. Promote angiogenesis
Mifune *et al.* [78]	Human ACL-derived CD34+ cells	Rats with ACL reconstruction using the autologous flexor digitorum longus tendon	1. Tendon graft 2. Tendon graft + cell injection 3. Tendon graft + cell sheet	1. Promote healing of tendon graft with higher mechanical strength 2. Promote angiogenesis 3. Promote angiogenesis and osteogenesis at the tendon-bone junction 4. Promote proprioceptive recovery
Lui *et al.* [18]	Allogeneic rat tendon-derived stem cells	Rats with ACL reconstruction using the autologous flexor digitorum longus tendon	1. Tendon graft 2. Tendon graft + cell sheet	1. Promote healing of tendon graft with higher mechanical strength 2. Promote osteointegration
Chang *et al.* [19]	Rabbit periosteal progenitor cell sheet	Rabbits with the extra-articular tendon-bone healing procedure	1. Tendon graft 2. Tendon graft + cell sheet	1. Enhanced tendon-bone junction healing
Liu *et al.* [79]	Autologous canine BM-MSCs	Canines with a full-thickness infraspinatus tendon injury	1. Suture repair 2. TFBC 3. TFBC + cell sheet	1. Promote tendon healing with higher mechanical strength 2. Promote graft integration at the tendon-bone junction

(Table 1) cont.....

Reference	Cells used to Prepare Cell Sheet	Animal Model	Grouping	Key Outcomes
Maruyama *et al.* [80]	Allogeneic rat BM-MSCs	Rats with Achilles tendon transection	1. Suture repair 2. Suture repair + cell sheet	1. Higher mechanical strength on day 5 and day 6
Zhao *et al.* [81]	Allogeneic rat BM-MSCs	Rats with Achilles tendon resection (7 mm)	1. PLGA mesh 2. PLGA mesh + bFGF-fibrin gel 3. PLGA + cell sheet 4. PLGA + bFGF-fibrin gel + cell sheet	1. Cell sheets promote tendon healing 2. Group 4 showed the best result with the highest mechanical strength
Zhou *et al.* [82]	Allogeneic rabbit BM-MSCs	Rabbits with partial patellectomy	1. No treatment 2. ATS 3. ATS + cell sheet	1. Promote the healing of bone-tendon interface injury

ACL- anterior cruciate ligament, BM-MSCs- bone marrow-derived mesenchymal stem cells, TFBC- tendon-fibrocartilage-bone composite, PLGA- poly(lactide-co-glycolide), bFGF- basic fibroblast growth factor, ATS- acellular tendon scaffold.

CONCLUSION

Advancement in science and technology has led to the introduction of more effective cell sheet fabrication techniques, which cause less damage to the cells. Additionally, these new techniques also preserve the matrix secreted by the cells. Preservation of secreted matrix is critical it has been found to influence cell*via*bility upon transplantation. Currently, cell sheet has yet to be widely utilised to promote tendon and ligament repair. Nonetheless, preliminary findings in animal models showed encouraging results. And we anticipate more studies, including clinical trials, will be conducted in the future to examine the efficacy of cell sheets in tendon and ligament repair.

ACKNOWLEDGEMENTS

This work was supported by research grants from Universiti Kebangsaan Malaysia Medical Centre (FF-2020-188 & FF-2020-096)

REFERENCES

[1]   Wu F, Nerlich M, Docheva D. Tendon injuries. EFORT Open Rev 2017; 2(7): 332-42.
[http://dx.doi.org/10.1302/2058-5241.2.160075] [PMID: 28828182]

[2]   Yang G, Rothrauff BB, Tuan RS. Tendon and ligament regeneration and repair: Clinical relevance and developmental paradigm. Birth Defects Res C Embryo Today 2013; 99(3): 203-22.
[http://dx.doi.org/10.1002/bdrc.21041] [PMID: 24078497]

[3]   Svensson RB, Heinemeier KM, Couppé C, Kjaer M, Magnusson SP. Effect of aging and exercise on

the tendon. J Appl Physiol 2016; 121(6): 1353-62.
[http://dx.doi.org/10.1152/japplphysiol.00328.2016] [PMID: 27150831]

[4]   Aicale R, Tarantino D, Maffulli N. Overuse injuries in sport: a comprehensive overview. J Orthop
Surg Res 2018; 13(1): 309.
[http://dx.doi.org/10.1186/s13018-018-1017-5] [PMID: 30518382]

[5]   Jung H-J, Fisher MB, Woo SL-Y. Role of biomechanics in the understanding of normal, injured, and
healing ligaments and tendons. Sports Med Arthrosc Rehabil Ther Technol 2009; 1(1): 9.
[PMID: 19457264]

[6]   Lim WL, Liau LL, Ng MH, Chowdhury SR, Law JX. Current progress in tendon and ligament tissue
engineering. Tissue Eng Regen Med 2019; 16(6): 549-71.
[http://dx.doi.org/10.1007/s13770-019-00196-w] [PMID: 31824819]

[7]   Yang J, Yamato M, Kohno C, *et al.* Cell sheet engineering: Recreating tissues without biodegradable
scaffolds. Biomaterials 2005; 26(33): 6415-22.
[http://dx.doi.org/10.1016/j.biomaterials.2005.04.061] [PMID: 16011847]

[8]   Moschouris K, Firoozi N, Kang Y. The application of cell sheet engineering in the vascularization of
tissue regeneration. Regen Med 2016; 11(6): 559-70.
[http://dx.doi.org/10.2217/rme-2016-0059] [PMID: 27527673]

[9]   Li M, Ma J, Gao Y, Yang L. Cell sheet technology: a promising strategy in regenerative medicine.
Cytotherapy 2019; 21(1): 3-16.
[http://dx.doi.org/10.1016/j.jcyt.2018.10.013] [PMID: 30473313]

[10]   Lu Y, Zhang W, Wang J, *et al.* Recent advances in cell sheet technology for bone and cartilage
regeneration: from preparation to application. Int J Oral Sci 2019; 11(2): 17.
[http://dx.doi.org/10.1038/s41368-019-0050-5] [PMID: 31110170]

[11]   Chen G, Qi Y, Niu L, *et al.* Application of the cell sheet technique in tissue engineering. Biomed Rep
2015; 3(6): 749-57.
[http://dx.doi.org/10.3892/br.2015.522] [PMID: 26623011]

[12]   Hafez P, Chowdhury SR, Jose S, *et al.* Development of an *in vitro* cardiac ischemic model using
primary human cardiomyocytes. Cardiovasc Eng Technol 2018; 9(3): 529-38.
[http://dx.doi.org/10.1007/s13239-018-0368-8] [PMID: 29948837]

[13]   Lim J, Razi ZRM, Law JX, *et al.* Mesenchymal stromal cells from the maternal segment of human
umbilical cord is ideal for bone regeneration in allogenic setting. Tissue Eng Regen Med 2018; 15(1):
75-87.
[http://dx.doi.org/10.1007/s13770-017-0086-6] [PMID: 30603536]

[14]   Hassan MNFB, Yazid MD, Yunus MHM, *et al.* Large-scale expansion of human mesenchymal stem
cells. Stem Cells Int 2020; 2020: 1-17.
[http://dx.doi.org/10.1155/2020/9529465] [PMID: 32733574]

[15]   Looi QH, Eng SP, Liau LL, *et al.* Mesenchymal stem cell therapy for sports injuries-From research to
clinical practice. Sains Malays 2020; 49(4): 825-38.
[http://dx.doi.org/10.17576/jsm-2020-4904-12]

[16]   Liau LL, Al-Masawa ME, Koh B, *et al.* The potential of mesenchymal stromal cell as therapy in
neonatal diseases. Front Pediatr 2020; 8: 591693.
[http://dx.doi.org/10.3389/fped.2020.591693] [PMID: 33251167]

[17]   Liau LL, Looi QH, Chia WC, Subramaniam T, Ng MH, Law JX. Treatment of spinal cord injury with
mesenchymal stem cells. Cell Biosci 2020; 10(1): 112.
[http://dx.doi.org/10.1186/s13578-020-00475-3] [PMID: 32983406]

[18]   Lui PPY, Wong OT, Lee YW. Application of tendon-derived stem cell sheet for the promotion of graft
healing in anterior cruciate ligament reconstruction. Am J Sports Med 2014; 42(3): 681-9.
[http://dx.doi.org/10.1177/0363546513517539] [PMID: 24451112]

[19]   Chang CH, Chen CH, Liu HW, *et al.* Bioengineered periosteal progenitor cell sheets to enhance tendon-bone healing in a bone tunnel. Biomed J 2012; 35(6): 473-80.
[http://dx.doi.org/10.4103/2319-4170.104412] [PMID: 23442360]

[20]   Lake SP, Liu Q, Xing M, *et al.* Chapter 54 - Tendon and ligament tissue engineering. In: Lanza R, Langer R, Vacanti JP, *et al.* (eds). Academic Press, 2020, pp. 989–1005.

[21]   Maffulli N, Wong J, Almekinders LC. Types and epidemiology of tendinopathy. Clin Sports Med 2003; 22(4): 675-92.
[http://dx.doi.org/10.1016/S0278-5919(03)00004-8] [PMID: 14560540]

[22]   Sharma P, Maffulli N. Biology of tendon injury: healing, modeling and remodeling. J Musculoskelet Neuronal Interact 2006; 6(2): 181-90.
[PMID: 16849830]

[23]   Baldino L, Maffulli N, Reverchon E. 14 - Bone–tendon interface. In: Nukavarapu SP, Freeman JW, Laurencin CTBT-RE of MT and I (eds). Woodhead Publishing, 2015, pp. 345–361.

[24]   Hoffmann A, Gross G. Tendon and ligament engineering in the adult organism: mesenchymal stem cells and gene-therapeutic approaches. Int Orthop 2007; 31(6): 791-7.
[http://dx.doi.org/10.1007/s00264-007-0395-9] [PMID: 17634943]

[25]   Derwin KA, Soslowsky LJ, Kimura JH, Plaas AH. Proteoglycans and glycosaminoglycan fine structure in the mouse tail tendon fascicle. J Orthop Res 2001; 19(2): 269-77.
[http://dx.doi.org/10.1016/S0736-0266(00)00032-2] [PMID: 11347701]

[26]   Iozzo RV, Murdoch AD. Proteoglycans of the extracellular environment: clues from the gene and protein side offer novel perspectives in molecular diversity and function. FASEB J 1996; 10(5): 598-614.
[http://dx.doi.org/10.1096/fasebj.10.5.8621059] [PMID: 8621059]

[27]   Connizzo BK, Yannascoli SM, Soslowsky LJ. Structure–function relationships of postnatal tendon development: A parallel to healing. Matrix Biol 2013; 32(2): 106-16.
[http://dx.doi.org/10.1016/j.matbio.2013.01.007] [PMID: 23357642]

[28]   Walden G, Liao X, Donell S, Raxworthy MJ, Riley GP, Saeed A. A Clinical, Biological, and Biomaterials Perspective into Tendon Injuries and Regeneration. Tissue Eng Part B Rev 2017; 23(1): 44-58.
[http://dx.doi.org/10.1089/ten.teb.2016.0181] [PMID: 27596929]

[29]   Riley G. Tendinopathy—from basic science to treatment. Nat Clin Pract Rheumatol 2008; 4(2): 82-9.
[http://dx.doi.org/10.1038/ncprheum0700] [PMID: 18235537]

[30]   Hauser RA, Dolan EE. Ligament injury and healing: an overview of current clinical concepts. *J prolotherapy* 2011; 3: 836–846.

[31]   September AV, Schwellnus MP, Collins M, Gibson W. Tendon and ligament injuries: the genetic component * COMMENTARY. Br J Sports Med 2007; 41(4): 241-6.
[http://dx.doi.org/10.1136/bjsm.2006.033035] [PMID: 17261551]

[32]   Snedeker JG, Foolen J. Tendon injury and repair – A perspective on the basic mechanisms of tendon disease and future clinical therapy. Acta Biomater 2017; 63: 18-36.
[http://dx.doi.org/10.1016/j.actbio.2017.08.032] [PMID: 28867648]

[33]   Rees JD, Wilson AM, Wolman RL. Current concepts in the management of tendon disorders. Rheumatology (Oxford) 2006; 45(5): 508-21.
[http://dx.doi.org/10.1093/rheumatology/kel046] [PMID: 16490749]

[34]   Keller TC, Hogan MV, Kesturu G, James R, Balian G, Chhabra AB. Growth/differentiation factor-5 modulates the synthesis and expression of extracellular matrix and cell-adhesion-related molecules of rat Achilles tendon fibroblasts. Connect Tissue Res 2011; 52(4): 353-64.
[http://dx.doi.org/10.3109/03008207.2010.534208] [PMID: 21250863]

[35] Liu CF, Aschbacher-Smith L, Barthelery NJ, Dyment N, Butler D, Wylie C. What we should know before using tissue engineering techniques to repair injured tendons: a developmental biology perspective. Tissue Eng Part B Rev 2011; 17(3): 165-76.
[http://dx.doi.org/10.1089/ten.teb.2010.0662] [PMID: 21314435]

[36] Leong NL, Kator JL, Clemens TL, James A, Enamoto-Iwamoto M, Jiang J. Tendon and Ligament Healing and Current Approaches to Tendon and Ligament Regeneration. J Orthop Res 2020; 38(1): 7-12.
[http://dx.doi.org/10.1002/jor.24475] [PMID: 31529731]

[37] Pasanen K, Ekola T, Vasankari T, *et al.* High ankle injury rate in adolescent basketball: A 3-year prospective follow-up study. Scand J Med Sci Sports 2017; 27(6): 643-9.
[http://dx.doi.org/10.1111/sms.12818] [PMID: 28033652]

[38] Rodrigues MT, Reis RL, Gomes ME. Engineering tendon and ligament tissues: present developments towards successful clinical products. J Tissue Eng Regen Med 2013; 7(9): 673-86.
[http://dx.doi.org/10.1002/term.1459] [PMID: 22499564]

[39] Rashidbenam Z, Jasman MH, Hafez P, *et al.* Overview of Urethral Reconstruction by Tissue Engineering: Current Strategies, Clinical Status and Future Direction. Tissue Eng Regen Med 2019; 16(4): 365-84.
[http://dx.doi.org/10.1007/s13770-019-00193-z] [PMID: 31413941]

[40] Zhang J. Engineered Tissue Patch for Cardiac Cell Therapy. Curr Treat Options Cardiovasc Med 2015; 17(8): 37.
[http://dx.doi.org/10.1007/s11936-015-0399-5] [PMID: 26122908]

[41] Yan Z, Yin H, Nerlich M, Pfeifer CG, Docheva D. Boosting tendon repair: interplay of cells, growth factors and scaffold-free and gel-based carriers. J Exp Orthop 2018; 5(1): 1.
[http://dx.doi.org/10.1186/s40634-017-0117-1] [PMID: 29330711]

[42] Vaquette C, Sudheesh Kumar PT, Petcu EB, Ivanovski S. Combining electrospinning and cell sheet technology for the development of a multiscale tissue engineered ligament construct (TELC). J Biomed Mater Res B Appl Biomater 2018; 106(1): 399-409.
[http://dx.doi.org/10.1002/jbm.b.33828] [PMID: 28170157]

[43] Matsumine H, Giatsidis G, Osada A, *et al.* Keratinocyte sheets prepared with temperature-responsive dishes show enhanced survival after *in vivo* grafting on acellular dermal matrices in a rat model of staged bi-layered skin reconstruction. Regen Ther 2019; 11: 167-75.
[http://dx.doi.org/10.1016/j.reth.2019.07.003] [PMID: 31388519]

[44] Venugopal B, Shenoy SJ, Mohan S, Anil Kumar PR, Kumary TV. Bioengineered corneal epithelial cell sheet from mesenchymal stem cells—A functional alternative to limbal stem cells for ocular surface reconstruction. J Biomed Mater Res B Appl Biomater 2020; 108(3): 1033-45.
[http://dx.doi.org/10.1002/jbm.b.34455] [PMID: 31400069]

[45] Imashiro C, Shimizu T. Fundamental Technologies and Recent Advances of Cell-Sheet-Based Tissue Engineering. Int J Mol Sci 2021; 22(1): 425. Epub ahead of print
[http://dx.doi.org/10.3390/ijms22010425] [PMID: 33401626]

[46] Yamato M, Okano T. Cell sheet engineering. Mater Today 2004; 7(5): 42-7.
[http://dx.doi.org/10.1016/S1369-7021(04)00234-2]

[47] Kushida A, Yamato M, Konno C, Kikuchi A, Sakurai Y, Okano T. Decrease in culture temperature releases monolayer endothelial cell sheets together with deposited fibronectin matrix from temperature-responsive culture surfaces. J Biomed Mater Res 1999; 45(4): 355-62.
[http://dx.doi.org/10.1002/(SICI)1097-4636(19990615)45:4<355::AID-JBM10>3.0.CO;2-7] [PMID: 10321708]

[48] Madathil BK, Anil Kumar PRA, Kumary TV. N-isopropylacrylamide-co-glycidylmethacrylate as a thermoresponsive substrate for corneal endothelial cell sheet engineering. BioMed Res Int 2014; 2014:

1-7.
[http://dx.doi.org/10.1155/2014/450672] [PMID: 25003113]

[49]   Lim YM, Jeun JP, Lee JH, *et al.* Cell sheet detachment from poly (N-vinylcaprolactam-c-
       -N-isopropylacrylamide) grafted onto tissue culture polystyrene dishes. J Ind Eng Chem 2007; 13: 21-
       6.

[50]   Nitschke M, Gramm S, Götze T, *et al.* Thermo□responsive poly(NiPAAm□ *co* □DEGMA) substrates
       for gentle harvest of human corneal endothelial cell sheets. J Biomed Mater Res A 2007; 80A(4):
       1003-10.
       [http://dx.doi.org/10.1002/jbm.a.31098] [PMID: 17187393]

[51]   Nakayama M, Yamada N, Kumashiro Y, Kanazawa H, Yamato M, Okano T. Thermoresponsive
       poly(N-isopropylacrylamide)-based block copolymer coating for optimizing cell sheet fabrication.
       Macromol Biosci 2012; 12(6): 751-60.
       [http://dx.doi.org/10.1002/mabi.201200018] [PMID: 22517674]

[52]   Doberenz F, Zeng K, Willems C, Zhang K, Groth T. Thermoresponsive polymers and their biomedical
       application in tissue engineering – a review. J Mater Chem B Mater Biol Med 2020; 8(4): 607-28.
       [http://dx.doi.org/10.1039/C9TB02052G] [PMID: 31939978]

[53]   Kobayashi Y, Cordonier CEJ, Noda Y, *et al.* Tailored cell sheet engineering using micro-
       stereolithography and electrochemical cell transfer. Sci Rep 2019; 9(1): 10415.
       [http://dx.doi.org/10.1038/s41598-019-46801-9] [PMID: 31320678]

[54]   Mochizuki N, Kakegawa T, Osaki T, *et al.* Tissue engineering based on electrochemical desorption of
       an RGD-containing oligopeptide. J Tissue Eng Regen Med 2013; 7(3): 236-43.
       [http://dx.doi.org/10.1002/term.519] [PMID: 22162306]

[55]   Enomoto J, Mochizuki N, Ebisawa K, *et al.* Engineering thick cell sheets by electrochemical
       desorption of oligopeptides on membrane substrates. Regen Ther 2016; 3: 24-31.
       [http://dx.doi.org/10.1016/j.reth.2015.12.003] [PMID: 31245469]

[56]   Enomoto J, Kageyama T, Osaki T, *et al.* Catch-and-Release of Target Cells Using Aptamer-
       Conjugated Electroactive Zwitterionic Oligopeptide SAM. Sci Rep 2017; 7(1): 43375.
       [http://dx.doi.org/10.1038/srep43375] [PMID: 28266533]

[57]   Mueller M, Rasoulinejad S, Garg S, Wegner SV. The Importance of Cell–Cell Interaction Dynamics in
       Bottom-Up Tissue Engineering: Concepts of Colloidal Self-Assembly in the Fabrication of
       Multicellular Architectures. Nano Lett 2020; 20(4): 2257-63.
       [http://dx.doi.org/10.1021/acs.nanolett.9b04160] [PMID: 31751141]

[58]   Patel NG, Zhang G. Responsive systems for cell sheet detachment. Organogenesis 2013; 9(2): 93-100.
       [http://dx.doi.org/10.4161/org.25149] [PMID: 23820033]

[59]   Yu ML, Yu MF, Zhu LQ, Wang TT, Zhou Y, Wang HM. The Effects of TiO$_2$ Nanodot Films with
       RGD Immobilization on Light-Induced Cell Sheet Technology. BioMed Res Int 2015; 2015: 1-10.
       [http://dx.doi.org/10.1155/2015/582359] [PMID: 26417596]

[60]   Na J, Heo JS, Han M, Lim H, Kim HO, Kim E. Harvesting of Living Cell Sheets by the Dynamic
       Generation of Diffractive Photothermal Pattern on PEDOT. Adv Funct Mater 2017; 27(10): 1604260.
       [http://dx.doi.org/10.1002/adfm.201604260]

[61]   Kim JD, Heo JS, Park T, Park C, Kim HO, Kim E. Photothermally induced local dissociation of
       collagens for harvesting of cell sheets. Angew Chem Int Ed 2015; 54(20): 5869-73.
       [http://dx.doi.org/10.1002/anie.201411386] [PMID: 25728742]

[62]   You J, Heo JS, Kim J, *et al.* Noninvasive photodetachment of stem cells on tunable conductive
       polymer nano thin films: selective harvesting and preserved differentiation capacity. ACS Nano 2013;
       7(5): 4119-28.
       [http://dx.doi.org/10.1021/nn400405t] [PMID: 23581994]

[63]   Li AE, Ito H, Rovira II, *et al.* A role for reactive oxygen species in endothelial cell anoikis. Circ Res

1999; 85(4): 304-10.
[http://dx.doi.org/10.1161/01.RES.85.4.304] [PMID: 10455058]

[64]   Kolesnikova TA, Kohler D, Skirtach AG, Möhwald H. Laser-induced cell detachment, patterning, and regrowth on gold nanoparticle functionalized surfaces. ACS Nano 2012; 6(11): 9585-95.
[http://dx.doi.org/10.1021/nn302891u] [PMID: 23066742]

[65]   Song H, Cha MJ, Song BW, *et al.* Reactive oxygen species inhibit adhesion of mesenchymal stem cells implanted into ischemic myocardium *via* interference of focal adhesion complex. Stem Cells 2010; 28(3): 555-63.
[http://dx.doi.org/10.1002/stem.302] [PMID: 20073042]

[66]   Koo MA, Lee MH, Kwon BJ, *et al.* Exogenous ROS-induced cell sheet transfer based on hematoporphyrin-polyketone film *via* a one-step process. Biomaterials 2018; 161: 47-56.
[http://dx.doi.org/10.1016/j.biomaterials.2018.01.030] [PMID: 29421562]

[67]   Guillaume-Gentil O, Semenov OV, Zisch AH, Zimmermann R, Vörös J, Ehrbar M. pH-controlled recovery of placenta-derived mesenchymal stem cell sheets. Biomaterials 2011; 32(19): 4376-84.
[http://dx.doi.org/10.1016/j.biomaterials.2011.02.058] [PMID: 21458856]

[68]   Kobayashi J, Kikuchi A, Aoyagi T, Okano T. Cell sheet tissue engineering: Cell sheet preparation, harvesting/manipulation, and transplantation. J Biomed Mater Res A 2019; 107(5): 955-67.
[http://dx.doi.org/10.1002/jbm.a.36627] [PMID: 30684395]

[69]   Wei Q, Reidler D, Shen MY, Huang H. Keratinocyte cytoskeletal roles in cell sheet engineering. BMC Biotechnol 2013; 13(1): 17.
[http://dx.doi.org/10.1186/1472-6750-13-17] [PMID: 23442760]

[70]   Osada A, Sekine H, Soejima K, Sakurai H, Shimizu T. Harvesting epithelial keratinocyte sheets from temperature-responsive dishes preserves basement membrane proteins and improves cell survival in a skin defect model. J Tissue Eng Regen Med 2017; 11(9): 2516-24.
[http://dx.doi.org/10.1002/term.2149] [PMID: 27061496]

[71]   Rovere MR, Rousselle P, Haftek M, *et al.* Preserving Basement Membranes during Detachment of Cultivated Oral Mucosal Epithelial Cell Sheets for the Treatment of Total Bilateral Limbal Stem Cell Deficiency. Cell Transplant 2018; 27(2): 264-74.
[http://dx.doi.org/10.1177/0963689717741140] [PMID: 29637812]

[72]   Ronfard V, Broly H, Mitchell V, *et al.* Use of human keratinocytes cultured on fibrin glue in the treatment of burn wounds. Burns 1991; 17(3): 181-4.
[http://dx.doi.org/10.1016/0305-4179(91)90099-3] [PMID: 1892546]

[73]   Itabashi Y, Miyoshi S, Kawaguchi H, *et al.* A new method for manufacturing cardiac cell sheets using fibrin-coated dishes and its electrophysiological studies by optical mapping. Artif Organs 2005; 29(2): 95-103.
[http://dx.doi.org/10.1111/j.1525-1594.2005.29020.x] [PMID: 15670278]

[74]   Shimizu K, Ito A, Lee JK, *et al.* Construction of multi-layered cardiomyocyte sheets using magnetite nanoparticles and magnetic force. Biotechnol Bioeng 2007; 96(4): 803-9.
[http://dx.doi.org/10.1002/bit.21094] [PMID: 16865728]

[75]   Ito A, Hibino E, Kobayashi C, *et al.* Construction and delivery of tissue-engineered human retinal pigment epithelial cell sheets, using magnetite nanoparticles and magnetic force. Tissue Eng 2005; 11(3-4): 489-96.
[http://dx.doi.org/10.1089/ten.2005.11.489] [PMID: 15869427]

[76]   Imashiro C, Hirano M, Morikura T, *et al.* Detachment of cell sheets from clinically ubiquitous cell culture vessels by ultrasonic vibration. Sci Rep 2020; 10(1): 9468.
[http://dx.doi.org/10.1038/s41598-020-66375-1] [PMID: 32528073]

[77]   Harada Y, Mifune Y, Inui A, *et al.* Rotator cuff repair using cell sheets derived from human rotator cuff in a rat model. J Orthop Res 2017; 35(2): 289-96.

[http://dx.doi.org/10.1002/jor.23289] [PMID: 27171575]

[78]   Mifune Y, Matsumoto T, Takayama K, *et al.* Tendon graft revitalization using adult anterior cruciate ligament (ACL)-derived CD34+ cell sheets for ACL reconstruction. Biomaterials 2013; 34(22): 5476-87.
[http://dx.doi.org/10.1016/j.biomaterials.2013.04.013] [PMID: 23632324]

[79]   Liu Q, Yu Y, Reisdorf RL, *et al.* Engineered tendon-fibrocartilage-bone composite and bone marrow-derived mesenchymal stem cell sheet augmentation promotes rotator cuff healing in a non-weigh--bearing canine model. Biomaterials 2019; 192: 189-98.
[http://dx.doi.org/10.1016/j.biomaterials.2018.10.037] [PMID: 30453215]

[80]   Maruyama M, Wei L, Thio T, Storaci HW, Ueda Y, Yao J. The Effect of Mesenchymal Stem Cell Sheets on Early Healing of the Achilles Tendon in Rats. Tissue Eng Part A 2020; 26(3-4): 206-13.
[http://dx.doi.org/10.1089/ten.tea.2019.0163] [PMID: 31608794]

[81]   Zhao T, Qi Y, Xiao S, *et al.* Integration of mesenchymal stem cell sheet and bFGF-loaded fibrin gel in knitted PLGA scaffolds favorable for tendon repair. J Mater Chem B Mater Biol Med 2019; 7(13): 2201-11.
[http://dx.doi.org/10.1039/C8TB02759E] [PMID: 32073579]

[82]   Zhou Y, Xie S, Tang Y, *et al.* Effect of book-shaped acellular tendon scaffold with bone marrow mesenchymal stem cells sheets on bone–tendon interface healing. J Orthop Translat 2021; 26: 162-70.
[http://dx.doi.org/10.1016/j.jot.2020.02.013] [PMID: 33437635]

CHAPTER 4

Cellulose Nanocrystals-Based Hydrogels for Drug Delivery

Wan Hafizi Wan Ishak[1] and **Ishak Ahmad**[1,*]

1 Department of Chemical Sciences, Faculty of Science and Technology, Universiti Kebangsaan Malaysia (UKM), 43600 Bangi Selangor, Malaysia

Abstract: Recently, cellulose nanocrystals (CNC) have gained attention from researchers around the world due to their favourable properties such as low cost, non-toxicity, biodegradability, biocompatibility, and as small, strong hydrophilic materials, which render them favourable candidates for the preparation of hydrogels. The incorporation of CNC within a hydrogel matrix enables the hydrogel to sustain its shape during swelling-deswelling. Besides absorbing and retaining large amounts of water, hydrogels also respond to specific external environmental factors, such as temperature, pH, the presence of ions, and concentration, making them appealing to be engineered for drug delivery applications. In addition, CNCs also confer high mechanical strength and thermal stability to the hydrogels, which expand their potential in biomedical applications. This chapter focuses on the synthesis of nano cellulose-based hydrogels for drug delivery applications, including the extraction of CNC from various sources, fabrication of hydrogels using chemical and radiation crosslinking, the chemical, physical, and 'smart' properties of the hydrogels, and their application in controlled drug delivery.

Keywords: CNC, Chemical crosslinking, Drug delivery, Gelatin, Radiation crosslinking.

INTRODUCTION

Cellulose Nanocrystals

In recent decades, the use of natural or naturally occurring polymers such as polysaccharides (cellulose, chitin, chitosan) has been paid serious attention by researchers around the globe. Among them, cellulose is known to be the most promising bio-material due to its abundance, renewability, degradability, strong mechanical properties, and cost efficiency [1]. Extensive efforts have been made to procure cellulose nanocrystals (CNC) under controlled conditions to improve

---

* **Corresponding author Ishak Ahmad:** Department of Chemical Sciences, Faculty of Science and Technology, Universiti Kebangsaan Malaysia (UKM), 43600 Bangi Selangor, Malaysia; E-mail: gading@ukm.edu.my

Mohd Fauzi Mh Busra, Daniel Law Jia Xian, Yogeswaran Lokanathan and Ruszymah Haji Idrus (Eds.)

their superior properties, such as high aspect ratio, dispersion, and good mechanical properties.

Cellulose can be extracted from various sources by alkali and bleaching treatments, such as kenaf, rice husk, agave, wood, sugar cane bagasse, and as agro-waste. Uniquely, cellulose is known as a semi-crystalline polymer as it is mainly made up of crystalline and amorphous regions plus hemicellulose, pectin, wax, and lignin [2]. The crystalline domain is structurally organised and dense compared to the amorphous region. Since the chemical structure of cellulose is rich in hydroxyl groups (OH), it is almost impossible to break the crystal part due to the strong hydrogen bonding between the hydroxyl groups in the structure [3]. Therefore, when a strong acid such as sulphuric acid (H_2SO_4) is added to cellulose under controlled conditions, the H^+ ions hydrolyse the disordered and low-density amorphous domains, leaving the individual crystalline part intact, made up of CNCs.

The rigid rod-needle-like CNCs, with a diameter (d) of 5–50 nm and length (L) of 100–200 nm, are the result of cleavage of native cellulose measuring micrometers. Removal of the amorphous part of cellulose not only reduces the size from micrometres to nanometres but also significantly improves the crystallinity and thermal stability of the CNCs produced. Furthermore, they are very crystalline with E-values of over ~100 GPa, thus resulting in good mechanical properties [3]. After sulphuric acid treatment, the CNCs possess negative charges on their surface, which improve their stability in an aqueous suspension [4]. The morphology of CNC relies on the cellulose source, acid conditions used, and the reaction time and it is commonly observed by transmission electron microscopy (TEM), as shown in Fig. (**1**).

Nanocellulose has emerged as one of the advanced nanotechnology prospects for biomedical applications such as tissue engineering, scaffolding, wound dressing, and drug delivery. The excellent properties of CNCs, such as non-toxicity, biocompatibility, high mechanical and thermal properties, renewability, and large surface area for better reactivity, employ a biomimetic approach in medical fields. With advances in technology, materials science, nanoparticle, and polymerisation techniques, the search for ideal drug delivery is widened, with numerous recent findings. The ultimate aim of drug delivery is to develop targeted drug delivery, controlled release, biocompatibility, and non-toxicity, as well as ensure safety with no undesirable side effects [6].

HYDROGELS

Hydrogels exist as three-dimensional networks of polymer with an ability to absorb and retain high amounts of water: up to thousands of times their dry weight. The affinity of hydrogels to absorb water is due to the presence of functional groups in their polymeric system that are strongly attracted to water ($-CONH_2$, $-COOH$, $-CONH-$, $-SO_3H$, and $-OH$). Instead of being dissolved into the aqueous surroundings, hydrogels show a swelling behavior due to the cross-linking in the polymeric network [7].

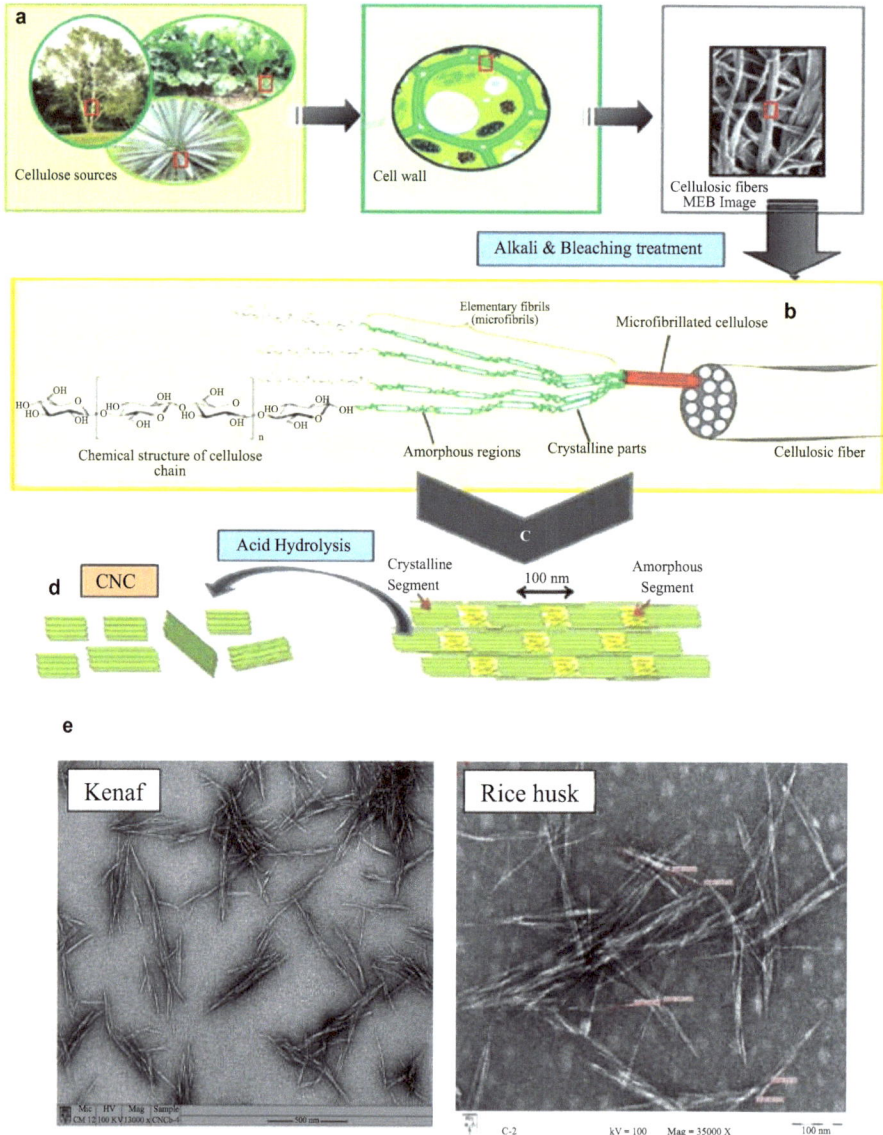

Fig. (1). Schematic route of nanocellulose extraction: (a) cellulosic sources; (b) cellulose structure; (c) cellulose microfibril bundles; and (d) cellulose nanocrystals. Reproduced from [5], copyright 2015 © permission from Elsevier. (e) TEM micrograph of CNC from kenaf and rice husk.

Hydrogels have aroused considerable interest in the medical and pharmaceutical fields due to their biodegradable and biocompatible properties. The labile bonds present within the backbone of biodegradable hydrogels can be broken, either chemically or enzymatically, under physiological conditions. In addition, the compatibility of hydrogels with the human immune system and their harmless degradation products that can be disposed of through excretion processes give them advantages in tissue engineering, wound healing, and drug delivery applications [8]. Therefore, the use of bio-materials such as gelatin, chitin, cellulose, carrageenan, chitosan, and others to synthesise hydrogels is crucial in maintaining these important characteristics. Riberio [9] synthesised chitosan hydrogels for wound dressing applications. The hydrogels prepared promoted cell adhesion and proliferation, and the degradation products were non-toxic [9]. Micro-moulded gelatin hydrogels have been prepared for engineered cardiac tissues with several advantages, such as extracellular gelatin proteins and longer spontaneous contractile activities that extend the culture life of the engineered tissues [10].

As unique polymers, hydrogels are also known for their promising 'smart material' or 'smart hydrogel' properties in their response to changes in the external environment, either chemical or physical. The physical and chemical conditions that induce changes in smart hydrogels include temperature, electric fields, solvent composition, pressure, concentration, pH, and the presence of ions [11]. Hydrogels with such 'sensor' properties or responsiveness to stimuli mimic biological systems where an external stimulus may result in volume or sol-gel phase transition, changes in conformation or solubility, and alteration of a hydrophilic or hydrophobic nature [11, 12]. These smart abilities extend the benefits of hydrogels for medical applications, especially for drug delivery and wound healing applications. For example, the changes in pH at the wound area prior to the healing process are notable, and smart hydrogels will show advantages in wound dressing. As for drug delivery, the different conditions or specific changes in internal organs, such as pH, concentration, the presence of ions, or temperature, will assist in the controlled release or targeted release of drugs entrapped within hydrogels. A schematic presentation of smart hydrogels is shown in Fig. (2).

HYDROGELS FOR BIOMEDICAL APPLICATIONS

The potential of hydrogels in biomedical and pharmaceutical applications has been noticed since the 1960s when the first soft contact lens was developed from hydrogels with high oxygen permeability. Other medical uses soon followed, including a drug delivery system in 1980, followed by wound dressing and tissue engineering applications [14].

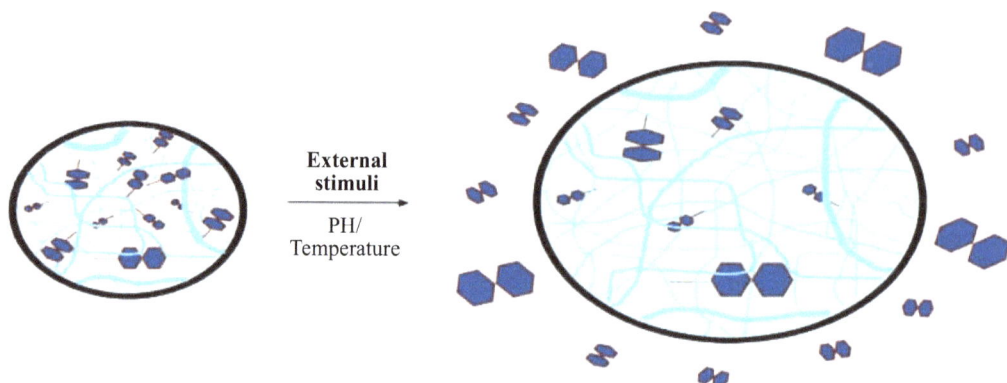

Fig. (2). Schematic representation of drug release from smart hydrogels. Reproduced from [13], copyright 2015©. Permission from Creative Commons Attribution-NonCommercial-ShareAlike-3.0 Licence.

Drug Delivery Systems

Hydrogels are known for their rapid and controllable diffusion rate, which is useful in drug delivery applications. The factor affecting drug release rate is mainly the hydrogel porosity, which can be easily manipulated by regulating the density of crosslinking, the amounts of reinforcing materials used, and the affinity of the hydrogel to swell in certain aqueous environments. Structured, rigid, and well-defined porosity helps drugs to penetrate the hydrogel matrix during drug loading and then permits drug release through the hydrogel network into the targeted organ at dependent rate coefficient diffusion [15].

There are several controlled-release mechanisms shown by hydrogels, such as chemical, diffusion and swelling-controlled mechanisms. Commonly, the kinetic drug release mechanisms of hydrogels are diffusion-controlled, based on Fick's diffusion theory for kinetic modeling where hydrogels might be acting as a matrix or reservoir. As a reservoir, the hydrogel's polymeric system surrounds and encapsulates the drug molecules so that the drug release obeys the first law of Fickian diffusion. The second law of Fickian diffusion explains the mechanism of release of homogeneously dispersed drug molecules from the matrix of a drug delivery system. For a swelling-controlled mechanism to occur, the drug diffusion rate must be higher than the swelling of the hydrogel, which fits a zero-order kinetic model. The glass transition temperature (T_g) will serve as the swelling-induced factor from a glassy to a rubbery phase that enhances the diffusion and release of the drug from the polymeric system. Chemical control describes the enzymatic or hydrolytic cleavage of the polymeric network within the hydrogel system, which leads to drug release. Polymeric chain cleavage could take place through either surface or bulk erosion that subsequently frees the drug molecules from the hydrogel [16]. A schematic representation of drug release mechanisms is illustrated in Fig. (**3**).

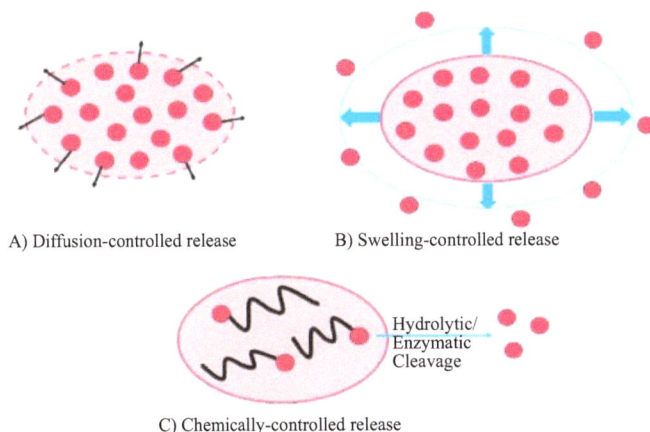

A) Diffusion-controlled release   B) Swelling-controlled release

C) Chemically-controlled release

Fig. (3).   Schematic illustration of drug release mechanism. Reproduced from [16], copyright 2019©. Permission from Creative Commons Licence Deed Attribution 4.0 International (CC BY 4.0).

Stimuli-responsive hydrogels have attracted great interest among both academic and industrial researchers. Among the stimuli studied, the focus has been on the development of pH-responsive systems. Generally, human body parts show variations of pH; even within the gastrointestinal t,ract the pH values vary widely: from the oral cavity (6.8–7.5) to the stomach (1.5–2.0), duodenum (5.6–8.0), small intestine (7.2–7.5) and colon (7.9–8.5). Hence, hydrogels with a pH-responsive ability will have the advantage of releasing the drug carried into the targeted organ. The swelling or de-swelling of pH-stimuli hydrogels in aqueous media of appropriate pH and ionic strength will take place due to the ionisation of pendant groups and development of charges on the polymer backbone, so generating the requisite electrostatic repulsive forces [17]. As a result, the charges will trigger the penetration of aqueous media into the polymer system and promote swelling, simultaneously opening up the pores of the hydrogel for drug release.

CROSSLINKING OF HYDROGELS

The dissolution of hydrogels into aqueous environments, especially during swelling, can be avoided by cross-linking. There are various crosslinking methods used in the preparation of hydrogels, such as physical, chemical, and radiation cross-linking. Physical crosslinking involves the curing of the polymer matrix by heating and cooling, where the interaction between the chains is weak. On the other hand, chemical crosslinking is commonly used since the formation of covalent bonds between the polymer chains enhances the thermal and mechanical properties of the hydrogel. This type of crosslinking uses crosslinking agents such as glutaraldehyde, genipin, formaldehyde, *etc.*, in order to initiate the formation of permanent covalent bonds [8]. Radiation crosslinking is an alternative to initiate crosslinking in hydrogels by using radiation such as electron beams, ultraviolet (UV), and gamma radiation. Unlike chemical crosslinking, this method does not involve any additive or chemical reagent [18].

Chemical Crosslinking of Gelatin and Nanocellulose-Based Hydrogels

Gelatin is a protein biopolymer extracted from the skin, bone, and cartilage of animals by collagen hydrolysis. Being a protein-based biopolymer, it has the advantages of biodegradability, biocompatibility, and non-toxicity, making it a promising materias in the pharmaceutical and biomedical fields, especially for drug delivery, wound dressing, and tissue engineering applications [19]. However, gelatin is unable to maintain its structural integrity or its mechanical properties at body temperature (37 °C), where a sol-gel transition takes place that limits its application. The thermal and mechanical limitations of gelatin can be improved by crosslinking and the use of reinforcing materials [20].

Chemical crosslinking is one of the common methods used to crosslink gelatin due to the abundant amine groups (NH) present in the chemical structures. Glutaraldehyde is used to crosslink gelatin chains, as it easily stabilises the collagen material. The absorption peak in the FTIR spectrum at about 1627 cm^{-1} shows an increase in intensity, which indicates the formation of covalent bonds between the gelatin chains Fig. (**4a**). As glutaraldehyde is present during the reaction, the dialdehyde reacts with the amine groups in the gelatin to form Schiff bases in the reaction between the carbonyl and amine groups, generating an imine as illustrated in Fig. (**4b**). The properties of gelatin hydrogels are improved by reinforcing with CNCs within the gelatin hydrogel matrix. However, the CNCs do not interact chemically with gelatin since there are no new peaks visible in the FTIR spectra of a CNC/gelatin hydrogel compared to that of a gelatin hydrogel Fig. (**4a**). Therefore, CNC/gelatin hydrogels exist as a semi-interpenetrating polymer network (semi-IPN), since the individual chemical structures of both materials are maintained, as illustrated in Fig. (**4b**) [21].

The high crystallinity of CNC can be observed in Fig. (**5a**) by three distinctive sharp and steep diffraction peaks at $2\theta = 16°$, $22°$ and $35°$ which are attributed to cellulose I. As for neat gelatin, the only peak observed is at $20°$, of low and broad structure; thus, the crystallinity is low. This peak is attributed to gelatin's triple-helix structure. The addition of CNCs to a gelatin hydrogel matrix successfully improves the overall crystallinity of the CNC/gelatin hydrogel, as the formation is observed of a peak at $16°$ together with the shifting of the gelatin peak at $20°$ towards $22°$, both as clear, sharp peaks. The impact of CNCs can clearly be observed in the thermal stability of CNC/gelatin hydrogels Fig. (**5b**). Based on derivative thermogravimetry (DTG), a significant degradation occurs at 250–400 °C due to degradation of the gelatin chains at high temperature. Neat gelatin hydrogels degrade readily at 325 °C, while the CNC/gelatin hydrogels with CNC loading of 5, 15 and 25% degrade at 330, 340 and 345 °C, respectively. The increase in thermal stability of gelatin hydrogels reinforced with CNCs is due to the formation of a rigid structure as more CNC is added. Besides the highly crystalline properties of CNCs, the good interfacial adhesion between CNCs and gelatin serve as the main factor in the greater thermal stability.

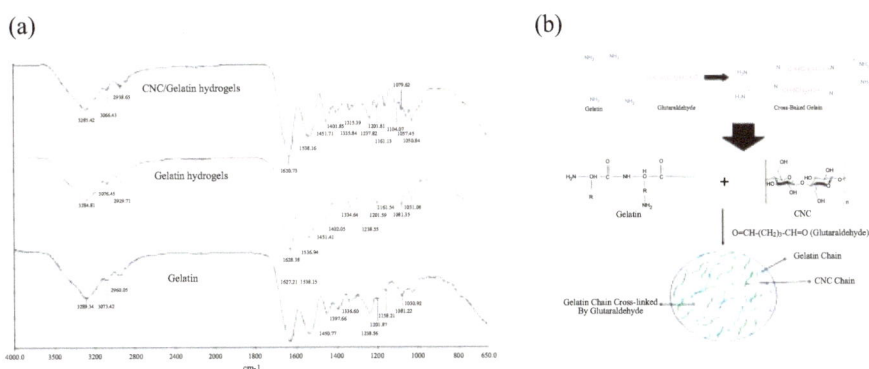

Fig. (4). (a) FTIR spectra of gelatin and gelatin and CNC/gelatin hydrogels; and (b) Mechanism of chemical crosslinking of gelatin and the formation of semi-IPN CNC/gelatin hydrogels. Reproduced from [21], copyright 2016© permission by Elsevier.

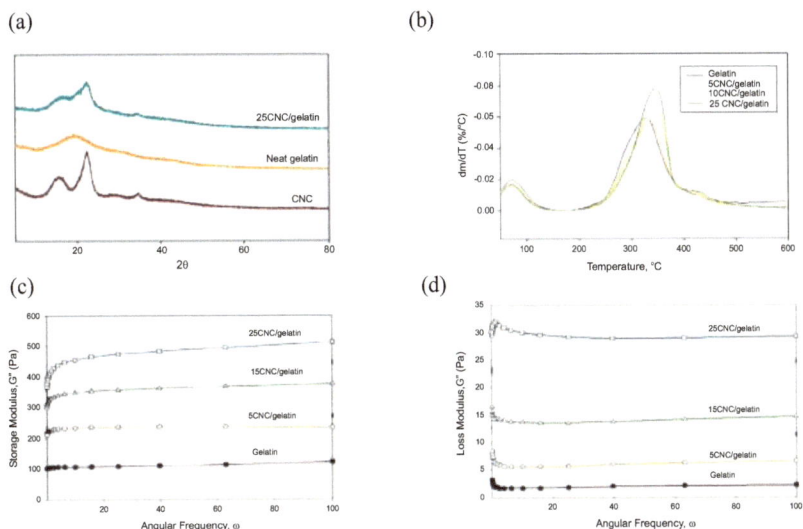

Fig. (5). (a) XRD pattern of CNC and hydrogels; (b) DTG thermogram; and (c) storage modulus and (d) loss modulus of hydrogels. Reproduced from [21], copyright 2016© permission by Elsevier.

Besides improving thermal stability, the reinforcement of gelatin hydrogels with CNCs also helps strengthen their mechanical properties. Rheological studies have been performed on hydrogels in order to understand their dynamic mechanical properties by analysing their storage modulus, G' (elasticity of material) and loss modulus, G" (viscosity of solid material). When subjected to shear, an elastic object will deform, while a viscous solid will preserve its shape. From (Fig. **5c**) and **5d**, it can be seen that the increase in CNC content successfully improves both G' and G". The overall stiffness of CNC/gelatin hydrogels is enhanced as G' increases; thus, solid-like hydrogels are formed. Again, the high crystallinity of CNCs is critical in increasing the stiffness of hydrogels by obstructing the movement of the gelatin chains, thereby enhancing the mechanical integrity [21].

The rigid structure of CNC/gelatin hydrogels can be observed in the SEM micrograph images (Figs. **6a** and **6b**), where the impact of CNC loading on the gelatin polymer network is revealed. With the addition of 5% CNC, a sturdy, well-built, and good void arrangement is observed as the movement of the chains is somewhat restricted. However, when more CNCs are added, the voids become smaller and more compact, with the formation of some agglomeration defects as a result of the significant hindrance in the movement of the polymer chains. This observation is consistent with the rheological properties of CNC/gelatin hydrogels, as discussed earlier. In addition, the formation of pores also affects the hydrogels' swelling capabilities. From Fig. (**6c**), it can be seen that the degree of swelling of gelatin hydrogels improves with the addition of CNCs up to 5% loading, although it decreases as more CNCs are added. As discussed earlier, the tough, large, and well-arranged pores formed with the optimum CNC content help the penetration of water or aqueous solutions into the hydrogel network. The high mechanical strength and crystallinity of CNCs reinforce the pores as the aqueous solution penetrates into the matrix, while the hydrophilic properties attract more water and lead to a high degree of swelling. However, when excess CNCs are present inside the system Fig. (**6b**), they restrict the ability of the chains to swell, and the CNC agglomerations close some of the pores and result in a low degree of swelling, as shown in Fig. (**6c**).

Since the demand for smart polymers has attracted great attention in the biomedical and pharmaceutical fields, the responsiveness of CNC/gelatin hydrogels toward different pH values has been studied. Based on (Fig. **6c**), the hydrogels show their highest degree of swelling at pH 3, followed by pH 11, 9, and 7, and the lowest absorption is at pH 5. Gelatin is an amphoteric polymer that acts as both acid and base due to the presence of amino and carboxyl groups on the side chains. Thus, the swelling performance of gelatin-based hydrogels will depend on the pH value of the aqueous solution. Since the isoelectric point of gelatin is at pH 4.9, the degree of swelling is the lowest at a value close to it (pH

5). At this point, the number of positive and negative charges on the gelatin chains is equal; thus, the electrical attraction between these opposite charges results in network collapse. The charge density in the network only increases with the degree of ionisation as the pH value of the aqueous solution moves further from the isoelectric point. Therefore, the degree of swelling increases. Gelatin forms a cationic gel below the isoelectric point (pH < 4.9) and an anionic gel above it (pH > 4.9). The highest degree of swelling is at pH 3 due to more amine groups present on the gelatin chain than carboxyl groups [22, 23]. Ionisation equations of gelatin in both anionic and cationic forms are shown in Equations (1) and (2):

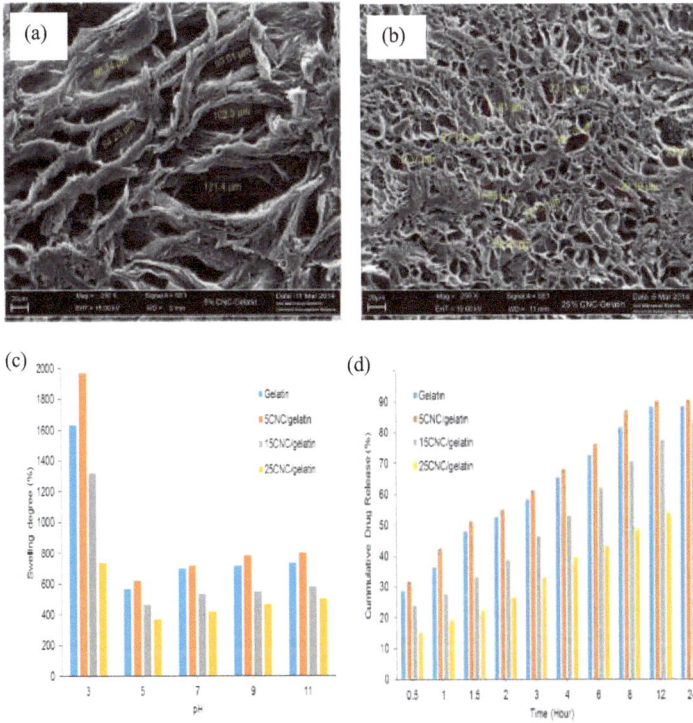

Fig. (6). (a) Degree of swelling of hydrogels at different pH; (b) Cumulative drug release of hydrogels. SEM images of (c) 5CNC/gelatin hydrogel and (d) 25CNC/gelatin hydrogel. Reproduced from [21], copyright 2016 © permission by Elsevier.

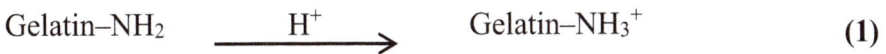

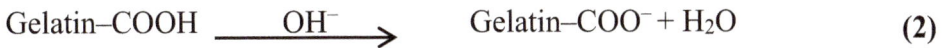

$$\text{Gelatin–NH}_2 \xrightarrow{\text{H}^+} \text{Gelatin–NH}_3^+ \qquad\qquad (1)$$

$$\text{Gelatin–COOH} \xrightarrow{\text{OH}^-} \text{Gelatin–COO}^- + \text{H}_2\text{O} \qquad\qquad (2)$$

The drug release profile in Fig. (**6d**) shows a gradually controlled drug release behaviour as a predesigned dose of theophylline diffuses out from the hydrogel network over a predetermined time. Over time, the performance of drug release can be divided into two stages: at the first stage (0.5 H), a burst effect occurs due to the rapid release of drug molecules present on the hydrogel surface. The second stage is known as the continuous effect, where a suitable level of drug molecules is released continuously over time. In this study, the in-vitro drug release mechanism was examined in simulated gastric fluid (SGF, pH 1.2) as the fabricated hydrogels show a higher degree of swelling at lower pH values, thus indicating this to be an optimum environment [21].

From Fig. (**6d**), the drug release profile can be seen to be coherent with the degree of swelling of all hydrogels: the 5CNC/gelatin hydrogels release the highest amount of theophylline, followed by neat gelatin, 15CNC/gelatin, and 25CNC/gelatin hydrogels [21]. This observation reveals that the morphology of hydrogels is important for drug delivery applications. In addition, the high crystallinity and high mechanical properties of CNC and the optimum CNC loading (5%) help in preserving the structure of the hydrogel voids as drugs diffuse out of the system. This study illustrates the potential application of CNC/gelatin hydrogels in the biomedical field, especially in drug delivery. However, further studies must be performed to ensure the safety and efficacy of the hydrogels.

Radiation Crosslinking of Gelatin and Nanocellulose-Based Hydrogels

Radiation crosslinking involves the use of high energy to induce crosslinking without the addition of additives or chemicals, thus being convenient and green for the preparation of biomedical materials. Generally, radiation has been used as a sterilisation tool for medical apparatus and food safety applications. However, with appropriately controlled conditions and the right materials, a three-dimensional network structure will form as a result of chemical bond formation between the macromolecular backbones of the materials during irradiation, while sterilisation occurs simultaneously [24]. This technique has advantages, especially in medical applications, since it reduces the consumption of chemical reagents and sterilises the materials, thus ensuring their safety and efficacy.

Several methods have been reported that are able to induce crosslinking of gelatin or collagen materials, such as ultraviolet (UV), electron beam, and gamma radiation [18]. Irradiation with UV is able to induce crosslinking only on the surface of the gelatin, as the radiation cannot penetrate the inner part of the material. Electron beam radiation is useful for the curing of materials; however, the energy is insufficient for penetration, as the samples are thicker. Therefore, gamma rays are more favourable since the energy is the strongest of all and thus easily crosslink the gelatin homogenously [24]. Gamma radiation is an important tool in improving the chemical resistance, thermal stability, and mechanical properties of gelatin through grafting, crosslinking, and degradation techniques [25]. (Fig. **7**) shows the synthesis of CNC/gelatin hydrogels using gamma radiation.

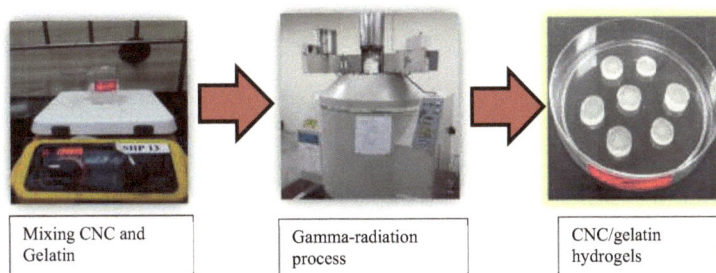

| Mixing CNC and Gelatin | Gamma-radiation process | CNC/gelatin hydrogels |

Fig. (7). Synthesis of gamma-irradiated CNC/gelatin hydrogels.

The FTIR spectrum of gelatin hydrogels shown in Fig. (**8a**) reveals the effect of gamma radiation on the molecular backbone, as more intense absorption appears compared to unirradiated gelatin due to gamma-radiation-induced crosslinking. According to Wisotzki [18], the shifting and reduction in the intensity of absorption peaks at around 3290 and 1550 cm^{-1}, which correspond to N–H stretching and bending, indicate the breakdown of these structures. As the intensity of these bands increases, crosslinking prevails and promotes the formation of more triple-helix networks. The intense band at 1637 cm^{-1} for gelatin hydrogels corresponds to C=O stretching (amide I) due to the organised configuration of helical structures as a result of crosslinking compared to the random configuration of unirradiated gelatin [26].

Based on the proposed mechanism in Fig. (**8b**), water acts as an initiator by absorbing most of the gamma radiation energy and undergoing water radiolysis to produce reactive radicals (proton (•H) and hydroxyl (•OH)). Propagation occurs as •OH removes H-atoms from the polypeptide chain, thus creating gelatin-derived radicals and H_2O. The gelatin radicals then recombine by covalent bonding to form new adjacent polypeptide chains as a termination step to complete the cross-linking process. Significantly, gamma radiation does not induce any crosslinking or grafting between CNC and gelatin, as both materials maintain their individual chemical structures since there are insignificant differences in the peaks Fig. (**8a**) between gelatin and CNC/gelatin hydrogels. Therefore, a semi-interpenetrating network of CNC/gelatin hydrogel is formed with the assistance of gamma-radiation crosslinking [26].

(a)   (b)

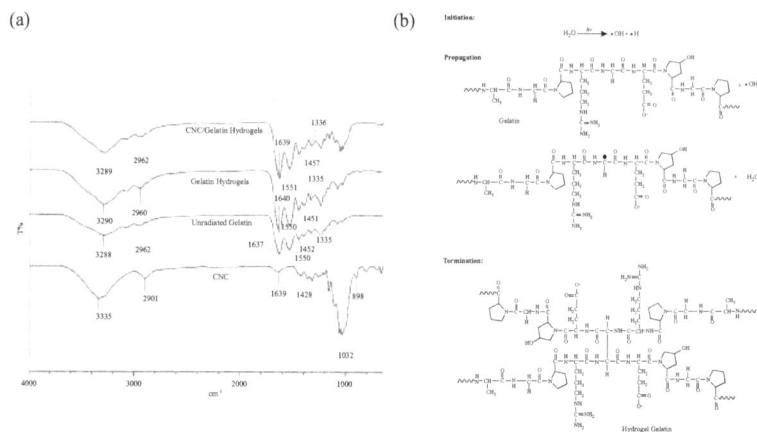

Fig. (8). (a) FTIR spectra of CNC, unirradiated gelatin, gelatin hydrogels and CNC/gelatin hydrogels; and (b) proposed mechanism of gelatin crosslinking by gamma radiation. Reproduced from [26], copyright 2018© permission from Creative Commons Licence Deed Attribution 4.0 International (CC BY 4.0).

The effect of gamma radiation on the dynamic mechanical properties of gelatin can be seen in Fig. (**9a**), where the storage modulus of gamma-irradiated gelatin (gelatin hydrogels) is higher than that of unirradiated gelatin. As discussed earlier, an increase in G' leads to a stiffer hydrogel, which makes it more solid-like. The gamma radiation crosslinks the gelatin molecular chains, creating ordered and more helical structures and thus obstructing the chain movement. In addition, the incorporation of reinforcing materials such as cellulose or CNCs results in improved storage modulus of both cellulose/gelatin and CNC/gelatin hydrogels compared to that of neat gelatin hydrogels. Although both are cellulosic materials, CNC/gelatin hydrogels display impressive storage modulus values, significantly higher than that of cellulose/gelatin hydrogels due to the higher crystallinity of CNC compared to cellulose Fig. (**9b**) [27]. Other than that, CNC also possesses formidable mechanical properties, with Young's modulus of over 100 GPa and large surface areas of several hundred m^2 g^{-1}, making them highly suitable reinforcing materials [28].

The morphologies of cellulose microfibrils, cellulose/gelatin hydrogels, CNC, and CNC/gelatin hydrogels are shown in Figs. (**10a, 10b, 10c,** and **10d**), respectively. It can be seen in Figs. (**10a** and **c**) that cellulose appears as large, long fibres while CNC consists) of individual fibres of needle-like appearance. When both materials are used to reinforce a gelatin matrix, the formation of pores shows significant differences: cellulose/gelatin hydrogels Fig. (**10b**) show an irregular, rough, and disordered pore shape and arrangement, while CNC/gelatin hydrogels (Fig. **10d**) show a smooth, regular, rigid and ordered arrangement of pores as a result of reinforcement with nano-sized CNCs. These morphology differences affect the swelling capabilities of the hydrogels, as displayed in Fig. (**10a**). A slight increase in the swelling ratio of cellulose/gelatin hydrogels over that of gelatin hydrogels is observed, as the addition of cellulose within the gelatin network improves the pore formation. However, the morphology of CNC/gelatin indicates the reason for the impressive swelling ratio of CNC/gelatin hydrogels, where CNC plays a role in sustaining pore integrity as a result of its high mechanical and crystalline properties as osmosis occurs.

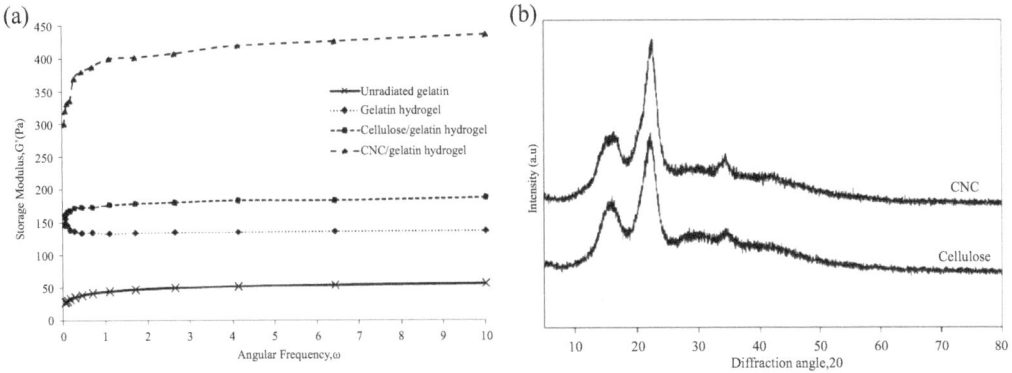

Fig. (9). (a) Storage modulus, G of unirradiated gelatin and hydrogels; (b) XRD of CNC and cellulose. Reproduced from [26], copyright 2018 © permission from Creative Commons Licence Deed Attribution 4.0 International (CC BY 4.0).

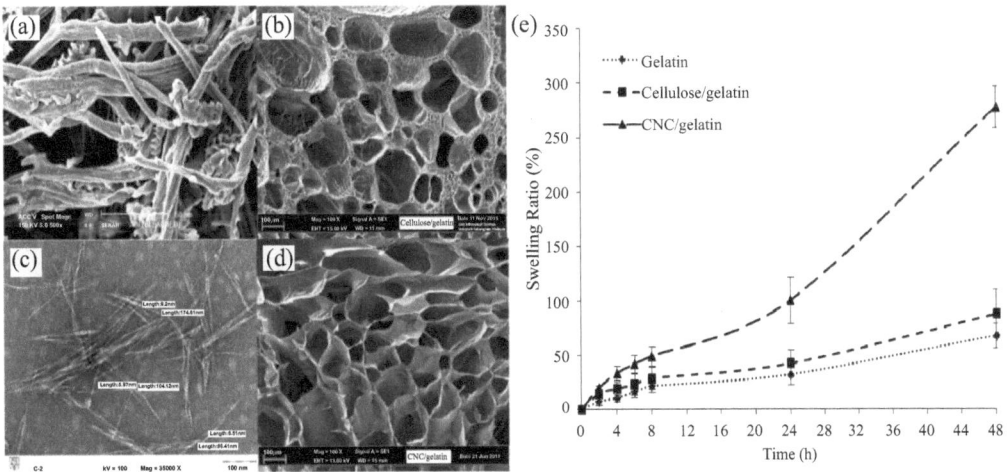

Fig. (10). SEM images of (a) cellulose fibre and (b) cellulose/gelatin hydrogels; (c) TEM image of CNC; (d) SEM image of CNC/gelatin hydrogels; and (e) swelling ratio of hydrogels. Reproduced from [26], copyright 2018 © permission from Creative Commons Licence Deed Attribution 4.0 International (CC BY 4.0).

The drug loading and release efficiency results in Fig. (**11**) show similar trends to the swelling ratio pattern, as CNC/gelatin hydrogels show higher drug loading and release efficiencies compared to gelatin hydrogels. For drug loading to occur, the hydrogels swell when immersed in riboflavin (drug) solution, allowing penetration of drug molecules through the pores to be entrapped within the hydrogel networks. The drug-entrapped hydrogels were then dried in order to remove the unbound water, leaving the drug molecules trapped within the polymer matrix. The drug release process was carried out by immersing the drug-entrapped hydrogels in simulated intestinal fluid (SIF, pH 7) where the hydrogels swelled and pore-opening was induced. The riboflavin molecules then diffused out of the polymer matrix into the SIF solution. This similar pattern reveals the dependence of the drug delivery mechanism on the pore formation, structural integrity and stiffness of hydrogels, as discussed earlier. The importance of radiation crosslinking and CNC reinforcement was reinforced, as the rigidity and sustainability of the hydrogels and their pores were required to uphold the osmotic driving force and the drug penetration mechanism in entering or exiting the hydrogel networks [26].

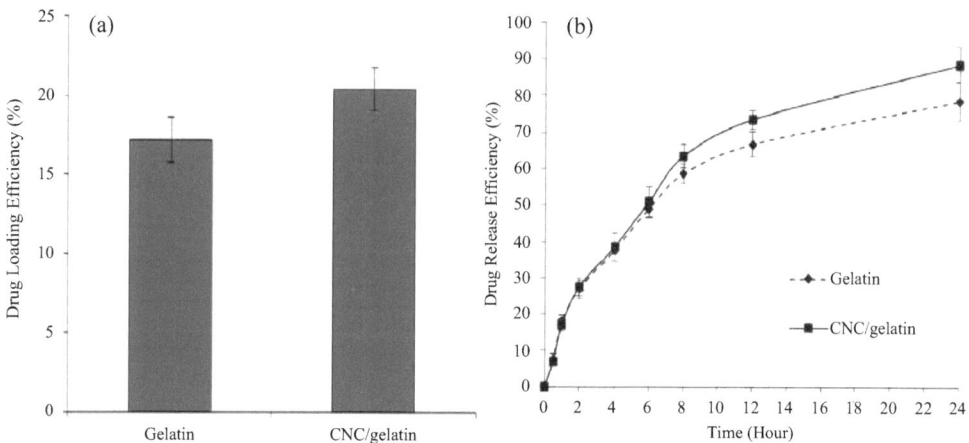

Fig. (11). (a) Drug loading efficiency and (b) drug release efficiency of hydrogels. Reproduced from [26], copyright 2018 © permission from Creative Commons Licence Deed Attribution 4.0 International (CC BY 4.0)

In order to understand the kinetic mechanism of drug release, a mathematical reasoning approach was used to analyse the data based on the Peppas-Sahlin Equation (3) [29].

$$\frac{M_t}{M_\infty} = K_1 t^n + K_2 t^{2n} \tag{3}$$

where M_t/M_∞ is the fraction of drug release at time t and n is the diffusional exponent, while the kinetic constants K_1 represent the contribution of Fickian diffusion and K_2 is attributed to polymer relaxation. The treated experimental data are recorded in Table 1. The regression coefficient (R^2) of the data must be higher than 0.90 in order to be evaluated by the Peppas-Sahlin model. Since the R^2 of the drug release data of this hydrogel is 0.97, they are fit to be elaborated with this model. This model expresses that the drug release mechanism follows the Fickian-type diffusion, as the n-value is 0.45, while non-Fickian or abnormal diffusion is indicated by an n-value greater than 0.45 but less than 1. The zero-order is seen when n = 1. Since the diffusional exponent n-values for both hydrogels are between 0.45 and 1, it is revealed that the kinetic mechanism of drug release in this study follows non-Fickian diffusion. Hence, the rate of drug diffusion depends on the drug concentration gradient (30). In addition, the higher value of K_1 over K_2 demonstrates the dominance of the swelling mechanism compared to the erosion mechanism as well as the high drug solubility [26].

Table 1. Results of experimental data treated by the Peppas-Sahlin equation. Reproduced from [26], copyright 2018© permission from Creative Commons Licence Deed Attribution 4.0 International (CC BY 4.0).

Hydrogel	Kinetic Constant (K_1)	Kinetic Constant (K_2)	Regression Coefficient (R^2)	n
Gelatin	95.85	0.45	0.97	0.68
CNC/Gelatin	100.62	0.48	0.97	0.75

CONCLUDING REMARKS

Cellulose nanocrystals show great potential as reinforcing materials in polymer hydrogels due to their high strength, rigidity, and large surface area. The abundance of CNCs is unquestionable, as they can be extracted from cellulose-based sources (wood, rice husk, corn, *etc.*) by alkali, bleaching, and acid hydrolysis treatments. In addition, the biocompatibility, biodegradability, and non-toxic characteristics of CNCs make them promising materials for drug delivery, wound dressing, and tissue engineering applications. This review summarises the application of CNCs as reinforcing materials in hydrogels for drug delivery applications. Hydrogels are known for their smart ability, by which they respond to changes in surroundings. Gelatin is one of the bio-functional materials used to develop smart hydrogels due to the amphoteric properties that render it sensitive to changes in pH. The combination of gelatin and CNC in a polymer matrix with appropriate crosslinking, particularly by the chemical and radiation techniques outlined in this review, has been shown to solve the limitations of gelatin as a polymer matrix. Furthermore, it also provides impressive thermal and mechanical properties, as well as improved drug delivery performance. Further studies must be performed to optimise the drug delivery application and ensure the safety of the products.

LIST OF ABBREVIATIONS

CNC	Cellulose nanocrystals
DTG	Derivative thermogravimetry
FTIR	Fourier-transform infrared
G'	Storage modulus
G"	Loss modulus
H_2SO_4	Sulphuric acid
NH	Amine group
OH	Hydroxyl groups
semi-IPN	Semi-interpenetrating polymer network
SGF	Simulated gastric fluid
SEM	Scanning electron microscopy
SIF	Simulated intestinal fluid
T_g	Glass transition temperature
TEM	Transmission electron microscopy
UV	Ultraviolet
XRD	X-ray diffraction

ACKNOWLEDGEMENTS

The authors would like to express their gratitude to the Ministry of Higher Education, Malaysia (MOHE), and Universiti Kebangsaan Malaysia (UKM) for financial support through research grants [GUP-2020-048] and [DIP-2018-037].

REFERENCES

[1]   Kargarzadeh H, Ahmad I, Thomas S, Dufresne A. Handbook of nanocellulose and cellulose nanocomposites. Wiley Online Library 2017.
[http://dx.doi.org/10.1002/9783527689972]

[2]   Li X, Tabil LG, Panigrahi S. Chemical treatments of natural fiber for use in natural fiber-reinforced composites: a review. J Polym Environ 2007; 15(1): 25-33.
[http://dx.doi.org/10.1007/s10924-006-0042-3]

[3]   Kim JH, Shim BS, Kim HS, *et al.* Review of nanocellulose for sustainable future materials. International Journal of Precision Engineering and Manufacturing-Green Technology 2015; 2(2): 197-213.
[http://dx.doi.org/10.1007/s40684-015-0024-9]

[4]   Peng BL, Dhar N, Liu HL, Tam KC. Chemistry and applications of nanocrystalline cellulose and its derivatives: A nanotechnology perspective. Can J Chem Eng 2011; 89(5): 1191-206.
[http://dx.doi.org/10.1002/cjce.20554]

[5]   Ng HM, Sin LT, Tee TT, *et al.* Extraction of cellulose nanocrystals from plant sources for application as reinforcing agent in polymers. Compos, Part B Eng 2015; 75: 176-200.
[http://dx.doi.org/10.1016/j.compositesb.2015.01.008]

[6]   Sunasee R, Hemraz UD, Ckless K. Cellulose nanocrystals: a versatile nanoplatform for emerging biomedical applications. Expert Opin Drug Deliv 2016; 13(9): 1243-56.
[http://dx.doi.org/10.1080/17425247.2016.1182491] [PMID: 27110733]

[7]   Hamidi M, Azadi A, Rafiei P. Hydrogel nanoparticles in drug delivery. Adv Drug Deliv Rev 2008; 60(15): 1638-49.
[http://dx.doi.org/10.1016/j.addr.2008.08.002] [PMID: 18840488]

[8]   Gulrez SKH, Al-Assaf S, Phillips GO. Hydrogels: methods of preparation, characterisation, and applications. Prog Mol Environ Bioeng Anal Model to Technol Appl 2011; pp. 117-50.

[9]   Ribeiro MP, Espiga A, Silva D, *et al.* Development of a new chitosan hydrogel for wound dressing. Wound Repair Regen 2009; 17(6): 817-24.
[http://dx.doi.org/10.1111/j.1524-475X.2009.00538.x] [PMID: 19903303]

[10]   McCain ML, Agarwal A, Nesmith HW, Nesmith AP, Parker KK. Micromolded gelatin hydrogels for extended culture of engineered cardiac tissues. Biomaterials 2014; 35(21): 5462-71.
[http://dx.doi.org/10.1016/j.biomaterials.2014.03.052] [PMID: 24731714]

[11]   Qiu Y, Park K. Environment-sensitive hydrogels for drug delivery. Adv Drug Deliv Rev 2001; 53(3): 321-39.
[http://dx.doi.org/10.1016/S0169-409X(01)00203-4] [PMID: 11744175]

[12]   Schmaljohann D. Thermo- and pH-responsive polymers in drug delivery. Adv Drug Deliv Rev 2006; 58(15): 1655-70.
[http://dx.doi.org/10.1016/j.addr.2006.09.020] [PMID: 17125884]

[13]   Ferreira P, Coelho JFJ, Almeida JF, Gil MH. Photocrosslinkable polymers for biomedical applications. Biomed Eng Challenges 2011; 1: 55-74.

[14]   Hoffman AS. Hydrogels for biomedical applications. Adv Drug Deliv Rev 2012; 64: 18-23.
[http://dx.doi.org/10.1016/j.addr.2012.09.010] [PMID: 11755703]

[15]   Hoare TR, Kohane DS. Hydrogels in drug delivery: Progress and challenges. Polymer (Guildf) 2008; 49(8): 1993-2007.
[http://dx.doi.org/10.1016/j.polymer.2008.01.027]

[16]   Ghasemiyeh P, Mohammadi-Samani S. Hydrogels as drug delivery systems; pros and cons. Trends Pharmacol Sci 2019; 5(1): 7-24.

[17]   Gupta P, Vermani K, Garg S. Hydrogels: from controlled release to pH-responsive drug delivery. Drug Discov Today 2002; 7(10): 569-79.
[http://dx.doi.org/10.1016/S1359-6446(02)02255-9] [PMID: 12047857]

[18]   Wisotzki EI, Hennes M, Schuldt C, *et al.* Tailoring the material properties of gelatin hydrogels by high energy electron irradiation. J Mater Chem B Mater Biol Med 2014; 2(27): 4297-309.
[http://dx.doi.org/10.1039/C4TB00429A] [PMID: 32261568]

[19]   Varghese JS, Chellappa N, Fathima NN. Gelatin–carrageenan hydrogels: Role of pore size distribution on drug delivery process. Colloids Surf B Biointerfaces 2014; 113: 346-51.
[http://dx.doi.org/10.1016/j.colsurfb.2013.08.049] [PMID: 24126319]

[20]   Haema K, Oyama TG, Kimura A, Taguchi M. Radiation stability and modification of gelatin for biological and medical applications. Radiat Phys Chem 2014; 103: 126-30.
[http://dx.doi.org/10.1016/j.radphyschem.2014.05.056]

[21]   Ooi SY, Ahmad I, Amin MCIM. Cellulose nanocrystals extracted from rice husks as a reinforcing material in gelatin hydrogels for use in controlled drug delivery systems. Ind Crops Prod 2016; 93: 227-34.

[http://dx.doi.org/10.1016/j.indcrop.2015.11.082]

[22]   Boral S, Gupta AN, Bohidar HB. Swelling and de-swelling kinetics of gelatin hydrogels in ethanol–water marginal solvent. Int J Biol Macromol 2006; 39(4-5): 240-9.
[http://dx.doi.org/10.1016/j.ijbiomac.2006.03.028] [PMID: 16687169]

[23]   Yang XJ, Zheng PJ, Cui ZD, Zhao NQ, Wang YF, De Yao K. Swelling behaviour and elastic properties of gelatin gels. Polym Int 1997; 44(4): 448-52.
[http://dx.doi.org/10.1002/(SICI)1097-0126(199712)44:4<448::AID-PI845>3.0.CO;2-M]

[24]   Zhang X, Xu L, Huang X, Wei S, Zhai M. Structural study and preliminary biological evaluation on the collagen hydrogel crosslinked by γ-irradiation. J Biomed Mater Res A 2012; 100A(11): 2960-9.
[http://dx.doi.org/10.1002/jbm.a.34243] [PMID: 22696280]

[25]   Islam MM, Zaman A, Islam MS, Khan MA, Rahman MM. Physico-chemical characteristics of gamma-irradiated gelatin. Prog Biomater 2014; 3(1): 21.
[http://dx.doi.org/10.1007/s40204-014-0021-z] [PMID: 29470724]

[26]   Wan Ishak W, Ahmad I, Ramli S, Mohd Amin M. Gamma irradiation-assisted synthesis of cellulose nanocrystal-reinforced gelatin hydrogels. Nanomaterials (Basel) 2018; 8(10): 749.
[http://dx.doi.org/10.3390/nano8100749] [PMID: 30241416]

[27]   Wan Ishak WH, Yong Jia O, Ahmad I. pH-Responsive Gamma-Irradiated Poly(Acrylic Acid)-Cellulose-Nanocrystal-Reinforced Hydrogels. Polymers (Basel) 2020; 12(9): 1932.
[http://dx.doi.org/10.3390/polym12091932] [PMID: 32867014]

[28]   Dufresne A. Nanocellulose: a new ageless bionanomaterial. Mater Today 2013; 16(6): 220-7.
[http://dx.doi.org/10.1016/j.mattod.2013.06.004]

[29]   Peppas NA, Sahlin JJ. A simple equation for the description of solute release. III. Coupling of diffusion and relaxation. Int J Pharm 1989; 57(2): 169-72.
[http://dx.doi.org/10.1016/0378-5173(89)90306-2]

[30]   Lim L, Rosli N, Ahmad I, Mat Lazim A, Mohd Amin M. Synthesis and swelling behavior of pH-sensitive semi-IPN superabsorbent hydrogels based on poly (acrylic acid) reinforced with cellulose nanocrystals. Nanomaterials (Basel) 2017; 7(11): 399.
[http://dx.doi.org/10.3390/nano7110399] [PMID: 29156613]

CHAPTER 5

Electrospun Nanofibers for Transdermal Drug Delivery: Current Scenarios

Renatha Jiffrin[1] and **Saiful Izwan Abd. Razak**[1,*]

[1] *Bio Inspired Device and Tissue Engineering Research Group, School of Biomedical Engineering and Health Science, Faculty of Engineering, Universiti Teknologi Malaysia, 81310 Skudai, Johor, Malaysia*

Abstract: Electrospinning is a commonly used approach to fabricate nanofibers of various morphologies. This method is highly effective and economically feasible, capable of producing flexible and scalable nanofibers from a wide variety of raw materials. To construct an ideal nanofiber with the desired morphological properties, electrospinning parameters involving the process, solution, and ambiance need to be fulfilled. Electrospun natural and synthetic polymeric nanofibers have recently proved to be a promising technique for drug delivery systems. Nanofiber-based drug delivery mechanisms can be utilised to transport drugs to specific locations and for a period of time to obtain the intended therapeutic outcomes. The use of electrospun nanofibers as drug carriers in biomedical applications, particularly in transdermal drug delivery systems, may be impressive in the future. Generally, in this kind of system, the active agent or drugs are delivered through the skin into the systemic circulation through a transdermal drug delivery mechanism that is distributed through the skin's surface. Therefore, by using electrospun nanofibers as the carrier of drugs for transdermal delivery, the system can enhance the drug's bioavailability and achieve controlled release.

Keywords: Controlled release, Drug carrier, Drug delivery, Electrospinning, Nanofibers, Transdermal.

INTRODUCTION

Electrospun Nanofibers

Over the past decade, many methods for nanotechnology fabrication have been discovered by researchers in order to study the eccentric characteristics and properties of nanomaterials. Nanoscaled biomaterials are fundamentally constructed according to their biological sources, which provide exclusive pro-

* **Corresponding author Saiful Izwan Abd. Razak:** Bio Inspired Device and Tissue Engineering Research Group, School of Biomedical Engineering and Health Science, Faculty of Engineering, Universiti Teknologi Malaysia, 81310 Skudai, Johor, Malaysia; E-mail: saifulizwan@utm.my

Mohd Fauzi Mh Busra, Daniel Law Jia Xian, Yogeswaran Lokanathan and Ruszymah Haji Idrus (Eds.)

perties different from the mass material. With the emergence of nanotechnology, electrospinning has become one of the most interesting developments in the field. Electrospinning allows polymers to be processed to form a nanoscaled material. The electrospinning method is identified as an extremely useful technique, as this method has the resilience and capability to construct continuous fiber on a huge scale. The diameter of this fiber can be modified from microns to nanometers, thus forming an unwoven construction [1].

Overview of Electrospun Nanofibers

Over the past few decades, nanotechnology has become a rising interdisciplinary area of scientific study. Nanotechnology is a field that includes science, engineering, and technology performed at a nanoscale of 1 to 100 nanometers. Predominantly, nanotechnology and nanoscience are the branches of study and application that work on minuscule matters. They are utilised throughout in other science disciplines. In nanotechnology research, the focus is constructing materials on the scale of atoms and molecules. The purpose is to modify the constructions of these materials at exceedingly tiny sizes to construct particular properties [2]. These developed materials are significantly stronger, lighter, more durable, more sieve,-like and have a lot of other nano traits. Nanotechnology has created a high number of benefits to everyday materials, as well as processes. These advantages have helped mankind in nanoscaled additives, nanoscaled materials, nano-bioengineering, nano-engineered materials, and nanoparticles.

Rather recently, nanotechnology expanded into the medical field, whereby it is broadly used in medical tools, knowledge, and therapies. The combination of nanotechnology and drug or diagnostic particles is identified as nanomedicine. Nanomedicine improves the compatibility of the constructed nanomaterial with targeted cells or tissues [3]. The materials utilised in nanomedicine are developed at nanoscaled sizes and are safe for administration into the human body. Imaging, diagnosis, and drug delivery are the applications that are employed for nanotechnology in medicine. Nevertheless, in efforts to further diversify and expand the use of nanotechnology in medicine, a branch of the science called nanomaterial holds potential.

The study of nanomaterials comprises nanofibers, nanorods, nanowires, nanotubes, nanofoams, and nanocrystals [4]. A variety of nanomaterials offer excellent potency of desirable characteristics comprising nanoscaled structures, excellent tensile strength, porosity, permeability, stability, and surface modification capability [5]. Nanomaterials are distinct from bulk materials of the same composition due to their eccentric physicochemical characteristics, for instance, macroscale surface area to mass ratio, minute size, and greater reactivity [6].

Nanofibers can be divided into two words which are 'nano' and 'fiber'. In Greek, 'nano' stands for extensively small, while fiber is a matter long in diameter. Nanofibers project great and extensive benefits as well as various applications in the biomedical area, textile industries, and filtration [5]. Nanofiber technology has been broadly used or integrated into various applications, whether in electronics, systems for energy transmission, aerospace structure composition, as well as in the medical field. These types of nanomaterials possess fibre-like structures with a diameter of 1 to 100 nanometres. Thus, this characteristic led to their utilisation in biomedical applications such as drug delivery systems, gene delivery, cell therapy, tissue engineering, cancer therapy, and rejuvenating medicine [7]. Lately, the use of nanofibers in biomedical applications has drastically increased due to their great mechanical strength, great porosity, and absence of difficulty in fabrication [8].

Several methods are used to produce nanofibers, including bicomponent extrusion, phase separation, template synthesis, melt-blowing, drawing, centrifugal spinning, and electrospinning. However, in comparison to the other methods, electrospinning is often cited and used due to its efficiency and simplicity in constructing nanofibers. For the past few decades, electrospinning has been acknowledged as a facile technique to produce polymer nanofibers in submicron diameters compared to the standard mechanical method [9]. It is also able to be functionally and effectively electrostatic in a nanometre-scaled diameter.

In electrospinning, the high-potential electric field plays an important role in the production of continuous polymer nanofibers. The electrospinning process has also gained the interests of researchers in tissue engineering and drug delivery for its ability to electrospun natural and biodegradable polymers. Natural and synthetic polymers have been utilised and researched over the length and breadth of the production of continuous nanofibers. Electrospinning is also the most favoured technique to produce biodegradable biopolymers or biocomposites with resemblance to collagen nanofibers of the extracellular matrix [9] and with porosity that allows cell movement for tissue rejuvenation [10].

The electrospinning process involves the extrusion of a liquid jet from the polymer solution with the help of a high voltage. This process enables the production of nanofibers with governable intrinsic pore construction. Thus, smaller pores and higher surface area favour the utilisation of electrospun nanofibers in numerous fields. The use of electrospinning has also spread to the field of biomedical engineering [11]

Important Features of the Electrospinning Process

Fundamentally, electrospinning is a spinning process that fabricates fine fiber with a smaller diameter and more extensive surface area compared to mainstream spinning methods. Electrospinning is also commonly accepted as a sovereign technique for the production of polymeric nanofibers and is an alternative method to electrospraying, which uses voltage to generate the production of liquid jets [12]. In contrast, electrospinning uses electrical forces on the droplet of a viscid polymer solution. This solution will compel polymer surface tension, thus generating jet formation. Before the jet reaches the metal collector, it will experience stretching, followed by the solidification of polymer solution on the metal collector in the form of nanofibers [12]. Numerous nanofibers with diameters varying from 3 nm to 5 μm have been effectively electrospun from natural and synthetic polymers [13].

Generally, there are four sequential steps to conduct the electrospinning process. The first step is the charging of liquid droplets followed by the construction of a Taylor cone. Next, the charged jet experiences elongation in a straight line. Next, with the existence of an electric field, the jet polymer experiences thinning and whipping instability. Lastly, the grounded metal collector plate collects the solidified jet in the form of nanofibers. The electrospinning process produces solid fiber from the evaporation of polymer solvent as the electrostatic forces stretch the solution [8]. The solidified fiber forms continuous nanofibers, which are collected to form a fibre mat.

The standard arrangement of the electrospinning apparatus is shown in Fig. (**1**). Predominantly, the electrospinning setup is composed of three crucial components: high voltage supplier, spinneret made from a capillary tube with a pipette tip or metal needle of a small diameter, and grounded metal collecting plate or rotating mandrel. The electrospinning process is commonly carried out at room temperature and atmospheric pressure. At present, vertical and horizontal setups are the two regular electrospinning configurations. Fig. (**1**) shows a horizontal setup of a commonly available and used electrospinning machine.

The majority of the polymers used in electrospinning are liquefied in a solvent and stirred for a period until a homogenous polymer solution is formed. The polymer solution is then inserted into the syringe and needle for the electrospinning process. In this process, the needle of a small diameter is flattened using sandpapering to ensure that the solidified solution disperses out as uniform nanofibers collected on the surface of the metal plate. The voltage power supply is attached from the metal needle tip to the metal collector plate. The power supply that is used in electrospinning includes a direct current (DC) or alternating current (AC) [14]. During electrospinning, the power supply is attached to the metal needle and metal collector to produce charges that induce repulsion surface charges of the solution [10]. Next, the concentrated charges at the metal needle of the syringe are forced out to the discharged and melting polymer towards an electric field. This leads to the formation of what is called a 'Taylor cone', which is a conical shaped-like droplet formed from the viscous polymer solution [15].

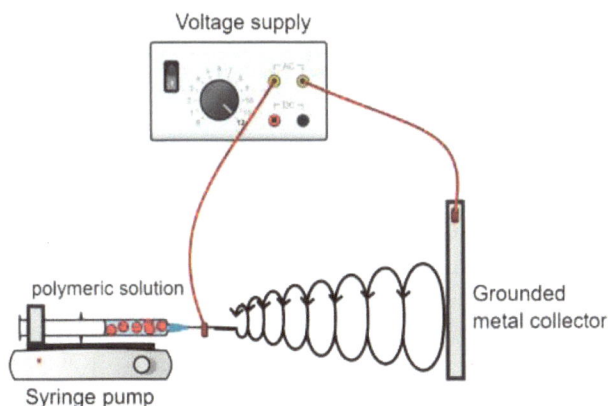

Fig. (1). Schematic of electrospinning setup.

The majority of the polymers used in electrospinning are liquefied in a solvent and stirred for a period until a homogenous polymer solution is formed. The polymer solution is then inserted into the syringe and needle for the electrospinning process. In this process, the needle of a small diameter is flattened using sandpapering to ensure that the solidified solution disperses out as uniform nanofibers collected on the surface of the metal plate. The voltage power supply is attached from the metal needle tip to the metal collector plate. The power supply that is used in electrospinning includes a direct current (DC) or alternating current (AC) [14]. During electrospinning, the power supply is attached to the metal needle and metal collector to produce charges that induce repulsion surface charges of the solution [10]. Next, the concentrated charges at the metal needle of the syringe are forced out to the discharged and melting polymer towards an electric field. This leads to the formation of what is called a 'Taylor cone', which is a conical shaped-like droplet formed from the viscous polymer solution [15].

The process continues with the evaporation of the polymer solution due to the relationship between the electric field and surface tension of the polymer solution, causing the jet stream to elongate. As a result, the solution experiences a whipping motion to form an evaporated solvent [12], that eventually becomes dried fiber deposited all over the metal collector plate [9]. During this process, the jet stream is constantly elongating in the form of hardened long and thin fibre that is collected on the surface of the oppositely charged metal plate, producing a uniform nanofiber sheet. It is vital to perform the electrospinning process at an appropriately high voltage supply because, at a low voltage, Rayleigh's instability would occur, whereby the polymer solution deforms to form spherical droplets [10]. Additionally, deposition time is another important factor. A short deposition time will cause greater jet elongation and solidification, producing longer and thinner nanofibers [10]. Increasing the distance from the spinneret to the metal collector is an approach to increase the deposition time. This creates bending instability during the elongation process [10].

Electrospinning Parameters

Numerous parameters essentially affect the electrospinning process in which they govern the characteristics and properties of the developed nanofibers. Operational parameters are especially crucial to comprehend the electrospinning process due to their ability to affect the nanofibers' morphological properties. Therefore, manipulation of the electrospinning functional parameters allows the design of the nanofibers' diameters and their morphologies to be easily targeted and possibly attained. The idyllic goals to fabricate polymers into nanofibers through the electrospinning process are shown in Fig. (**2**).

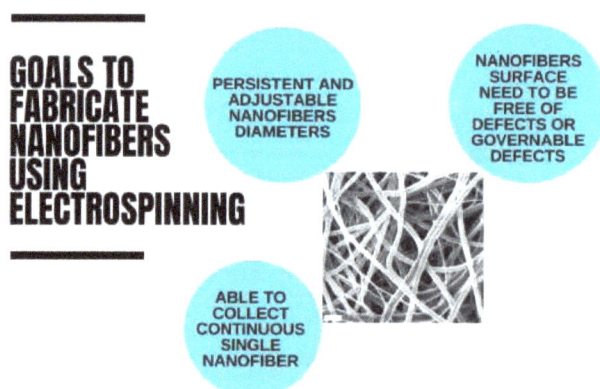

Fig. (2). Goals to fabricate nanofibers using electrospinning.

In electrospinning, the nanofiber's diameter is one of the vital quantities, followed by the diameter's consistency [12]. The essential, commonly utilised, and researched functional parameters of electrospinning can be categorised into processing, solution, and ambient parameters [9]. The parameters that influence the electrospinning process are further illustrated in Fig. (**3**).

CONCERNED PARAMETERS

PROCESSING PARAMETERS	SOLUTION PARAMETERS	AMBIENT PARAMETERS
Flow rate or feeding rate	Viscosity	Humidity
	Concentration	Temperature
Applied voltage	Molecular weight	
Distance between needle tip-metal collector	Surface tension	
	Conductivity	

Fig. (3). Parameters concerning the electrospinning process.

Factors that influence each of the listed parameters are discussed in further detail:

Processing Parameters

The Flow Rate or Feeding Rate

Adjustment to the flow rate or feeding rate of the polymer extrusion controls the material delivering rate and speed of the jet [12]. The feeding rate determines the charge density of the solution [16]. Electrospinning jet that experiences secondary bending instabilities when a great charge density occurs results in the formation of nanofibers with small diametres [17].

Increasing the flow rate equivalently increases the diameters of the nanofibers. Thus, when the feeding rate of the solution is set at a very high value, it causes the formation of beads on the fibers [16]. Zuo *et al.* explain that as more solution is jetted out from the needle tip, as the feeding rate increases, the electric field force is unable to adequately stretch the jet. Consequently, beads are formed from the surplus solution as a result of the presence of surface tension [18]. Beads and pores are the two critical defects that develop in polymer nanofibers formed through electrospinning [19].

Applied Voltage

The applied voltage to the solution during electrospinning is another critical contributing factor that needs to be considered. The applied voltage requires a baseline voltage to be exceeded to ensure the charged jets are extruded from the Taylor cone. Electrospinning is initiated when the baseline voltage is achieved, triggering changes in the solution and electric field, thus developing fiber [12].

This parameter affects the jet flow, thus affecting the diameter of the nanofibers and their morphology. The solution experiences more vigorous stretching as a high voltage is applied. This phenomenon occurs because of the higher columbic forces in the jet and greater electric field that causes the fibre's diameter to decrease and the solvent to evaporate faster [20].

Distance between the Needle Tip and Metal Collector

In electrospinning, the distance between the needle tip and the metal collectors plays a vital role, although it might show less notable effects on the fibre morphology and diameters. A minimal distance between the needle tip and a metal collector is needed to ensure the solvent has ample time to evaporate before the nanofibers land on the surface of the metal collector [16]. If the distance is too short, the fibre will not have sufficient time to evaporate and solidify before reaching the surface of the collector [21]. On the other hand, if the distance is too wide, beads form on the fiber [21].

Solution Parameters

Viscosity

Solution viscosity acts as a vital element affecting the size and morphological properties of the nanofibers. Sukigara *et al*. proved that a low viscosity could not help develop continuous and smooth fiber [21]. Contrarily, at the highest viscosity, the jet struggles to be extruded from the solution, thus achieving an optimum and appropriate viscosity to electrospun the polymer solution [21]. Furthermore, divergent polymer-solvent systems and types of polymers exhibit exceptional viscosity levels [22]. In addition, regulation of the polymer solution's concentration allows simultaneous governing of the solution's viscosity [21].

Concentration

Solution concentration is another vital element that affects the diameter and morphology of nanofibers. The polymer solution's concentration is strongly correlated to the viscosity of the solution. Due to the differences in viscosity and surface tension, the solution's concentration determines the limiting conditions in producing electrospun nanofibers [23]. Dietzel *et al*. researched the effects of processing variables on the morphology of electrospun nanofibers and textiles. Uncontrolled processing variables produced fiber tainted with droplets [24]. However, when a highly concentrated solution is electrospun, nanofibers with regularity, cylindrical morphology, uniform structure, and higher density are produced [24].

Molecular Weight

Polymer molecular weight affects the morphological properties of the electrospun nanofibers in addition to influencing viscosity, surface tension, conductivity, and dielectric strength [24]. Most often, high molecular weight polymer solutions could generate a desirable viscosity to fabricate nanofibers [20]. Polymer solution with a low molecular weight is prone to form beads at a fixed concentration, while a high molecular weight solution produces fiber with averagely larger diameters [20].

Surface Tension

Surface tension crucially correspondents to the characteristics of the solvent rather than the polymer [9] Surface tension of the polymer solution can be diverse, as it depends on the solvent's quantity and the mutual relationship between polymer and solvent [9]. Commonly, the electrospinning process initiated by a high solution surface tension produces jet instability and droplets in spray form [25]. This factor influences the production of droplets, beads, and fiber. Haghi and Akbari state that by lowering the surface tension of the polymeric solution, fibers with fewer beads can be fabricated [26]. However, a solvent with lower surface tension does not always lead to its utilisation in electrospinning. Additionally, when all parameters are fixed, upper and lower boundaries depend on the solution's surface tension [26].

Conductivity

Polymers are commonly conductive, in which charged ions in the polymeric solution are essential in producing the jet during electrospinning. The conductivity of a polymeric solution is normally contemplated by the type of polymer and solvent used and the presence of ionisable salts [20]. Adding a small quantity of ionic salts, namely sodium chloride (NaCl), lithium chloride (LiCl), or selenide chloride (R_4NCl), into the electrospinning solution causes enhancement of the electrospinning solution's conductivity [27]. This lowers the chances of beads being present on the nanofibers [27]. Salts that are soluble in an organic solvent are commonly utilised to increase the solution's electrical conductivity to ensure that jets can withstand a higher current. Huang *et al.* researched to improve the conductivity of nylon solutions in formic acid. These researchers used pyridine, an organic base, to enhance conductivity. The base reacted with the formic acid, causing the escalation of the formation of organic salts from a weak acid and weak base [27]. The nylon nanofibers developed from the pyridine-added solution revealed the absence of beads on the nanofibers' surfaces [27].

Ambient Parameters

In addition to processing and solution parameters, ambient parameters that comprise temperature and humidity are important factors. Numerous studies and research have been carried out to investigate the post-effects of ambient parameters on the electrospinning process, especially on the morphological properties of the nanofibers. Nezarati *et al.* found that at low relative humidity, the nanofibers of polyethylene glycol (PEG) experienced breakage. A low humidity causes the increase of the jet's stretching during whipping after adequate evaporation of the solvent to maintain the nanofiber's morphology [28]. In addition, at relatively high humidity, nanofibers experience breakage as well as morphological degeneration. This is a result of water absorption and PEG dissolution in water [28]. Temperature works inversely to viscosity. By increasing the surrounding temperature, the viscosity of the electrospinning solution decreases, producing a smaller nanofiber diameter [5].

Electrospun Nanofiber for Drug Delivery

Over the last few years, the design and production of controlled drug delivery systems (DDS) have gained a lot of focus. Commonly, DDS is used to enhance the clinical effectiveness and safety of medications by supplying them to a targeted site at a pace determined by the physiological condition throughout therapy. A controlled DDS has various benefits, for instance, enhancing therapeutic effectiveness and transporting drugs at a controlled rate to minimise toxicity that may be present with a regular dosage [29].

Electrospun nanofibers are fibrous carriers also capable of transporting drugs to a specific location of the human body. It also allows for more drugs to be directly loaded into the fibrous carrier. For over a decade, electrospun nanofiber scaffolds have been utilised as carriers for various medications, genomes, and growth factors, with their release profile, precisely regulated by varying morphology, porosity, and composition [21]. Therefore, nanofiber composition and its internal structures are vital to accomplishing unique drug-release profiles.

The hierarchical structures of electrospun nanofibers, including higher surface area, intertwined pore structure, and biocompatible components, aid in drug delivery [10]. In addition, the structure and concentration of shell polymers, the solvents used, drug concentration, surface additives, electrospinning environments, and solubility properties of bioactive agents also influence the drug release profiles [15]. Nanofibers that release drugs quickly usually have a plain, homogenous construction involving a drug and a polymer or polymer blends.

Since electrospun scaffolds are able to deliver site-specific drugs to the human body, they are promising for potential biomedical applications. These are specifically to inhibit post-surgical adhesions and infections, for postoperative local chemotherapy, and in bone and skin tissue engineering [21]. The biochemical characteristics of the encapsulation system are tailored to obtain the required release profiles for a given targeted tissue, which allows the polymeric DDS to deliver therapeutic agents in a coordinated and constant manner [30]. In a DDS, hingeing on the characteristics of the polymer, the drug is released through diffusion or distribution. The former is applied for non-degradable polymers, while the latter is for degrading systems [9].

In addition, to minimise the risk of local drug accumulation, the degradation rate of the polymer specifies the type of drug that will be embedded into the DDS [9]. Thus, significant research has been done on controlling drug release and polymer degradation speeds. DDS with polymer nanofibers highly depends on the surface area of the drug. A larger drug surface area leads to a higher dissolution rate [19]. To ensure ideal selection of polymer nanofibers to achieve an extended drug release, the nanofibers should be made of biodegradable or swellable polymers, which degrade slowly and swell in a biological condition.

To attain polymers with desirable properties, a mixture or blend may be useful [31]. Core-shell nanofibers are a type of DDS with a unique feature. This system consists of several drug-loaded layers or an outer polymer layer that acts as a rate-controlling constriction for drug release, thus encouraging extended drug release [32]. In addition, another method that is used to prolong drug delivery is a sand-wich-type nanofiber mesh. They are constructed by sequential electro spinning of various polymer solutions [33]. Controlling the diameters of the bead in the polymeric nanofibers is also a method to lengthen drug release [34].

Electrospun Nanofiber for Transdermal Drug Delivery

In order to apply electrospun nanofibers in transdermal drug delivery is the first key to understanding the human skin anatomy. The stratum corneum has a thickness of between 25 to 25 μm and is the outermost layer of the skin which has a significant responsibility in absorption and protection against foreign materials [35]. Owing to blood vessels and dendritic cells covering hair follicles, the follicles may be utilised as alternate routes for drug entry through the skin. As a result, permeability is achieved by cosmetics and skin-associated drugs to the circulatory system. The skin thus offers the desired media for drug absorption and penetration into the vascular system [36].

In transdermal drug transport through diffusion, a variety of polymers are functionalised as gelatinisation agents in gel systems and stabilisers in emulsions and creams. These polymers are fabricated to develop scaffolds in the form of patch matrices and wound dressings [37]. Meanwhile in transdermal systems, these polymers play the role of skin adhesives to improve the permeability of medications, and enhance treatment efficacy [38].

Phase separation, prototype synthesis, self-assembly, and electrospinning are some of the techniques used to fabricate polymeric nanofibers. Antibiotics, antitumor medications, anti-inflammatory drugs, proteins, and nucleic acids are some of the pharmaceutical products typically administered using electrospun polymeric scaffolds [39]. Nonetheless, the bulk of experiments has been focused on implantable scaffolds or wound dressings, while researchers have paid little attention to transdermal patches. The few experimental data are very impressive and exciting in terms of potential functional applications. Commonly, polymeric nanofibers are widely used to distribute active pharmaceutical agents, which researchers have classified into two categories. The first category is that of nanofibers which are primed and characterised with encapsulated drugs. This nanofiber-based system is used for external therapy, such as transdermal drug delivery and wound dressings [40].

Transdermal Delivery

Overview of Drug Delivery System

Using a system to deliver drugs is a method of prescribing a medicinal compound to humans or animals by one of the traditional administration routes for a therapeutic result [41]. The administration of the medicine, the release of its active compounds, and subsequent transfer through biological membranes to the site of action are processes of DDS [42]. Systemic adverse effects are common with traditional DDS and are primarily due to their vague and general biodistribution and unmanageable drug release features. Therefore, improvements in the medication's effectiveness and safety through its method of administration are critical aspects in the field.

Additionally, to improve clinical effects and minimise post-effects, activated drug compounds need to aggregate at the specific pathological region while having high controllability for an extended period [43]. To develop better systems, numerous drug delivery and drug targeting systems are being designed and fabricated to minimise drug deterioration and loss, avoid adverse after-effects, improve drug bioavailability, and reach optimal concentration at a targeted site. Researchers have also been developing advanced controlled DDS to allow drug compounds to be released in a restrained manner.

As DDS consists of the therapeutic compound and the delivery system, their differences are a crucial criterion used by drug or pharmacy enforcement agencies to assess the product. There is a broad and case-by-case distinction and categorisation between the drugs and their delivery devices. The active ingredients of a medication can only be released into the targeted region of the body; therefore, the drug's release over time can be primarily regulated by its composition without contact with the host's defensive system. The route of administration is a key factor in ensuring these properties.

The assortment of the route varies based on three factors: the desired result, type of illness, and, finally, the type of substance [41]. Drugs can be directly prescribed to the diseased organ or routinely and specifically to the affected organ. The following are the most generally used drug administration pathways:

• Oral: The reasons for this choice are self-evident since they are simple to administer and widely accepted by patients.
• Parenteral: Parenteral refers to injecting drugs into the bloodstream by pathways other than the gastrointestinal tract. It refers to injection through subcutaneous, intramuscular, intravenous, and intra-arterial routes.
• Transdermal: The release of medications *via* the skin or mucous membranes is known as transdermal drug delivery. This route of administration is strongly correlated to a local effect rather than a systemic. In addition, active ingredients will be precisely distributed to the systemic circulation, bypassing gastrointestinal and liver metabolism [41].
• Inhalation: For this route, drugs or medications would immediately enter the lungs, making it the best option to avoid systemic effects.

Transdermal Drug Delivery System

Conventional transdermal drug delivery systems (TDDS) and transdermal patches release drugs through permeability. Transdermal drug delivery is a promising alternative to oral drug delivery, which could soon be a viable alternative to hypodermic injection [44]. Transdermal delivery also has benefits against hypodermic injections that are uncomfortable, produce hazardous medical wastes, and create a risk for disease transmission through needle re-use [45]. Furthermore, transdermal devices are non-invasive, self-administrable, and able to release drugs for more extended periods. They often help patients comply with their treatment plans, and the services are mostly affordable.

Reservoir systems, matrix systems without a rate-controlling membrane, and matrix systems with a rate-controlling membrane are the three types of transdermal drug distribution systems [38]. The medication reservoir, rate-controlling membrane, and adhesive are the three main components of each reservoir system [38]. The medication and excipients are typically found in the drug reservoir. The drug is stored in the adhesive in a matrix structure, then makes its way through the membrane and adhesive to the blood. The adhesive acts both as a base and an adhesive for the product, while a rate-controlling membrane is present between the drug-matrix structures of the adhesive layers.

Transdermal Delivery Using Electrospun Nanofibers

Electrospinning produces nanofibers of microns and nanometres in size using electrostatic energy [46]. Table (1) lists the examples of commonly used polymers for electrospinning. The type of polymers that are predominantly safe for humans are biopolymers and synthetic polymers.

Table 1. Selected polymers formed by electrospinning.

Polymer	Type of polymer	Solvent	Reference
Polyvinyl alcohol (PVA)	Biopolymer	Distilled water	[47]
Poly(caprolactone)	Biopolymer	Tri-fluoroethanol	[48]
Chitosan	Biopolymer	Acetic acid	[49]
Gelatine	Biopolymer	Concentrated formic acid	[50]
Cellulose acetate	Biopolymer	Tri-fluoroethanol	[51]
Polyurethane	Synthetic polymer	N,N-Dimethylformamide (DMF), dimethylsulfoxide (DMSO), N-Methylpyrrolidone, tetrahydrofuran (THF).	[52]
Poly (vinyl chloride)	Synthetic polymer	Tetrahydrofuran (THF), Diemthylformamide (DMF)	[53]

In transdermal DDS, the drug is delivered to the skin's surface, preventing unintended drug dissemination and providing exceptional skin permeability. Transdermal patches are now commercially available for treating local tissue areas. Table (2) shows a selection of goods.

In a DDS made of electrospun nanofibers as the drug carrier, drug loading can be accomplished through a few methods. The first method is post-spining modifications. This technique requires post-adsorption of a drug, accomplished by the covalent interaction of the electrospun polymer nanofibers or altered polymer surface [9]. The other method for loading drugs into electrospun nanofibers is by electrospinning a blended solution of polymers and drug or polymer and nanoparticles. Kenawy *et al.* used this method to load ketoprofen into polyurethane/polycaprolactone electrospun nanofiber by blending the drug with the polymer solution [29]. Zhang *et al.* and colleagues blended captopril with a polymer solution of poly(l-lactic acid) (PLLA), poly(lactide-co-glycolide) (PLGA); and poly(lactide-co-glycolide) (PLGA). These blended solutions were then electrospun to form nanofibers loaded with drugs [55]. Fig. (**4**) is the illustration of a drug loading method into a polymeric solution. Here, the drug-polymer solution will be fabricated into electrospun nanofibers through the electrospinning process. Another method used to load drugs is core-shell electrospinning using a co-axial setup. Research conducted by Yu *et al.* used this method to encapsulate ketoprofen in electrospun cellulose acetate (CA) as the core-shell [56].

Table 2. Drugs used in transdermal products [54].

Active Ingredient	Type of Delivery System	Name	Concentration	Dose and Application	Uses
Capsaicin	Topical patch (drug in adhesive)	Qutenza®	8%	For a 60 minutes application, four patches (maximum) can be implemented every three months. Administration by healthcare professional and local topical anaesthetic may be necessary.	Neuropathic pain
Diclofenac epolamine	Topical patch (drug in adhesive)	Flector®	1.3%	Patch of 10 × 14cm loaded with 180 mg. Two times a day administration.	Pain relief
Lidocaine	Topical patch (drug in adhesive)	Lidoderm®	5%	Patch of 10 × 14cm loaded 70 mg/patch, in 24 hour period, three patches are applied at one time for 12 hours.	Postherpetic neuralgia
Menthol and methyl salicylate	Topical patch	Salonpas® Arthritis pain	31.5 mg menthol, 105 mg methyl salicylate	For daily usage, a patch can be used up to four times.	Arthritis associated pain
Salicylic acid	Topical patch	Trans-Ver-Sal®	15%	6 - 20 mm patch	Acne vulgaris, hyperkeratotic psoriasis and removal of wart

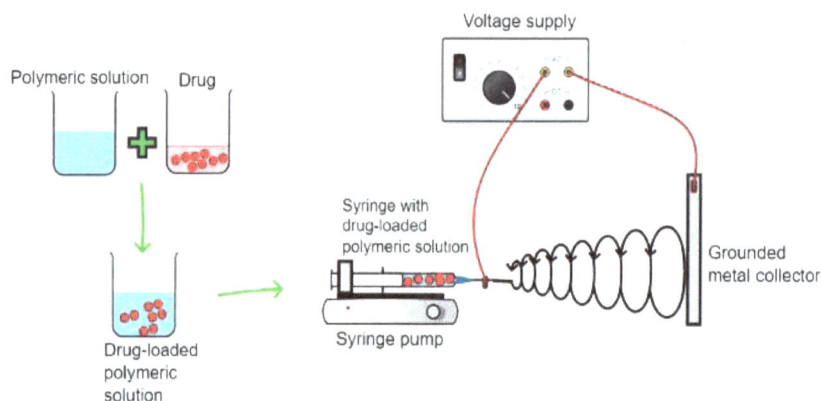

Fig. (4). Schematic diagram of an electrospinning setup for drug-loaded polymeric solutions.

Electrospun scaffolds have been made from a variety of polymers. Example of natural polymers is those originating from collagen, chitosan, gelatin, and hyaluronic acid, whereas polylactic acid (PLA), polycaprolactone (PCL), polyethylene oxide (PEO), polyvinyl alcohol (PVA) and other related co-polymers are synthetic polymers. However, biodegradable polymers are more frequently used for electrospun nanofibers for use as drug delivery carriers.

Fig. (**5**) illustrates the two methods used to load biodegradable polymers, which are corrosion and diffusion. In terms of the speed ratio of both techniques, drug release from these polymers can be regulated *in vivo* by a combination of the two. The majority of biodegradable polymers used in drug delivery are hydrolysable, but specific polymers are regulated by enzymatic catalytic activity [57]. It is also key to note that drug release occurs concurrently with the breakdown of biodegradable polymers. This may result in toxicity due to a sudden build-up of the drug in the body [58]. Therefore, the composition of the drug, polymer fibre content, and rate of drug release, as well as both polymer degradation and biodegradation rates, should be concurrently optimised [57]. Additionally, further consideration must be made of the skin's biology.

With the increment of drug absorption into the skin, the patches should be amorphous or non-ionic [58]. Fig. (**6**) illustrates the drug penetration into the dermal capillary network occurring mostly between cells. This route is known as an intercellular transport, while the shunting route alternatively allows the penetration of electrospun nanofibers into the skin. The transportation of drugs happens when electrospun drug-loaded nanofibers come into contact with the skin's surface. The drug enters through three possible pathways: sweat ducts, hair follicles, and sebaceous glands.

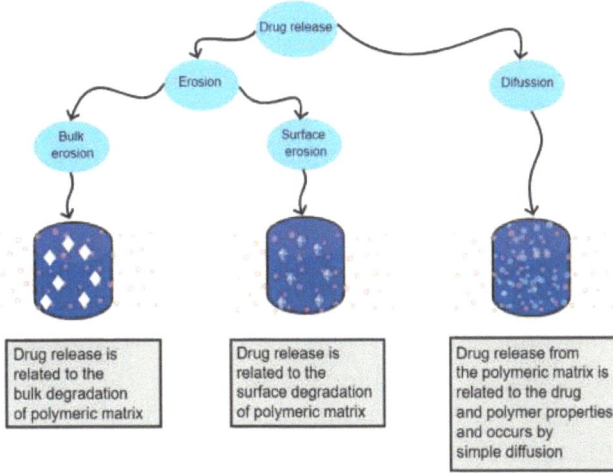

Fig. (5). Kinds of drug release [58].

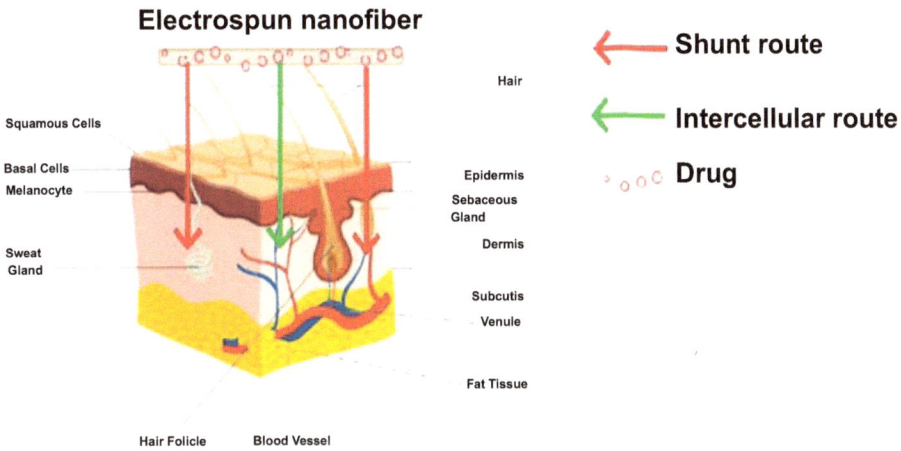

Fig. (6). Drug-loaded electrospun nanofiber for transdermal administration of drugs.

Furthermore, two methods are available to study the characteristics of drug-loaded electrospun nanofibers to identify drug release characteristics. These methods are known as total immersion and transdermal diffusion through pig skin [57]. In the total immersion approach, drug-loaded electrospun nanofibers of a circular disc shape of approximately 2.8 cm in diameter are immersed in 40 ml of the acetate buffer solution at 37 °C. After a specific diffusion period, 0.5 ml of the buffer solution is drawn out [57]. On the other hand, the drug-loaded electrospun nanofiber is placed on a fresh piece of pig skin positioned on top of the acetate buffer solution on a modified Franz diffusion cell. After the required diffusion time, 0.3 ml of the buffer solution is extracted [57]. The amount of drug in the extracted solutions is evaluated using an ultraviolet (UV) spectrophotometer at wavelengths of 296, 282, 272, and 321 nm for sodium salicylate (SS), diclofenac sodium (DS), naproxen (NAP), and indomethacin (IND). Absorbance readings are then compared to a pre-set calibration curve for every model of the drug [57].

CONCLUSION

Electrospinning is a cost-effective technique to fabricate nanofibrous matrices of differing nanofiber diameters from an array of materials. Emergence of the electrospinning technique and the accessibility to a broad range of natural, synthetic, and semisynthetic polymers have led to the successful electrospinning of numerous drugs and polymers into nanofibers. These very fine fibers are nanoscaled with tunable diameters and morphologies. These constructed matrices can be utilised to create multiscaled biomimetic constructions that accommodate a tuneable distribution pattern and broad functionality.

Using electrospinning to construct nanofibers is likely to create a personalised microenvironment depending on the biomedical applications required. In tissue engineering, electrospun nanofibers are utilised in tissue regeneration, whereby several drugs are loaded into the nanofiber's frameworks for a programmed release. To make sure a personalised microenvironment is achieved, it is essential to identify and tailor key and associated parameters to electrospun desired nanofibers of the selected materials. Electrospun nanofibers have already been broadly used in DDS. In recent years, nanofibers have been utilised in transdermal DDS in which nanofibers are loaded with drugs for delivery through the skin's surface. Finally, electrospinning has been shown to be very useful in a broad range of biomedical applications as well as in research due to its simplicity, cost-effectiveness, ease of use, and fabrication, even with limited financial resources.

LIST OF ABBREVIATIONS

AC	Alternating Current
CA	Cellulose Acetate
DC	Direct Current
DDS	Drug Delivery Systems
DMF	N-Dimethylformamide
DMSO	Dimethylsulfoxide
DS	Diclofenac Sodium
IND	Indomethacin
LiCl	Lithium Chloride
NaCl	Sodium Chloride

NAP	Naproxen
PEG	Polyethylene Glycol
PVA	Polyvinyl Alcohol
PLLA	Poly(l-lactic Acid)
PLGA	Poly(lactide-co-glycolide)
PLA	Polylactic Acid
PCL	Polycaprolactone
PEO	Polyethylene Oxide
R₄NC	Selenide Chloride
SS	Sodium Salicylate
TDDS	Transdermal Drug Delivery Systems
THF	tetrahydrofuran
UV	Ultraviolet

REFERENCES

[1]   Maheshwari R, Joshi G, Mishra DK, Tekade RK. Bionanotechnology in Pharmaceutical Research. 2019; 449-71.

[2]   Initiative USNN. https://www.nano.gov/node/639

[3]   Research   GT.   https://www.medicaldevice-network.com/comment/nanotechnology-medici-e-technology/#:~:text=Nanomedicine

[4]   Almetwally AA, El-Sakhawy M, Elshakankery MH, Kasem MH. Technology of nano-fibers: Production techniques and properties - Critical review. J Text Assoc 2017; 78(1): 5-14.

[5]   Jain R, Shetty S, Yadav KS. Unfolding the electrospinning potential of biopolymers for preparation of nanofibers. J Drug Deliv Sci Technol 2020; 57: 101604.
        [http://dx.doi.org/10.1016/j.jddst.2020.101604]

[6]   Chen S, Zhang Q, Hou Y, Zhang J, Liang XJ. Nanomaterials in medicine and pharmaceuticals: nanoscale materials developed with less toxicity and more efficacy. Eur J Nanomed 2013; 5(2): 61-79.
        [http://dx.doi.org/10.1515/ejnm-2013-0003]

[7]   Ramalingam M, Ramakrishna S. Introduction to nanofiber Composites. Nanofiber Composites for Biomedical Applications 2017; pp. 3-29.

[8]   Sabra S, Ragab DM, Agwa MM, Rohani S. Recent advances in electrospun nanofibers for some biomedical applications. Eur J Pharm Sci 2020; 144: 105224.
        [http://dx.doi.org/10.1016/j.ejps.2020.105224] [PMID: 31954183]

[9]   Rogina A. Electrospinning process: Versatile preparation method for biodegradable and natural polymers and biocomposite systems applied in tissue engineering and drug delivery. Appl Surf Sci 2014; 296: 221-30.
        [http://dx.doi.org/10.1016/j.apsusc.2014.01.098]

[10]   Badmus M, Liu J, Wang N, Radacsi N, Zhao Y. Hierarchically electrospun nanofibers and their applications: A review. Nano Materials Science 2021; 3(3): 213-32.
        [http://dx.doi.org/10.1016/j.nanoms.2020.11.003]

[11]   Yang J, Wang K, Yu DG, Yang Y, Bligh SWA, Williams GR. Electrospun Janus nanofibers loaded with a drug and inorganic nanoparticles as an effective antibacterial wound dressing. Mater Sci Eng C

2020; 111: 110805.
[http://dx.doi.org/10.1016/j.msec.2020.110805] [PMID: 32279788]

[12]   Karakaş H. Electrospinning of nanofibers and their applications. Istanbul Technical University, Textile Technologies and Design Faculty 2015.

[13]   Sridhar R, Sundarrajan S, Venugopal JR, Ravichandran R, Ramakrishna S. Electrospun inorganic and polymer composite nanofibers for biomedical applications. J Biomater Sci Polym Ed 2013; 24(4): 365-85.
[http://dx.doi.org/10.1080/09205063.2012.690711] [PMID: 23565681]

[14]   Xue J, Wu T, Dai Y, Xia Y. Electrospinning and electrospun nanofibers: Methods, materials, and applications. Chem Rev 2019; 119(8): 5298-415.
[http://dx.doi.org/10.1021/acs.chemrev.8b00593] [PMID: 30916938]

[15]   Cleeton C, Keirouz A, Chen X, Radacsi N. Electrospun nanofibers for drug delivery and biosensing. ACS Biomater Sci Eng 2019; 5(9): 4183-205.
[http://dx.doi.org/10.1021/acsbiomaterials.9b00853] [PMID: 33417777]

[16]   Shi X, Zhou W, Ma D, *et al.* Electrospinning of nanofibers and their applications for energy devices. J Nanomater 2015; 2015: 1-20.
[http://dx.doi.org/10.1155/2015/140716]

[17]   Rošic R, Kocbek P, Baumgartner S, Kristl J. Electro-spun hydroxyethyl cellulose nanofibers: the relationship between structure and process. J Drug Deliv Sci Technol 2011; 21(3): 229-36.
[http://dx.doi.org/10.1016/S1773-2247(11)50031-0]

[18]   Zuo W, Zhu M, Yang W, Yu H, Chen Y, Zhang Y. Experimental study on relationship between jet instability and formation of beaded fibers during electrospinning. Polym Eng Sci 2005; 45(5): 704-9.
[http://dx.doi.org/10.1002/pen.20304]

[19]   Huang Z, Zhang Y, Kotaki M, Ramakrishna S. A review on polymer nanofibers by electrospinning and their applications in nanocomposites 2003; 63: 2223-53.

[20]   Bhardwaj N, Kundu SC. Electrospinning: A fascinating fiber fabrication technique. Biotechnol Adv 2010; 28(3): 325-47.
[http://dx.doi.org/10.1016/j.biotechadv.2010.01.004] [PMID: 20100560]

[21]   Li Z, Wang C. One-dimensional nanostructures: electrospinning technique and unique nanofibers. 2013.

[22]   Tiwari SK, Venkatraman SS. Importance of viscosity parameters in electrospinning: Of monolithic and core–shell fibers. Mater Sci Eng C 2012; 32(5): 1037-42.
[http://dx.doi.org/10.1016/j.msec.2012.02.019]

[23]   Subbiah T, Bhat GS, Tock RW, Parameswaran S, Ramkumar SS. Electrospinning of nanofibers. J Appl Polym Sci 2005; 96(2): 557-69.
[http://dx.doi.org/10.1002/app.21481]

[24]   Deitzel JM, Kleinmeyer J, Harris D, Beck Tan NC. The effect of processing variables on the morphology of electrospun nanofibers and textiles. Polymer (Guildf) 2001; 42(1): 261-72.
[http://dx.doi.org/10.1016/S0032-3861(00)00250-0]

[25]   Hohman MM, Shin M, Rutledge G, Brenner MP, Rutledge G. Electrospinning and electrically forced jets II Applications Electrospinning and electrically forced jets II. Applications 2001; p. 2221.

[26]   Haghi AK, Akbari M. Trends in electrospinning of natural nanofibers. Phys Status Solidi, A Appl Mater Sci 2007; 204(6): 1830-4.
[http://dx.doi.org/10.1002/pssa.200675301]

[27]   Huang C, Chen S, Lai C, *et al.* Electrospun polymer nanofibres with small diameters. Nanotechnology 2006; 17(6): 1558-63.
[http://dx.doi.org/10.1088/0957-4484/17/6/004] [PMID: 26558558]

[28]   Nezarati RM, Eifert MB, Cosgriff-Hernandez E. Effects of humidity and solution viscosity on electrospun fiber morphology. Tissue Eng Part C Methods 2013; 19(10): 810-9.
[http://dx.doi.org/10.1089/ten.tec.2012.0671] [PMID: 23469941]

[29]   Kenawy E, Abdel-hay FI, El-newehy MH, Wnek GE. Processing of polymer nanofibers through electrospinning as drug delivery systems 2009.

[30]   Ghafoor B, Aleem A, Najabat Ali M, Mir M. Review of the fabrication techniques and applications of polymeric electrospun nanofibers for drug delivery systems. J Drug Deliv Sci Technol 2018; 48: 82-7.
[http://dx.doi.org/10.1016/j.jddst.2018.09.005]

[31]   Zupančič Š, Sinha-Ray S, Sinha-Ray S, Kristl J, Yarin AL. Long-term sustained ciprofloxacin release from PMMA and hydrophilic polymer blended nanofibers. Mol Pharm 2016; 13(1): 295-305.
[http://dx.doi.org/10.1021/acs.molpharmaceut.5b00804] [PMID: 26635214]

[32]   Acevedo F, Hermosilla J, Sanhueza C, *et al.* Gallic acid loaded PEO-core/zein-shell nanofibers for chemopreventive action on gallbladder cancer cells. Eur J Pharm Sci 2018; 119: 49-61.
[http://dx.doi.org/10.1016/j.ejps.2018.04.009] [PMID: 29630938]

[33]   Laha A, Sharma CS, Majumdar S. Sustained drug release from multi-layered sequentially crosslinked electrospun gelatin nanofiber mesh. Mater Sci Eng C 2017; 76: 782-6.
[http://dx.doi.org/10.1016/j.msec.2017.03.110] [PMID: 28482590]

[34]   Li T, Ding X, Tian L, Hu J, Yang X, Ramakrishna S. The control of beads diameter of bead-on-string electrospun nanofibers and the corresponding release behaviors of embedded drugs. Mater Sci Eng C 2017; 74: 471-7.
[http://dx.doi.org/10.1016/j.msec.2016.12.050] [PMID: 28254320]

[35]   Prausnitz MR, Langer R. Transdermal drug delivery. Nat Biotechnol 2008; 26(11): 1261-8.
[http://dx.doi.org/10.1038/nbt.1504] [PMID: 18997767]

[36]   Zamani M, Prabhakaran MP, Ramakrishna S. Advances in drug delivery *via* electrospun and electrosprayed nanomaterials. Int J Nanomedicine 2013; 8: 2997-3017.
[PMID: 23976851]

[37]   Kontogiannopoulos KN, Assimopoulou AN, Tsivintzelis I, Panayiotou C, Papageorgiou VP. Electrospun fiber mats containing shikonin and derivatives with potential biomedical applications. Int J Pharm 2011; 409(1-2): 216-28.
[http://dx.doi.org/10.1016/j.ijpharm.2011.02.004] [PMID: 21316431]

[38]   Wokovich AM, Prodduturi S, Doub WH, Hussain AS, Buhse LF. Transdermal drug delivery system (TDDS) adhesion as a critical safety , efficacy and quality attribute 2006; 64: 1-8.

[39]   Pillay V, Dott C, Choonara YE, *et al.* A review of the effect of processing variables on the fabrication of electrospun nanofibers for drug delivery applications. 2013.
[http://dx.doi.org/10.1155/2013/789289]

[40]   Shen X, Yu D, Zhu L, Branford-White C, White K, Chatterton NP. Electrospun diclofenac sodium loaded Eudragit® L 100-55 nanofibers for colon-targeted drug delivery. Int J Pharm 2011; 408(1-2): 200-7.
[http://dx.doi.org/10.1016/j.ijpharm.2011.01.058] [PMID: 21291969]

[41]   Abdul B, Hassan R. Overview on Drug Delivery System 2012; 3(10): 4172.

[42]   Jain KK. Drug delivery systems - an overview. Methods Mol Biol 2008; 437: 1-50.
[http://dx.doi.org/10.1007/978-1-59745-210-6_1] [PMID: 18369961]

[43]   Liu D, Yang F, Xiong F, Gu N. The Smart Drug Delivery System and Its Clinical Potential. 2016.

[44]   Prausnitz MR, Mitragotri S, Langer R. Current status and future potential of transdermal drug delivery. Nat Rev Drug Discov 2004; 3(2): 115-24.
[http://dx.doi.org/10.1038/nrd1304] [PMID: 15040576]

[45]   Miller MA, Pisani E. The cost of unsafe injections. Bull World Health Organ 1999; 77(10): 808-11. [PMID: 10593028]

[46]   Sill TJ, von Recum HA. Electrospinning: Applications in drug delivery and tissue engineering. Biomaterials 2008; 29(13): 1989-2006. [http://dx.doi.org/10.1016/j.biomaterials.2008.01.011] [PMID: 18281090]

[47]   Sa'adon S, Abd Razak SI, Ismail AE, Fakhruddin K. Drug-loaded poly-vinyl alcohol electrospun nanofibers for Transdermal Drug Delivery: Review on factors affecting the drug release. Procedia Comput Sci 2019; 158: 436-42. [http://dx.doi.org/10.1016/j.procs.2019.09.073]

[48]   Chatterjee K. Fabrication of poly (Caprolactone) nanofibers by electrospinning. J Polym Biopolym Phys Chem 2014; 2(4): 62-6.

[49]   Zarghami A, Irani M, Mostafazadeh A, Golpour M. 2015.

[50]   Topuz F, Uyar T. Electrospinning of gelatin with tunable fiber morphology from round to flat/ribbon. Mater Sci Eng C 2017; 80: 371-8. [http://dx.doi.org/10.1016/j.msec.2017.06.001] [PMID: 28866176]

[51]   Omollo E, Zhang C, Mwasiagi JI, Ncube S. Electrospinning cellulose acetate nanofibers and a study of their possible use in high-efficiency filtration. J Ind Text 2016; 45(5): 716-29. [http://dx.doi.org/10.1177/1528083714540696]

[52]   Ahmet ÇA, Kumbasar EP, Akduman Ç. Effects of solvent mixtures on the morphology of electrospun thermoplastic polyurethane nanofibres. Textile and Apparel 2015; 25(1): 38-46.

[53]   ElMessiry M, Fadel N. The tensile properties of electrospun Poly Vinyl Chloride and Cellulose Acetate (PVC/CA) bi-component polymers nanofibers. Alex Eng J 2019; 58(3): 885-90. [http://dx.doi.org/10.1016/j.aej.2019.08.003]

[54]   Paudel KS, Milewski M, Swadley CL, Brogden NK, Ghosh P, Stinchcomb AL. Challenges and opportunities in dermal/transdermal delivery. Ther Deliv 2010; 1(1): 109-31. [http://dx.doi.org/10.4155/tde.10.16] [PMID: 21132122]

[55]   Zhang H, Lou S, Williams GR, *et al.* A systematic study of captopril-loaded polyester fiber mats prepared by electrospinning. Int J Pharm 2012; 439(1-2): 100-8. [http://dx.doi.org/10.1016/j.ijpharm.2012.09.055] [PMID: 23043960]

[56]   Yu DG, Yu JH, Chen L, Williams GR, Wang X. Modified coaxial electrospinning for the preparation of high-quality ketoprofen-loaded cellulose acetate nanofibers. Carbohydr Polym 2012; 90(2): 1016-23. [http://dx.doi.org/10.1016/j.carbpol.2012.06.036] [PMID: 22840034]

[57]   Taepaiboon P, Rungsardthong U, Supaphol P. Drug-loaded electrospun mats of poly(vinyl alcohol) fibres and their release characteristics of four model drugs. Nanotechnology 2006; 17(9): 2317-29. [http://dx.doi.org/10.1088/0957-4484/17/9/041]

[58]   Rahmani M, Arbabi Bidgoli S, Rezayat S. Electrospun polymeric nanofibers for transdermal drug delivery. Nanomed J 2017; 4(2): 61-70.

CHAPTER 6

Naturally-Derived Biomaterials for Oral and Dental Tissue Engineering

Fan Ying Zhen[1], Hasan Subhi Azeez[2], Mohd Nor Ridzuan Abd Mutalib[1] and Asma Abdullah Nurul[1,*]

[1] *School of Health Sciences, Universiti Sains Malaysia, 16150 Kubang Kerian, Kelantan, Malaysia*

[2] *School of Dental Sciences, Universiti Sains Malaysia, 16150 Kubang Kerian, Kelantan, Malaysia*

Abstract: Damage to different body tissues may occur as a result of trauma, injury, or disease, which requires therapies to aid their healing through repair or regeneration. Tissue engineering aims to repair, sustain or recover the function of injured tissue or organs by producing biological substitutes. Advances in different approaches of dental tissue engineering, ranging from conventional triad (stem cells, scaffold, and regulatory signals-based tissue engineering) to modern technologies (3D printing and 4D printing), further emphasize that there are promising treatment approaches offered by the dental tissue engineering field to a variety of orofacial disorders, specifically through the design and manufacture of materials, application of appropriate regulatory signals and the enhanced knowledge of stem cells application. Inspired by their unique properties, scaffolds of natural origins, such as chitosan, cellulose, alginate, collagen, silk, and gelatin, have become a popular source of materials manufacturing that would simulate the biological environment. Future research should focus on translating laboratory findings into feasible therapies, *i.e.*, directing basic sciences discovered in dental tissue engineering into contemporary clinically applicable therapies for orofacial disorders.

Keywords: Biomaterials, Chitosan, Dental tissue engineering, Polymer, Polysaccharide-based biomaterials, Protein-based biomaterial.

INTRODUCTION

Tissue engineering is a multidisciplinary field that is related to regenerative medicine. It employs principles of engineering, life sciences, and cellular and molecular biology to design and manufacture new healthy tissues which would repair, restore or replace the damaged ones [1]. Tissue engineering aims to utilise

---

* **Corresponding author Asma Abdullah Nurul:** School of Health Sciences, Universiti Sains Malaysia, 16150 Kubang Kerian, Kelantan, Malaysia; E-mail: nurulasma@usm.my

Mohd Fauzi Mh Busra, Daniel Law Jia Xian, Yogeswaran Lokanathan and Ruszymah Haji Idrus (Eds.)

patient's own cells in generating functional tissue or even organs, providing an alternative for grafts or transplants. This method has achieved popularity among oral and dental disciplines as it offers a new option for teeth reconstruction, periodontal tissues, bones, oral mucosa, temporomandibular joint, both bone and cartilage, nerves, muscles, tendons, and blood vessels [2]. Furthermore, the availability of unlimited bioengineered materials does not necessitate the suppression of the immune system [3]. Traditionally, tissue engineering is based on three key foundations: (a) Stem/progenitor cells, which synthesise new tissue matrix; (b) Signaling or growth factors, which stimulate the functionalities; and (c) Biomaterial scaffolds, which act as an extracellular matrix (ECM) and they are required for cell differentiation, multiplication, and biosynthesis. The biomaterial scaffolds serve as templates for tissue regeneration and as growth guides for new tissues formation [4, 5]. Human stem/progenitor cells interact with their surroundings by using a variety of components to repair damaged tissues after being seeded with appropriate scaffold biomaterials. Tissue engineering requires the presence of a combination of any of these three elements to regenerate or replace damaged tissues which would allow it to function similarly to the original tissue [6, 7]. Scaffolds and biomaterials are critical components in dental tissue regeneration. They serve as attachment sites for surrounding regenerative cells templates for tissue regeneration, as well as the source of bioactive compounds, particularly growth factors that enhance regenerative ability [8, 9]. Biomaterials are any materials that interact with the biological systems, whether they are natural or synthetic, alive or dead. A range of biomaterials, including natural organic, synthetic organic, and inorganic materials, are utilized to regenerate the oral and maxillofacial tissues. Each of these biomaterials has its benefits and drawbacks. Peptides (collagen or gelatin) and polysaccharides (alginate, chitosan, agarose) are examples of natural organic compounds. Poly(lactic acid) (PLA), poly(caprolactone) (PCL), poly(lactic-co-glycolic acid) (PLGA), and poly(glycolic acid) (PGA) are the most often used synthetic organic compounds [10]. These materials are frequently used in medical and dental applications to supplement or substitute natural functions. This chapter discusses bio-based materials used in dental tissue engineering, specifically protein-based and polysaccharide-based materials, with an emphasis on their properties and applications.

DENTAL DISORDERS AND THERAPY APPROACHES

Several causes can induce the inflammation of the dental pulp, including caries, attrition, abrasion, erosion, congenital defects, coronal cracks, and fractures [11]. Dental caries is a localized dissolution of a tooth-hard structure. Dental caries is caused primarily by bacteria found in dental plaque (biofilm) that demineralizes, enamel, dentin, and cementum, resulting in tooth cavities. The acid is formed when the microorganisms, containing dental plaque, are exposed to fermentable carbohydrate. However, when dental plaque is not exposed on a regular basis, a natural defense mechanism can re-mineralize the affected areas through saliva, therefore, prevent the production of cavities [11, 12]. The bacterial irritation causes pulp inflammation when it reaches the area, which subsequently would spread to other parts of the pulp. Even though the bacteria may not penetrate the pulp, irritation can still occur when the toxins and enzymes released by bacteria pass through the dentinal tubules. The intensity of inflammation, however, is related to the severity of bacterial irritation and closeness to the pulp [13, 14]. The pulpal degeneration and necrosis would then occur, followed by infection of the periapical tissues, which lead to acute or chronic abscess [11].

Pulp inflammation is referred to as pulpitis, and it is classified into reversible and irreversible pulpitis based on the symptoms, pulp response, radiographic and clinical tests, and the presence of caries or restorations. Reversible pulpitis indicates a mild inflammation condition of the pulp, which can be reversed and healed by removing the cause through appropriate therapy such as dental restoration or indirect pulp capping. Whereas irreversible pulpitis refers to a more severe inflammation of the pulp that is unlikely to return to its normal condition after the removal of the irritant [11]. The treatment includes vital pulp therapy, such as direct pulp capping and pulpotomy, as well as pulp tissue extirpation [15, 16]. The vital pulp therapy aims to regenerate the damaged dentin-pulp complex through reactionary dentinogenesis in indirect pulp capping, and reparative dentinogenesis in direct pulp capping and pulpotomy [17].

As the infection spreads apically, the periapical bone is replaced by soft tissue, resulting in bone resorption and periapical lesion formation. Apical periodontitis is categorized into the apical granuloma, apical cyst, and apical abscess [11]. Apical granuloma is formed as a result of the local inflammatory response to various irritants [18]. The lesion is characterized by granulation tissue and bone loss as well as inflammatory cells [19, 20]. An apical abscess lesion forms when a necrotic area within a granuloma is encompassed by an intense inflammatory cellular response. The growth of Mallassez epithelial that is resting inside the granuloma causes an apical cyst lesion. Mallassez epithelial cells are originated from the Hertwig epithelial root sheath, which is important in root development [11]. Apical periodontitis would resolve once the microbial irritants are eliminated, which can be accomplished through tooth extraction or by decreasing the microbial irritants with non-surgical or surgical endodontic therapy. Non-surgical treatment includes root canal treatment, while surgical treatment includes apicoectomy (known as root-end filling). The repair of a periapical lesion is a complex process which involves the regeneration of periodontal ligament, cementum and alveolar bone [17].

Apexification is described as the process of calcified barrier development in a root with an open apex or the continuation of the apical growth of an incompletely formed root in the teeth with necrotic pulps [17]. The therapy includes the removal of the necrotic tissue and the application of a biocompatible material to stimulate the development of an apical hard tissue barrier [21], which is described as a cementum-like tissue or osteodentin [22, 23] through the reparative process of dentin-pulp complex [17]. The bacteria in the dental plaque induce a non-destructive inflammatory disease of the gum along the gingival margin called gingivitis. Untreated gingivitis can advance to periodontitis, in which the infection would spread to the tooth-supporting tissues (*i.e.*, the periodontium) thus resulting in their destruction and eventually tooth loss if it is not treated [12]. The healing of periodontal wound is a complex process due to the unique composition of the periodontium, comprising gingiva, underlying connective tissue, cementum, periodontal ligament, and alveolar bone [24]. The current therapies of periodontal disease aim to arrest the disease progression by reducing the inflammation and microbial level in the periodontium by cleaning the root surface and removing the diseased tissues. These treatments include a non-surgical approach through sub-gingival debridement or a surgical approach by open flab debridement [25]. These techniques are useful in preventing further disease development and ultimately, tooth loss, but they can only achieve limited periodontal repair, which is not considered a true regeneration [26]. Recently, periodontal regenerative medicine attempted to regenerate the damaged periodontium by applying the tissue engineering principle through the interaction of progenitor/stem cells, bioactive molecules, and scaffold [27 - 33]. As effective results have been achieved, these regenerative strategies through the application of growth factors and the potential of scaffold to deliver cells are encouraged, as they offer a promising therapeutic approach in dentistry.

DENTAL TISSUE ENGINEERING AND REGENERATION

Over the past decade, tissue engineering has been experiencing a massive expansion in the regenerative medicine. The term "tissue engineering" was first emerged in the late 1980s. The development of biological alternatives applies the principles of life sciences and engineering with the aim of restoring, preserving or improving the function of targeted organs and tissues [34]. As an alternative, preceding transplantation of integrating cells embedded onto biomaterial can regenerate and restore the cells' function from the defected or injured area [35]. It also intends to stimulate tissues and organs' regenerative properties by either constructing substitutes *in vitro* or biomaterial implantation *in vivo* [36]. The tissue engineering triad comprises stem/progenitor cells, scaffolds, and regulatory signals to regenerate operational biological tissues [37] (Fig. **1**). Dental tissue engineering aims to explore various factors affecting tooth development since birth and restore damaged or missing tooth components such as dentin, enamel and dental pulp. A suitable choice of cells is required to be applied with the scaffolds and regulatory signals to stimulate new dental tissue formation, which is favorable to the surrounding tissues [38].

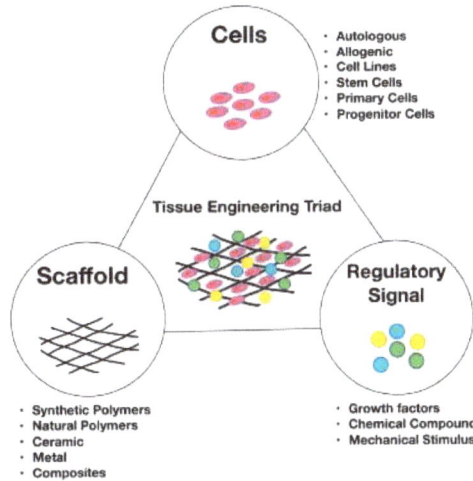

Fig. (1). Tissue Engineering Triad.

Tissue engineering in dentistry has grabbed the interest of others as it is capable of providing a biologically centered treatment and stimulating tooth maturation in injured teeth [39]. The objective of regenerative dentistry is to apply the principle of tissue engineering into clinical settings, which provides effective approaches in order to manage dental and oral health issues in the future. For example, the regenerative endodontics procedures were designed to restore damaged root structures, dentin, and dentin-pulp complex with live tissues, ideally from a similar source, which were efficient in restoring the physiological function of dentin-pulp complex [40]. The clinical and scientific success of regenerative dentistry was inspired by knowledge of minimizing unfavorable regeneration environments, such as bacterial contamination and chronic inflammatory management, as well as tissue damage reduction in any restorative surgical intervention [41]. Lately, nanoscale topography and geometry have demonstrated a significant influence on the differentiation of cells, 3-dimensional (3D) regeneration enhancement, and behavior in periodontal nanotechnology tissue engineering [42]. The development of nanotechnology provides strategies for the treatment of periodontitis-induced bone loss and bone deficiencies in the oral cavity [43]. This chapter will further elaborate on the properties and applications of bio-based materials, as well as some cutting-edge technologies for dental tissue engineering.

BIO-BASED MATERIALS FOR DENTAL TISSUE ENGINEERING

As most tissue engineering research aim to improve biomaterials, the advancements in scaffold development in the area of regenerative medicine are becoming more popular. The term scaffold refers to a 3D porous solid biomaterial with surface characteristics that are intended to promote and facilitate cell attachment [44]. It can be categorized into synthetic or natural biomaterials as their fundamental function is to stimulate tissue regeneration by promising a satisfactory function of the surrounding cells [45]. Scaffolds play an important role in tissue engineering by supplementing growth factors and nutrients to promote repair mechanisms or initiate regeneration activities in various tissues [44]. The biomaterials should possess a suitable degradability rate [46] and high biocompatibility properties to avoid rejection or inflammatory response by the host tissues [47]. Scaffold components or degradation products must not induce any adverse biological response, and they should provide chemical stability to prevent chemical alterations during the regenerative process [48]. The surface characteristics of biomaterial scaffolds must support cell adhesion, proliferation, and differentiation to stimulate and guide the regenerative process [46]. To stimulate successful tissue engineering, the regulatory signals must be involved in the regenerative process by stimulating the release of growth factors from the tissue matrix or incorporating desired growth factors in the biomaterial used.

Synthetic polymers are alternatives to natural materials that can produce well-defined and modifiable mechanical and chemical properties. Several benefits of synthetic scaffolds are found over natural scaffolds in which the former are able to have tailored structures and properties based on the polymer functional groups designed according to the specific applications [49]. For example, the degradation rate of synthetic polymer can be changed by altering its molecular weight, chemical composition, and polymer crystallinity [50]. A number of synthetic scaffolds have been explored in the majority of tissue engineering applications [51]; among the most used scaffolds are polycaprolactone (PCL), polylactide (PLA/PLLA), poly(lactide-co-glycolide) (PLGA) and poly(ethylene glycol) (PEG) [51].

Natural scaffolds generally include bio-functional molecules that can ensure natural remodelling and bioactivity and provide a biomimetic surface. These scaffolds mainly comprise two types of polymers, which are proteins-based (silk, collagen, and gelatin) and polysaccharides-based (chitosan, cellulose, and alginate). The scaffolds that have been developed from these polymers are bioactive, able to support cell attachment, biocompatible, and can provide a suitable environment for cell function [49]. Besides, the degradation products are less toxic and far more metabolically accessible as compared to the synthetic scaffolds. However, natural scaffolds have some drawbacks, such as chemical heterogeneity, high dispersity, inconsistency of mechanical and structural properties, and varying degradability rates [49].

Polysaccharide-Based Scaffolds

Chitosan

The application of chitosan as a unique bio-based polymer in tissue engineering attracts the attention of researchers. Chitosan (poly-(β-1/4)-2-amino-2--eoxy-D-glucopyranose) is a semi-crystalline, biocompatible, bioactive, natural, non-toxic linear biopolymer that originates from chitin and it is comprised of N-acetyl glucosamine and N-acetyl-D-glucosamine bonds and β bonds (1-4) (Fig. **2**) [52].

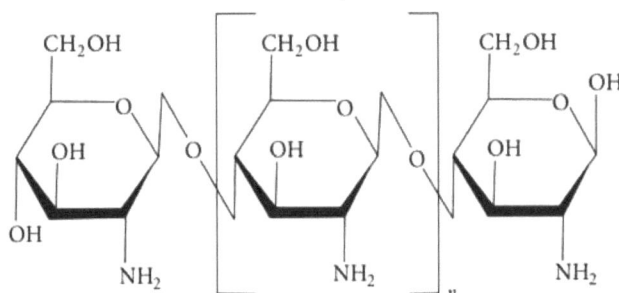

Fig. (2). A chemical structure of chitosan.

The chemical modification of chitosan enables the formation of hydrogels and composites that enhance its properties for a variety of biomedical applications. Chitosan hydrogel is produced by creating a cross-linked network with a high composition of hydrophilic groups, demonstrating its water super absorbency but insolubility in water [53]. Chitosan hydrogels can be shaped and molded into various forms. They are primarily used in tissue engineering [54], drug delivery, and wound healing [55]. Nanoparticles are materials with sizes ranging from 1 to 100 nm. They exhibit favourable characteristics when compared to their bulk equivalents due to their reduction in dimension to the atomic level [56]. Chitosan nanoparticles combine the properties of both chitosan and nanoparticles. Chitosan nanoparticles are employed in various biomedical applications, which include tissue engineering, cancer diagnosis, drug delivery, enzyme immobilization support, antioxidant activity, and antibacterial agent [56].

Chitosan applications in dentistry, such as dental tissue engineering, have received a lot of attention. Chitosan has been studied as a direct pulp capping material, with a chitosan bilayer-microsphere construct containing TGF-1 inducing 3-6 times more reparative dentin in dogs than in a control model [57]. Another study showed that nanocomplexes of carboxymethyl chitosan/amorphous calcium phosphate (CMC/ACP) are a potential material for indirect pulp capping to re-mineralize the demineralized dentin in deep caries management [58]. In addition, chitosan nanofiber membrane and chitosan-collagen membrane [59] enhanced bone formation, and they were suggested to be used as guided bone regeneration [60]. The implantation of chitosan/collagen scaffold combined with Ad-BMP-7 around implant defects showed a greater bone formation than control at 4 or 8 weeks [61]. In a previous study, chitosan-based accelerated portland cement (APC-CT) was evaluated for endodontic applications; the material was shown to be non-toxic, promoted cell attachment, and had good physicochemical and mechanical properties [62].

Chitosan-gelatin scaffolds were prepared for bone tissue engineering supported rat BMMSCs attachment and osteogenic differentiation [63]. For perforation repair of the TMJ disc, the fibrin/chitosan hybrid scaffold combined with rat TMJ-SDSCs cell was implanted into the rat TMJ defect. The study revealed more cartilage ECM formation in the fibrin/chitosan scaffold, indicating the regenerative potential of this scaffold for TMJ disc perforation repair [64]. Furthermore, chitosan has some advantages in periodontal tissue regeneration. Chitosan/tricalcium phosphate (TCP) sponges were suggested as a scaffold to grow osteoblast in a 3D structure for transplantation into the defective site [65]. They were also found to be suitable as a delivery system of PDGF-BB growth factor in calvarial defects of rats [66]. As a membrane for guided bone and tissue regeneration, a nanocomposite membrane, which consists of chitosan (CHT) and bioactive glass nanoparticles (BG-NPs), could effectively be used in periodontal regeneration [67]. Chitosan should be utilised to develop chitosan-based products in various aspects of dentistry as it has been effectively used as an anti-plaque agent in mouthwashes [68] and toothpaste to inhibit dental plaque [69]. Chitosan also has been used as a hemostatic agent in oral surgery [70]. Due to its antibacterial activity, chitosan has exhibited favourable results when incorporated with different dental materials to enhance their antibacterial potential [70 - 75].

Cellulose

Cellulose and its derivatives are considered highly abundant natural polymers in the environment. They can be found in the cell walls of green plants as well as certain types of algae and are supplied by bacteria [76]. Although cellulose is easily accessible, there are major challenges in its refinement which in turn makes it a poor alternative as a natural biomaterial. Based on Mi Young *et al.*, there is a lack of physiological or pharmaceutical applications regarding cellulose use [77]. Presently, research is emphasizing the production of cellulose derivatives like bacterial cellulose (BC) as a biomaterial and BC-based biomaterial as a promising scaffold in tissue regeneration [78]. Besides being non-toxic, biodegradative, and biocompatible, BC exhibits several advantages over plant cellulose, including high purity and porosity, better liquid and gas permeability, increased water uptake capacity, and mechanical strength [79].

Several types of research have demonstrated BC's applicability in dental tissue engineering, despite the fact that BC is currently underdeveloped in the area. Prior applications in dentistry were connected to guide tissue regeneration (GTR) techniques that focused on the treatment of periodontal disease. Novaes Jr *et al.* demonstrated a successfully treated class II furcation lesion in a patient, employing a non-resorbable BC membrane by applying the GTR technique. The defect closure was evaluated clinically by re-entry process, attachment level, and radiographs [80]. Further study was also done by Novaes Jr *et al.*, where a similar group of class II furcation lesion was treated using the same membrane in dogs with periodontitis [81].

Carvalho *et al.* in 2020 successfully developed nanostructured patches comprised of bacterial nanocellulose (BNC), hyaluronic acid (HA), and diclofenac (DFC). The biomaterial aimed to trigger the healing of aphthous ulcers in recurrent aphthous stomatitis (RAS), was a form of ordinary mucosal ulcer in the mouth and achieved a pain-relieving effect [82]. This type of sore can be tremendously unpleasant, causing local inflammation and stinging pain as it needs spontaneous healing in several days. Thus, the membrane patches were created by simply diffusing DCF and HA aqueous solutions into a 3D porous network of wet BNC [82]. The patches exhibited a positive effect on the targeted aphthous stomatitis in addition to its thermal stability, which was up to 200 °C with good dynamic properties as well [82].

Manzine Costa *et al.* proposed using otolith/BC nanocomposite (OTL) in dental pulp capping therapy to regenerate dentin [83]. The histological response of exposed tooth pulp in dogs after 21 days showed that this material could be used as a dental pulp capping material in the future [83]. Another study by Voicu *et al.* developed a new family of composites based on biocellulose membrane and mineral binder powder, with the combination demonstrated excellent potential in regenerative endodontics [84]. The nanocomposite exhibited shorter setting time, no cytotoxic effects, and enhanced cell adhesion, proliferation, and mineralization activity, thus indicating that it had great potential in regenerative endodontic therapies, particularly in root perforations, dentin remineralisation, and root canal filling [84].

Alginate

Alginate is a biocompatible natural polysaccharide. Alginate is also known as an alginic acid salt, which also refers to the alginic acid derivatives and original alginic acid. Alginate is the most abundant biopolymer available after cellulose [85, 86]. Alginates such as alginic acid and its calcium, potassium, ammonium salts, and propylene glycol alginate are the most common sources of alginate. Alginates are polysaccharide-based biomaterials with structural components that are identical to the cell walls of brown microalgae Phaeophyceae, and they exist as divalent alginic acid salts. Commercial alginates are derived from a variety of species, including Macrocystis, Sargassum, Laminaria, Lessonia, Ascophyllum, Durvillea, and Eclonia [87, 88]. Although brown seaweed is the most common source of alginate, it can also be produced by bacteria such as Azotobacter and Pseudomonas, which are abundant in the vegetative growing cells. Alginates formed from algae have a wide molecular weight range, whereas those derived from bacteria have large molar weights and a high degree of polymerization.

Table 1. An overview of the main advantages of bacterial cellulose in the dental and oral disciplines.

Dental and Oral Treatment	Potential Use	Advantages
Periodontal treatment	Barrier membrane using guided-tissue regeneration technique [80, 81]	Enables cell attachment and proliferation. Class II furcation lesions can be treated. Aesthetics restoration of the oral function.
Wound patches	Heal aphthous ulcers in recurrent aphthous stomatitis [82]	Thermal resistant. Reduce and heal RAS discomfort. Permit HA and DFC delivery.
Treatment of dental pulp tissue	Potential scaffold for regenerative endodontic treatment [83, 84]	Reduces the setting time of biomaterial Mimics extracellular matrix Stimulates mineralised barrier Promotes apical closure and cell adhesion Does not indicate the cytotoxic effect

Alginate-based biomaterials are used in wound healing and wound dressing [89]. Alginate has low mechanical rigidity and an uncontrollable breakdown rate *in vivo* [89]. To improve mechanical strength, the calcium concentration and crosslinking density can be increased [89]. In addition, stable covalent cross-linking provides better mechanical strength than ionic cross-linking in alginate hydrogels [90]. The addition of arginine-glycine-aspartic acid (RGD) to an alginate hydrogel would enhance cell attachment, spreading, proliferation, and differentiation [91]. Alginate hydrogels provide a suitable matrix for the regeneration of dentin-pulp complex and periodontal tissues, and they may also be efficient for the delivery of growth factors such as TGF to promote the regenerative capacity of the dental pulp. TGF-containing and acid-treated alginate hydrogels would increase the secretion of dentin matrix and promote odontoblast-like cell differentiation in conjunction with regular tubular dentin matrix secretion [91]. Human periodontal ligament fibroblasts (hPDLF) grown on alginate/bioglass composite scaffolds adhere and proliferate well, and the addition of nano bioactive glass-ceramic (nBGC) promotes alkaline phosphatase (ALP) activity [92]. Due to its non-toxicity, the grafted copolymer of alginate has a variety of functions in biomedical, pharmaceuticals, and tissue engineering [93].

Protein-Based Scaffolds

Collagen

Collagen is the most abundant structural protein found in connective tissue extracellular matrix, including bone, cartilage, tendon, muscle, and skin [94]. It has been widely investigated in dental regeneration research due to the similarities in its structural and chemical to the major structural protein that is present in the extracellular matrix of many tooth tissues. Its biocompatibility and bioactivity promote cell adhesion, migration, and growth, and it may be destroyed by enzymes and collagenase with just a moderate inflammatory response [94]. Collagen has a high tensile strength and can be woven or twisted into the desired shape [94]. Despite the fact that its physical strength is not considered great, it is adequate enough for pulp regeneration [94]. The mechanical and physical properties of collagen can be altered through the cross-linking method. For example, cross-linking by using glutaraldehyde or diphenylphosphoryl azide enhances mechanical stiffness, but it may have an impact on cell viability and biocompatibility [95]. The development of hybrid scaffolds from βTCP/poly-ethylene and HA would enhance the mechanical properties and bone conductivity [96]. Collagen scaffolds also exhibited promising cellular properties by promoting dental pulp stem cell attachment and proliferation (DPSCs) [97]. The study also showed that the combination of DPSCs, collagen scaffold, and DMP-1 had resulted in the formation of a structured matrix that was comparable to that of pulpal tissue, therefore demonstrating its ability to generate hard tissue. Another study [52] found that pulp tissue was formed in the cavities of canine teeth implanted with 220 ng of BMP-2 or collagen, as well as in teeth implanted with 4 g of BMP-4 with collagen. The formed pulp tissue was most likely to be osteodentin, suggesting that BMP-2 and BMP-4 stimulated the formation of osteodentin when combined with collagen as a carrier. In another study, the implantation of collagen scaffolds containing basic fibroblast growth factor (bFGF), vascular endothelial growth factor (VEGF), and/or platelet derived growth factor (PDGF) into the endodontically treated root canals in mouse dorsum demonstrated re-cellularised and revascularised dental pulp tissue which integrated to the native dentinal wall in root canals with new dentin formation [98]. Collagen sponges are often utilised for bone regeneration, whereas collagen membranes are used for guided bone and tissue regeneration in clinical settings. Pulp cells, on the other hand, are known to cause substantial collagen contraction [99]. Therefore, this problem must be addressed when employing collagen scaffolds to regenerate pulp.

Silk

Silk-based biomaterials have been widely used in soft and hard tissue engineering due to their diverse physical properties, biocompatibility, and capability to enhance the adhesion, proliferation, and differentiation of various cell types [100]. The silk gel material is effective in periodontal and maxillofacial treatments because it can augment long-term soft tissue repair [100]. The regeneration properties of hexafluoroisopropanol(HFIP)-based silk are superior to those of aqueous-based silk, as they promote the development of soft tooth pulp and mineralised tissue, thus indicating the scaffolds' potential for osteodentin formation [101]. This material also can stimulate hBMSC differentiation and bone-like tissue formation, therefore indicating that it may be employed in bone tissue engineering [102].

Silk fibroin (SF) is a biocompatible, enzymatically degradable material that can be made into water-insoluble implants through biomimetic procedures that are developed from the silkworm and spider silk spinning processes [103, 104]. The process involved in the production of SF requires minimal use of organic solvents [105, 106]. Sericin-free SF has been shown to be as biocompatible as collagen and PLGA *in vitro* and *in vivo* [107]. The β-sheet structure of silk can remarkably affect the degradation rate, tensile properties, and elasticity of scaffolds. As a result, by modifying its structure *via* a cross-linking procedure, the properties of the scaffold can be changed [108]. Consequently, the biocompatibility and degradation rate of silk materials can be modified by using different methods [109]. Although PLGA scaffold was employed for dental pulp tissue engineering, its slow degradation had a detrimental impact on the regenerated pulp-like tissue quality; thus, the use of silk scaffold was suggested to overcome this drawback [110]. Due to the effectiveness of silk properties in hard tissue engineering, four scaffolds with or without RGD peptide were developed from biomaterial silk protein with different degrees of porosity, ranging from 250 to 550 mm. These scaffolds were subsequently implanted with tooth bud cells, resulting in mineralised tissue regeneration in rats [111].

Gelatin

Gelatin is a biodegradable, biocompatible, low antigenicity, and entirely absorbable biopolymer that is derived from the partial degradation of collagen fibres [112 - 114]. It contains the integrin recognition motif Arg-Gly-Asp (RGD) sequence found in the natural extracellular matrix (ECM), where it enhances cell attachment, proliferation, and spreading within the biomimetic matrix [112, 113]. Gelatin has been commonly used in regenerative tissue engineering due to its advantages, including its biological nature, hydrogel properties, and high commercial availability at a comparatively minimal cost [114, 115]. Based on a study by Vagropoulou *et al.*, a hybrid gelatin/chitosan/nanohydroxyapatite scaffold for odontogenic differentiation and mineralisation achieved high porosity and biocompatibility. The scaffold was also found to be beneficial for cell attachment, differentiation, and long-term preservation of DPSCs. The study concluded that a biomimetic approach with the addition of exogenous inductive factors could be a potential candidate for dental tissue engineering [116].

Ribeiro *et al.* developed an injectable chlorhexidine (CHX)-loaded nanotube-modified gelatin methacryloyl (GelMA) hydrogel. It was biodegradable, cytocompatible, and able to deliver CHX for dental infection ablation [70]. The injectable GelMA-based hydrogel displayed minimal localized inflammatory responses and excellent biocompatibility *in vivo,* indicating that it can offer prolonged intracanal drug delivery [117]. Monteiro *et al.* optimized a new technique for photopolymerizing GelMA with a visible light dental curing (DL) unit and compared it to ultraviolet light (UV) [118]. According to the studies, both DL and UV photo-crosslinked hydrogels resulted in a significant percentage of cell viability, showing that the proposed method had turned out to be successful and established a chair-side technique in regenerative dental therapy. DPSCs seeded on biomimetic chitosan/gelatin scaffolds showed the significant formation of a hydroxyapatite-rich nanocrystalline calcium phosphate phase [119]. In addition, *in vivo* analysis revealed the nanocrystalline and mineralised matrix formation with increased quantities of osteoid, thus indicating a potential approach for orofacial bone tissue engineering. Gelatin-based hemostatic hydrogels demonstrated better performance than fibrin-based hemostatic hydrogels which included higher cell viability, favourable root development and newly mineralised tissue deposited in the root canal system [120]. A recent study described the development of alginate-gelatine/nanohydroxyapatite microcapsules which showed promising bone regenerative properties by promoting cell proliferation and osteogenic differentiation [121]. A summary of various natural-based biomaterials and their properties in dental tissue engineering applications is summarised in Table **2**.

Table 2. Natural-based biomaterials and their biological effects.

Material	Type of Study	Biological Effect	Reference
Chitosan/β-glycerophosphate (CS/β-GP) hydrogel	*In vitro.* CS/β-GP hydrogel was synthesised by a sol-gel method for reparative dentine.	CS/β-GP hydrogel enhanced adhesion and proliferative activity of DPSCs. The addition of VEGF in CS/β-GP hydrogel promoted the odontogenic differentiation of DPSCs.	Wu *et al.* (2019) [122]
Chitosan (CS), β-sodium glycerophosphate (β-GP), and gelatin hydrogel	*In vitro* and *in vivo.* Injectable and thermosensitive CS/β-GP/gelatin hydrogel for periodontium regeneration.	The CS/-GP/gelatin hydrogels exhibited high biocompatibility and were effective in controlling inflammation and periodontal regeneration.	Xu *et al.* (2019) [123]
Chitosan-aniline oligomer/polyvinyl alcohol	*In vitro.* Chitosan was synthesised by coupling with aniline oligomers and fabricated using the electrospinning method.	Chitosan-aniline oligomer/polyvinyl alcohol exhibited on-demand drug release and higher biocompatibility.	Bagheri *et al.* (2020) [124]
Elastin-like protein–hyaluronic acid (ELP–HA) hydrogel	*In vitro.* ELP-HA was synthesised using dynamic covalent crosslinking for tissue engineering.	ELP-HA produced a shear-thinning hydrogel that protected cells from mechanically disruptive forces during the injection. The cells encapsulated in the hydrogel showed their ability to differentiate into multiple lineages, including chondrogenic, adipogenic, and osteogenic cell types.	Wang *et al.* (2017) [125]
Hyaluronic acid (HA), cellulose nanocrystals (CNCs), and platelet lysate (PL) hydrogel	*In vitro* and *ex vivo.* HA was formed in situ, reinforced with CNCs, and enriched with PL for dentin-pulp complex regeneration.	HA/CNC/PL enhanced the chemotactic and pro-angiogenic activity of hDPSCs by promoting hDPCs recruitment and cell sprouting in hDPCs/human umbilical vein endothelial cell co-cultures.	Silva *et al.* (2018) [126]

Material	Type of Study	Biological Effect	Reference
Hyaluronic acid (HA) and platelet lysate (PL) hydrogel	*In vitro.* HAPL hydrogel was prepared by photocrosslinking of methacrylated HA (Met-HA) for the pulp/dentin tissue and endodontics regeneration.	HAPL supported the recruitment, adhesion, and proliferation of hDPCs. The HAPL also enhanced cellular metabolism and mineralized matrix deposition by hDPSCs.	Almeida *et al.* (2018) [127]
Alginate (Alg) and hydroxyapatite (HAp) composite scaffold	*In vitro.* Alg and HAp were mixed in water using the calcium release method. Alg-HAp-based nanocomposite scaffolds were prepared for bone tissue engineering.	Alg-HAp increased the expression of osteogenic differentiation markers and promoted calcium deposition and mineralization on DPSCs.	Sancilio *et al.* (2018) [128]
Collagen and alginate composite scaffold	*In vitro.* Collagen and alginate were mixed and cast into a sodium alginate mould to produce a gutta-percha point-like cone for endodontics regeneration.	Human stem cells from the apical papilla (SCAPs) seeded into Col-Alg composite scaffold were able to spread, proliferate and differentiate into osteoblasts.	Devillard *et al.* (2017) [129]
Gelatin methacryloyl (GelMA) hydrogel	*In vitro.* GelMA hydrogel was synthesised using a UV crosslinked method for dental-pulp tissue engineering.	GelMA hydrogel increased the spreading, proliferation, and viability of odontoblast-like cells (OD21). In the root canal model, OD21 cells showed enhanced spreading and proliferation near the dentin walls, while endothelial colony-forming cells (ECFCs) formed endothelial monolayers with active angiogenic sprouts.	Athirasala *et al.* (2017) [130]
Chitin-poly(lactic-co-glycolic acid) (PLGA) and nano bioactive glass-ceramic (nBGC)	*In vitro* and *in vivo.* Chitin–PLGA/nBGC was produced in a tri-layered nanocomposite hydrogel scaffold to incorporate cementum protein 1 as the cementum layer, fibroblast growth factor 2 as the periodontal ligament layer, and platelet-rich plasma-derived growth factors as the alveolar bone layer for periodontal regeneration.	The tri-layered Chitin–PLGA/nBGC nanocomposite hydrogel scaffold was compatible and induced cementogenic, fibrogenic, and osteogenic differentiation of human dental follicle stem cells. *In vivo*, the scaffold demonstrated complete defect closure and healing with new cancellous-like tissue formation *e.g.* cementum, fibrous PDL, and alveolar bone.	Sowmya *et al.* (2017) [131]

(Table 2) cont.....

Material	Type of Study	Biological Effect	Reference
Dentin, collagen, and peptide fibrillary scaffolds	*In vitro.* A 3D periodontal model was generated by assembling dentin, collagen hydrogel, and self-assembling peptide.	The 3D periodontal model coated with collagen 1 and enamel matrix protein (EMP) increased the viability of human periodontal ligament fibroblasts (HPLF) and showed a positive effect on periodontal regeneration.	Koch *et al.* (2020) [132]
Silk fibroin and hydroxyapatite scaffold	*In vitro.* Nanofibrous silk fibroin (SF) scaffolds containing hydroxyapatite (HAp) nanoparticles were fabricated by using the freeze-drying method for dental pulp repair.	SF-HAp scaffold exhibited good hemocompatibility and biocompatibility when tested using dental pulp stem cells.	Zhang *et al.* (2019) [133]

THREE-DIMENSIONAL (3D) AND 4D PRINTING

The advancement of manufacturing technology enables the printing of biofunctional scaffolds which are identical to ECM to serve as a milieu for cell adhesion, proliferation, and differentiation [134, 135]. Additive manufacturing (also known as 3D printing) of biomaterials presents a potential perspective for the biomedical engineering field because of its ability to supply high structural complexity, patient-specific designs, as well as quick on-demand manufacturing [136]. The earliest document on 3D printing was recorded by the Japanese inventor Hideo Kodama in 1981 through the additive process. Kodama developed a device that employed ultraviolet lights to solidify polymers. It was a stepping stone to the stereolithography (SLA) technology which was invented three years later by Charles Hull. The 3D printing that is based on the SLA technology would allow designers to create 3D models by using digital data, which can subsequently be used to create a physical object. The additive manufacturing techniques for tissue engineering are classified into two types: techniques that involve live cell printing along with materials (3D bioprinting) [72] and non-cellular fabrication techniques. The 3D bioprinting principle is performed through the layer-by-layer deposition of biological components and biochemical and live cells to allow on-demand printing of organs, tissues, and cells [137, 138] for tissue engineering applications [139]. Tissue-engineered constructs may be customized to attain the desired structures and properties by integrating various bioprinting techniques [140, 141]. 3D printing has shown to be successful in the production of biomaterial scaffolds with custom-designed geometries, and it is rapidly becoming an important technology for tissue engineering [142]. Previously, tissue manufacturing had depended on scaffold fabrication techniques which had limited ability to reproduce tissue complexity. Today, 3D printing offers significant advantages, such as the capacity to produce various shapes to fully match any tissue defect, as well as to replicate intricate internal tissue architecture and heterogeneity with a precise arrangement of different materials and/or cell types [143, 144]. For hard tissue engineering, 3D printing of bone transplant scaffolds would involve techniques that utilised natural and synthetic biomaterials [145, 146] built in a biomimetic scaffold [147]. There have been various specialties in dentistry such as endodontics, orthodontics, prosthodontics, craniofacial, and oral and maxillofacial surgery that have successfully utilized 3D objects [148].

Several studies have reported the use of bio-based materials prepared by 3D bioprinting technology. A 3D-printed alginate/gelatin hydrogel enhanced hDPSC proliferation and adhesion while promoting osteogenic/odontoblastic differentiation, as shown by increasing the formation of bone-like nodules and mineralisation activity [149]. Athirasala *et al.* developed a novel bio-ink by combining printable alginate hydrogels and the soluble and insoluble fractions of the dentin matrix, which demonstrated cytocompatibility and enhanced odontogenic differentiation of stem cells from the apical papilla, which could be used to experiment fabricate scaffolds with complex 3D microarchitectures for regeneration of dental tissues [150]. A recent study showed that a 3D-printed hybrid biodegradable hydrogel which was composed of alginate, gelatin, and cellulose nanocrystals, demonstrated enhanced cell proliferation, mineralisation activity, and increased expression of osteogenic-specific gene markers, as well as improved bone formation in the calvaria critical-sized defects model [151].

3D bioprinting simply evaluates the printed object's original state and it is considered an inanimate and static scaffold; nevertheless, printing biocompatible materials and cells is inadequate to construct a tissue or organ [152]. With 4D printing, however, the resultant 3D shape may morph into many shapes in response to the environmental stimuli, with the 4th dimension being the time-dependent shape change following printing [153]. 4D bioprinting is applied in tissue engineering applications because it allows the fabrication of delicate and complex structures. 4D printing is determined by five key factors: the additive manufacturing process, stimulus-responsive material types, interaction mechanism, stimuli, and the mathematical modeling of material transformation [154]. There are a limited number of studies that reported the use of 4D printing as it is a relatively new technique, and it is still in an exploration stage, especially in dental tissue engineering. Several bio-based responsive materials that have been applied as printing materials for 4D printing include nano-fibrillated cellulose [155] and soybean oil epoxidized acrylate [156]. These smart materials are used to create 4D scaffolds in response to a variety of stimuli and adapt to their microenvironment by altering their conformation or other properties.

CONCLUSION AND PERSPECTIVE

Dental tissue regeneration is a challenging endeavor due to the diversity and complexity of tissues in the oral and maxillofacial regions. Advances in different approaches of dental tissue engineering, ranging from conventional triad (stem cell-, scaffold-, and regulatory signal-based tissue engineering) to modern technologies (3D and 4D printings), further emphasize that the dental tissue engineering field offers promising treatment approaches to a variety of orofacial disorders through the design and manufacture of materials, application of appropriate regulatory signals, and the enhanced knowledge of stem cells application. Currently, there is a renewed interest in the fabrication of biocompatible and biodegradable scaffolds from natural sources. Scaffolds of natural origin, such as chitosan, cellulose, alginate, collagen, silk, and gelatin, have unique biological activities, which make them a prevalent source for materials manufacturing in different aspects of dental tissue engineering. Future work should focus on translating laboratory outcomes into viable therapies. For that, dental practitioners should be conscious of these advances in the field of dental tissue engineering and contribute in the development of new tissue engineering-based technologies to provide more efficient clinical treatments and improve the quality of life.

CONSENT FOR PUBLICATION

All authors consent to the publication of the manuscript should the article be accepted by the Editor-in-chief upon completion of the refereeing process.

ACKNOWLEDGEMENTS

This work was supported by the Prototype Research Grant Scheme with project code: PRGS/1/2022/SKK0/USM/02/1 from the Ministry of Higher Education Malaysia.

REFERENCES

[1]   Stoltz JF, Decot V, Huseltein C, *et al.* Introduction to regenerative medicine and tissue engineering. Biomed Mater Eng 2012; 22(1-3): 3-16.
[http://dx.doi.org/10.3233/BME-2012-0684] [PMID: 22766697]

[2]   Rai R, Raval R, Khandeparker RVS, Chidrawar SK, Khan AA, Ganpat MS. Tissue engineering: step ahead in maxillofacial reconstruction. J Int oral Heal. 2015; 7(9): 138.

[3]   Borrelli MR, Hu MS, Longaker MT, Lorenz HP. Tissue engineering and regenerative medicine in craniofacial reconstruction and facial aesthetics. J Craniofac Surg 2020; 31(1): 15-27.
[http://dx.doi.org/10.1097/SCS.0000000000005840] [PMID: 31369496]

[4]   Zhang K, Wang S, Zhou C, *et al.* Advanced smart biomaterials and constructs for hard tissue engineering and regeneration. Bone Res 2018; 6(1): 31.
[http://dx.doi.org/10.1038/s41413-018-0032-9] [PMID: 30374416]

[5]   Upadhyay RK. Role of biological scaffolds, hydro gels and stem cells in tissue regeneration therapy. Advances in Tissue Engineering & Regenerative Medicine: Open Access 2017; 2(1): 121-35.
[http://dx.doi.org/10.15406/atroa.2017.02.00020]

[6]   Gao ZH, Hu L, Liu GL, *et al.* Bio-root and implant-based restoration as a tooth replacement alternative. J Dent Res 2016; 95(6): 642-9.
[http://dx.doi.org/10.1177/0022034516639260] [PMID: 26976131]

[7]   Guan X, Avci-Adali M, Alarçin E, Cheng H, Kashaf SS, Li Y, *et al.* Development of hydrogels for regenerative engineering. Biotechnology Journal. Wiley-VCH Verlag 2017; Vol. 12.

[8]   Baranova J, Büchner D, Götz W, Schulze M, Tobiasch E. Tooth Formation: Are the Hardest Tissues of Human Body Hard to Regenerate? Int J Mol Sci 2020; 21(11): 4031.
[http://dx.doi.org/10.3390/ijms21114031] [PMID: 32512908]

[9]   Tonk C, Witzler M, Schulze M, Tobiasch E. 2020. https://link.springer.com/content/pdf/10.1007/978-3-030-33923-4.pdf

[10]   Marin E, Boschetto F, Pezzotti G. Biomaterials and biocompatibility: An historical overviewof the Art of Antibacterial Materials and Coatings View project 3D mapping of residual stresses and crystallographic structures on zirconia toughened alumina retrivals View project Biomaterials and biocompatibility: an historical overview. Artic J Biomed Mater Res Part A [Internet]. 2020 Aug 1 [cited 2021 Jun 26];108(8):1617–33. Available from: https://www.researchgate.net/publication/340068302

[11]   Fouad AF, Khan AA. Etiology and Pathogenesis of Pulpitis and Apical Periodontitis. Essent Endodontology Prev Treat Apical Periodontitis 2019; pp. 59-90.
[http://dx.doi.org/10.1002/9781119272014.ch3]

[12]   Bratthall D, Petersen PE, Stjernswärd JR, Brown LJ. Oral and craniofacial diseases and disorders. 2nd ed., Dis Control Priorities Dev Countries 2006.

[13]   Mjör IA, Tronstad L. Experimentally induced pulpitis. Oral Surg Oral Med Oral Pathol 1972; 34(1): 102-8.
[http://dx.doi.org/10.1016/0030-4220(72)90278-2] [PMID: 4624753]

[14]   Reeves R, Stanley HR. The relationship of bacterial penetration and pulpal pathosis in carious teeth. Oral Surg Oral Med Oral Pathol 1966; 22(1): 59-65.
[http://dx.doi.org/10.1016/0030-4220(66)90143-5] [PMID: 5220026]

[15]   Eghbal MJ, Asgary S, Baglue RA, Parirokh M, Ghoddusi J. MTA pulpotomy of human permanent molars with irreversible pulpitis. Aust Endod J 2009; 35(1): 4-8.
[http://dx.doi.org/10.1111/j.1747-4477.2009.00166.x] [PMID: 19335509]

[16]   Asgary S, Eghbal MJ, Ghoddusi J. Two-year results of vital pulp therapy in permanent molars with irreversible pulpitis: an ongoing multicenter randomized clinical trial. Clin Oral Investig 2014; 18(2): 635-41.
[http://dx.doi.org/10.1007/s00784-013-1003-6] [PMID: 23712823]

[17]   Lin LM, Rosenberg PA. Repair and regeneration in endodontics. Int Endod J 2011; 44(10): 889-906.
[http://dx.doi.org/10.1111/j.1365-2591.2011.01915.x] [PMID: 21718337]

[18]   Márton IJ, Kiss C. Protective and destructive immune reactions in apical periodontitis. Oral Microbiol Immunol 2000; 15(3): 139-50.
[http://dx.doi.org/10.1034/j.1399-302x.2000.150301.x] [PMID: 11154396]

[19]   Piattelli A, Artese L, Rosini S, Quaranta M, Musiani P. Immune cells in periapical granuloma: Morphological and immunohistochemical characterization. J Endod 1991; 17(1): 26-9.
[http://dx.doi.org/10.1016/S0099-2399(07)80157-9] [PMID: 1895036]

[20]   Kabashima H, Nagata K, Maeda K, Iijima T. Involvement of substance P, mast cells, TNF-$α$ and ICAM-1 in the infiltration of inflammatory cells in human periapical granulomas. J oral Pathol \&

Med 2002; 31(3): 175-80.

[21] Rafter M. Apexification: a review. Dent Traumatol 2005; 21(1): 1-8.
[http://dx.doi.org/10.1111/j.1600-9657.2004.00284.x] [PMID: 15660748]

[22] Dylewski JJ. Apical closure of nonvital teeth. Oral Surg Oral Med Oral Pathol 1971; 32(1): 82-9.
[http://dx.doi.org/10.1016/0030-4220(71)90253-2] [PMID: 4996614]

[23] Baldassari-Cruz LA, Walton RE, Johnson WT. Scanning electron microscopy and histologic analysis
of an apexification "cap". Oral Surg Oral Med Oral Pathol Oral Radiol Endod 1998; 86(4): 465-8.
[http://dx.doi.org/10.1016/S1079-2104(98)90375-4] [PMID: 9798233]

[24] Könönen E, Gursoy M, Gursoy U. Periodontitis: A multifaceted disease of tooth-supporting tissues. J
Clin Med 2019; 8(8): 1135.
[http://dx.doi.org/10.3390/jcm8081135] [PMID: 31370168]

[25] Han J, Menicanin D, Gronthos S, Bartold PM. Stem cells, tissue engineering and periodontal
regeneration. Aust Dent J 2014; 59 (Suppl. 1): 117-30.
[http://dx.doi.org/10.1111/adj.12100] [PMID: 24111843]

[26] Narayanan AS, Bartold PM. Biochemistry of periodontal connective tissues and their regeneration: a
current perspective. Connect Tissue Res 1996; 34(3): 191-201.
[http://dx.doi.org/10.3109/03008209609000698] [PMID: 9023048]

[27] Sigurdsson TJ, Fu E, Tatakis DN, Rohrer MD, Wikesjö UME. Bone morphogenetic protein-2 for peri-
implant bone regeneration and osseointegration. Clin Oral Implants Res 1997; 8(5): 367-74.
[http://dx.doi.org/10.1034/j.1600-0501.1997.080503.x] [PMID: 9612141]

[28] Teare JA, Ramoshebi LN, Ripamonti U. Periodontal tissue regeneration by recombinant human
transforming growth factor-β 3 in Papio ursinus. J Periodontal Res 2008; 43(1): 1-8.
[PMID: 18230100]

[29] Nevins M, Garber D, Hanratty JJ, *et al.* Human histologic evaluation of anorganic bovine bone
mineral combined with recombinant human platelet-derived growth factor BB in maxillary sinus
augmentation: case series study. Int J Periodontics Restorative Dent 2009; 29(6): 583-91.
[PMID: 20072735]

[30] Hakki SS, Bozkurt B, Hakki EE, *et al.* Bone morphogenetic protein-2, -6, and -7 differently regulate
osteogenic differentiation of human periodontal ligament stem cells. J Biomed Mater Res B Appl
Biomater 2014; 102(1): 119-30.
[http://dx.doi.org/10.1002/jbm.b.32988] [PMID: 23853066]

[31] Hakki SS, Foster BL, Nagatomo KJ, *et al.* Bone morphogenetic protein-7 enhances cementoblast
function in vitro. J Periodontol 2010; 81(11): 1663-74.
[http://dx.doi.org/10.1902/jop.2010.100074] [PMID: 20681807]

[32] Cochran DL, Oh TJ, Mills MP, *et al.* A randomized clinical trial evaluating rh-FGF-2/βS-TCP in
periodontal defects. J Dent Res 2016; 95(5): 523-30.
[http://dx.doi.org/10.1177/0022034516632497] [PMID: 26908630]

[33] Carmagnola D, Pellegrini G, Dellavia C, Rimondini L, Varoni E. Tissue engineering in
periodontology: Biological mediators for periodontal regeneration. Int J Artif Organs 2019; 42(5):
241-57.
[http://dx.doi.org/10.1177/0391398819828558] [PMID: 30935276]

[34] Woodfield T, Lim K, Morouço P, Levato R, Malda J, Melchels F. 5.14 biofabrication in tissue
engineering. Compr Biomater II 2017; 5: 236-66.

[35] Abbasi E, Milani M, Fekri Aval S, *et al.* Silver nanoparticles: Synthesis methods, bio-applications and
properties. Crit Rev Microbiol 2016; 42(2): 173-80.
[PMID: 24937409]

[36] Brouwer KM, Lundvig DMS, Middelkoop E, Wagener FADTG, Von den Hoff JW. Mechanical cues

in orofacial tissue engineering and regenerative medicine. Wound Repair Regen 2015; 23(3): 302-11.
[http://dx.doi.org/10.1111/wrr.12283] [PMID: 25787133]

[37]   Murphy CM, O'Brien FJ, Little DG, Schindeler A. Cell-scaffold interactions in the bone tissue engineering triad. Eur Cell Mater 2013; 26: 120-32.
[http://dx.doi.org/10.22203/eCM.v026a09] [PMID: 24052425]

[38]   Yen AHH, Sharpe PT. Stem cells and tooth tissue engineering. Cell Tissue Res 2008; 331(1): 359-72.
[http://dx.doi.org/10.1007/s00441-007-0467-6] [PMID: 17938970]

[39]   Kim SG, Kahler B, Lin LM. Current developments in regenerative endodontics. Curr Oral Health Rep 2016; 3(4): 293-301.
[http://dx.doi.org/10.1007/s40496-016-0109-8]

[40]   Murray PE, Garcia-Godoy F, Hargreaves KM. Regenerative endodontics: a review of current status and a call for action. J Endod 2007; 33(4): 377-90.
[http://dx.doi.org/10.1016/j.joen.2006.09.013] [PMID: 17368324]

[41]   Lanza R, Langer R, Vacanti JP, Atala A. Principles of tissue engineering. 2020.

[42]   Bartold PM, Gronthos S, Ivanovski S, Fisher A, Hutmacher DW. Tissue engineered periodontal products. J Periodontal Res 2016; 51(1): 1-15.
[http://dx.doi.org/10.1111/jre.12275] [PMID: 25900048]

[43]   Larsson L, Decker AM, Nibali L, Pilipchuk SP, Berglundh T, Giannobile WV. Regenerative Medicine for Periodontal and Peri-implant Diseases. J Dent Res 2016; 95(3): 255-66.
[http://dx.doi.org/10.1177/0022034515618887] [PMID: 26608580]

[44]   Roi A, Ardelean LC, Roi CI, Boia ER, Boia S, Rusu LC. Oral bone tissue engineering: advanced biomaterials for cell adhesion, proliferation and differentiation. Materials (Basel) 2019; 12(14): 2296.
[http://dx.doi.org/10.3390/ma12142296] [PMID: 31323766]

[45]   Lizarbe MA. Tissue substitutes: from biomaterials to tissue engineering Rev R Acad Cienc Exact Fís Nat 2007; 101(1): 227-49.

[46]   Rodriguez-Vázquez M, Vega-Ruiz B, Ramos-Zúñiga R, Saldaña-Koppel DA, Quiñones-Olvera LF. Chitosan and its potential use as a scaffold for tissue engineering in regenerative medicine Biomed Res Int 2015 2015.

[47]   Jagur-Grodzinski J. Biomedical application of functional polymers. React Funct Polym 1999; 39(2): 99-138.
[http://dx.doi.org/10.1016/S1381-5148(98)00054-6]

[48]   Foda NH, El-laithy HM, Tadros MI. Implantable biodegradable sponges: effect of interpolymer complex formation of chitosan with gelatin on the release behavior of tramadol hydrochloride. Drug Dev Ind Pharm 2007; 33(1): 7-17.
[http://dx.doi.org/10.1080/03639040600975188] [PMID: 17192246]

[49]   Dash B, Xu Z, Lin L, *et al.* Stem cells and engineered scaffolds for regenerative wound healing. Bioengineering (Basel) 2018; 5(1): 23.
[http://dx.doi.org/10.3390/bioengineering5010023] [PMID: 29522497]

[50]   Stoppel WL, Ghezzi CE, McNamara SL, Iii LDB, Kaplan DL. Clinical applications of naturally derived biopolymer-based scaffolds for regenerative medicine. Ann Biomed Eng 2015; 43(3): 657-80.
[http://dx.doi.org/10.1007/s10439-014-1206-2] [PMID: 25537688]

[51]   Chocholata P, Kulda V, Babuska V. Fabrication of scaffolds for bone-tissue regeneration. Materials (Basel) 2019; 12(4): 568.
[http://dx.doi.org/10.3390/ma12040568] [PMID: 30769821]

[52]   Bansal V, Sharma PK, Sharma N, Pal OP, Malviya R. Applications of Chitosan and Chitosan Derivatives in Drug Delivery. Biol Res 2011; 5(1): 28-37.

[53]   Bhattarai N, Gunn J, Zhang M. Chitosan-based hydrogels for controlled, localized drug delivery. Adv

Drug Deliv Rev 2010; 62(1): 83-99.
[http://dx.doi.org/10.1016/j.addr.2009.07.019] [PMID: 19799949]

[54]   Jin R, Moreira Teixeira LS, Dijkstra PJ, *et al.* Injectable chitosan-based hydrogels for cartilage tissue engineering. Biomaterials 2009; 30(13): 2544-51.
[http://dx.doi.org/10.1016/j.biomaterials.2009.01.020] [PMID: 19176242]

[55]   Liu H, Wang C, Li C, *et al.* A functional chitosan-based hydrogel as a wound dressing and drug delivery system in the treatment of wound healing. RSC Advances 2018; 8(14): 7533-49.
[http://dx.doi.org/10.1039/C7RA13510F] [PMID: 35539132]

[56]   Divya K, Jisha MS. Chitosan nanoparticles preparation and applications. Environ Chem Lett 2018; 16(1): 101-12.
[http://dx.doi.org/10.1007/s10311-017-0670-y]

[57]   Li X, Wang X, Zhao T, *et al.* Guided bone regeneration using chitosan-collagen membranes in dog dehiscence-type defect model. J Oral Maxillofac Surg 2014; 72(2): 304.e1-304.e14.
[http://dx.doi.org/10.1016/j.joms.2013.09.042] [PMID: 24438600]

[58]   Chen Z, Cao S, Wang H, *et al.* Biomimetic remineralization of demineralized dentine using scaffold of CMC/ACP nanocomplexes in an in vitro tooth model of deep caries. PLoS One 2015; 10(1): e0116553.
[http://dx.doi.org/10.1371/journal.pone.0116553] [PMID: 25587986]

[59]   Shin SY, Park HN, Kim KH, *et al.* Biological evaluation of chitosan nanofiber membrane for guided bone regeneration. J Periodontol 2005; 76(10): 1778-84.
[http://dx.doi.org/10.1902/jop.2005.76.10.1778] [PMID: 16253101]

[60]   Li F, Liu X, Zhao S, Wu H, Xu HHK. Porous chitosan bilayer membrane containing TGF-β1 loaded microspheres for pulp capping and reparative dentin formation in a dog model. Dent Mater 2014; 30(2): 172-81.
[http://dx.doi.org/10.1016/j.dental.2013.11.005] [PMID: 24332410]

[61]   Zhang Y, Song J, Shi B, *et al.* Combination of scaffold and adenovirus vectors expressing bone morphogenetic protein-7 for alveolar bone regeneration at dental implant defects. Biomaterials 2007; 28(31): 4635-42.
[http://dx.doi.org/10.1016/j.biomaterials.2007.07.009] [PMID: 17664001]

[62]   Subhi H, Husein A, Mohamad D, Nurul AA. Physicochemical, mechanical and cytotoxicity evaluation of chitosan-based accelerated portland cement. J Mater Res Technol 2020; 9(5): 11574-86.
[http://dx.doi.org/10.1016/j.jmrt.2020.07.108]

[63]   Miranda SCCC, Silva GAB, Hell RCR, Martins MD, Alves JB, Goes AM. Three-dimensional culture of rat BMMSCs in a porous chitosan-gelatin scaffold: A promising association for bone tissue engineering in oral reconstruction. Arch Oral Biol 2011; 56(1): 1-15.
[http://dx.doi.org/10.1016/j.archoralbio.2010.08.018] [PMID: 20887975]

[64]   Wu Y, Gong Z, Li J, Meng Q, Fang W, Long X. The pilot study of fibrin with temporomandibular joint derived synovial stem cells in repairing TMJ disc perforation Biomed Res Int 2014 2014.

[65]   Lee YM, Park YJ, Lee SJ, *et al.* Tissue engineered bone formation using chitosan/tricalcium phosphate sponges. J Periodontol 2000; 71(3): 410-7.
[http://dx.doi.org/10.1902/jop.2000.71.3.410] [PMID: 10776928]

[66]   Lee YM, Park YJ, Lee SJ, *et al.* The bone regenerative effect of platelet-derived growth factor-BB delivered with a chitosan/tricalcium phosphate sponge carrier. J Periodontol 2000; 71(3): 418-24.
[http://dx.doi.org/10.1902/jop.2000.71.3.418] [PMID: 10776929]

[67]   Mota J, Yu N, Caridade SG, *et al.* Chitosan/bioactive glass nanoparticle composite membranes for periodontal regeneration. Acta Biomater 2012; 8(11): 4173-80.
[http://dx.doi.org/10.1016/j.actbio.2012.06.040] [PMID: 22771458]

[68]   Sano H, Shibasaki KI, Matsukubo T, Takaesu Y. Effect of chitosan rinsing on reduction of dental

plaque formation. Bull Tokyo Dent Coll 2003; 44(1): 9-16.
[http://dx.doi.org/10.2209/tdcpublication.44.9] [PMID: 12772581]

[69]   Mohire N, Yadav A. Chitosan-based polyherbal toothpaste: As novel oral hygiene product. Indian J Dent Res 2010; 21(3): 380-4.
[http://dx.doi.org/10.4103/0970-9290.70808] [PMID: 20930349]

[70]   Azargoon H, Williams BJ, Solomon ES, Kessler HP, He J, Spears R. Assessment of hemostatic efficacy and osseous wound healing using HemCon dental dressing. J Endod 2011; 37(6): 807-11.
[http://dx.doi.org/10.1016/j.joen.2011.02.023] [PMID: 21787494]

[71]   Kim J-S, Shin D-H. Inhibitory effect on Streptococcus mutans and mechanical properties of the chitosan containing composite resin Restor Dent \& Endod 2013; 38(1): 36-42.

[72]   del Carpio-Perochena A, Kishen A, Shrestha A, Bramante CM. Antibacterial properties associated with chitosan nanoparticle treatment on root dentin and 2 types of endodontic sealers. J Endod 2015; 41(8): 1353-8.
[http://dx.doi.org/10.1016/j.joen.2015.03.020] [PMID: 25958178]

[73]   Ibrahim MA, Neo J, Esguerra RJ, Fawzy AS. Characterization of antibacterial and adhesion properties of chitosan-modified glass ionomer cement. J Biomater Appl 2015; 30(4): 409-19.
[http://dx.doi.org/10.1177/0885328215589672] [PMID: 26079388]

[74]   Debnath A, Kesavappa SB, Singh GP, Eshwar S, Jain V, Swamy M. *et al.* Comparative evaluation of antibacterial and adhesive properties of chitosan modified glass ionomer cement and conventional glass ionomer cement: an in vitro study. J Clin diagnostic Res JCDR. 2017; 11(3): ZC75..

[75]   Loyola-Rodr\'\iguez JP, Torres-Méndez F, Espinosa-Cristobal LF, Garc\'\ia-Cortes JO, Loyola-Leyva A, González FJ, et al. Antimicrobial activity of endodontic sealers and medications containing chitosan and silver nanoparticles against Enterococcus faecalis. J Appl Biomater \& Funct Mater. 2019; 17(3) 2280800019851771.

[76]   Domozych DS, Ciancia M, Fangel JU, Mikkelsen MD, Ulvskov P, Willats WGT. The cell walls of green algae: A journey through evolution and diversity. Front Plant Sci 2012; 3(MAY): 82.
[http://dx.doi.org/10.3389/fpls.2012.00082] [PMID: 22639667]

[77]   Eo MY, Fan H, Cho YJ, Kim SM, Lee SK. Cellulose membrane as a biomaterial: from hydrolysis to depolymerization with electron beam. Biomater Res 2016; 20(1): 16.
[http://dx.doi.org/10.1186/s40824-016-0065-3] [PMID: 27418974]

[78]   Wang B, Lv X, Chen S, *et al.* Use of heparinized bacterial cellulose based scaffold for improving angiogenesis in tissue regeneration. Carbohydr Polym 2018; 181: 948-56.
[http://dx.doi.org/10.1016/j.carbpol.2017.11.055] [PMID: 29254059]

[79]   Portela R, Leal CR, Almeida PL, Sobral RG. Bacterial cellulose: a versatile biopolymer for wound dressing applications. Microb Biotechnol 2019; 12(4): 586-610.
[http://dx.doi.org/10.1111/1751-7915.13392] [PMID: 30838788]

[80]   Novaes Júnior AB, de Moraes NH, Novaes AB. Uso do BioFill como membrana biológica no tratamento da lesao de furca com e sem a utilizaçao da hidroxiapatita porosa. Rev Bras Odontol 1990; 29-32.

[81]   Gengiflex, an alkali-cellulose membrane for GTR: histologic observations. Braz Dent J 1993; 4(2): 65-71.

[82]   Carvalho JPF, Silva ACQ, Bastos V, *et al.* Nanocellulose-based patches loaded with hyaluronic acid and diclofenac towards aphthous stomatitis treatment. Nanomaterials (Basel) 2020; 10(4): 628.
[http://dx.doi.org/10.3390/nano10040628] [PMID: 32231070]

[83]   Costa LMM, Olyveira GM, Basmaji P, *et al.* Novel otoliths/bacterial cellulose nanocomposites as a potential natural product for direct dental pulp capping. J Biomater Tissue Eng 2012; 2(1): 48-53.
[http://dx.doi.org/10.1166/jbt.2012.1031]

[84]   Voicu G, Jinga SI, Drosu BG, Busuioc C. Improvement of silicate cement properties with bacterial cellulose powder addition for applications in dentistry. Carbohydr Polym 2017; 174: 160-70.
[http://dx.doi.org/10.1016/j.carbpol.2017.06.062] [PMID: 28821055]

[85]   Kanasan N, Adzila S, AzimahMustaffa N, Gurubaran P. AzimahMustaffa N, Gurubaran P. The effect of sodium alginate on the properties of hydroxyapatite. Procedia Eng 2017; 184: 442-8.
[http://dx.doi.org/10.1016/j.proeng.2017.04.115]

[86]   Dey P, Ramanujam R, Venkatesan G, Nagarathnam R. Sodium alginate potentiates antioxidant defense and PR proteins against early blight disease caused by Alternaria solani in Solanum lycopersicum Linn. PLoS One 2019; 14(9): e0223216.
[http://dx.doi.org/10.1371/journal.pone.0223216] [PMID: 31568481]

[87]   Pawar SN, Edgar KJ. Alginate derivatization: A review of chemistry, properties and applications. Biomaterials 2012; 33(11): 3279-305.
[http://dx.doi.org/10.1016/j.biomaterials.2012.01.007] [PMID: 22281421]

[88]   Aprilliza M. Characterization and properties of sodium alginate from brown algae used as an ecofriendly superabsorbent iopscience.iop.org2016.https://iopscience.iop.org/article/10.1088/1757-899X/188/1/012019/meta

[89]   Varaprasad K, Jayaramudu T, Kanikireddy V, Toro C, Sadiku ER. Alginate-based composite materials for wound dressing application:A mini review. Carbohydr Polym 2020; 236: 116025.
[http://dx.doi.org/10.1016/j.carbpol.2020.116025] [PMID: 32172843]

[90]   Sakai S, Kawakami K. Synthesis and characterization of both ionically and enzymatically cross-linkable alginate. Acta Biomater 2007; 3(4): 495-501.
[http://dx.doi.org/10.1016/j.actbio.2006.12.002] [PMID: 17275429]

[91]   Dobie K, Smith G, Sloan AJ, Smith AJ. Effects of alginate hydrogels and TGF-β 1 on human dental pulp repair in vitro. Connect Tissue Res 2002; 43(2-3): 387-90.
[http://dx.doi.org/10.1080/03008200290000574] [PMID: 12489186]

[92]   Srinivasan S, Jayasree R, Chennazhi KP, Nair SV, Jayakumar R. Biocompatible alginate/nano bioactive glass ceramic composite scaffolds for periodontal tissue regeneration. Carbohydr Polym 2012; 87(1): 274-83.
[http://dx.doi.org/10.1016/j.carbpol.2011.07.058] [PMID: 34662961]

[93]   Sahoo DR, Biswal T. Alginate and its application to tissue engineering. SN Applied Sciences 2021; 3(1): 30.
[http://dx.doi.org/10.1007/s42452-020-04096-w] [PMID: 34901750]

[94]   Karami A, Tebyanian H, Sayyad Soufdoost R, Motavallian E, Barkhordari A, Nourani MR. Extraction and Characterization of Collagen with Cost-Effective Method from Human Placenta for Biomedical Applications. World J Plast Surg 2019; 8(3): 352-8.
[PMID: 31620338]

[95]   Wu X, Black L, Santacana-Laffitte G, Patrick CW Jr. Preparation and assessment of glutaraldehyde-crosslinked collagen–chitosan hydrogels for adipose tissue engineering. J Biomed Mater Res A 2007; 81A(1): 59-65.
[http://dx.doi.org/10.1002/jbm.a.31003] [PMID: 17109417]

[96]   Wahl DA, Sachlos E, Liu C, Czernuszka JT. Controlling the processing of collagen-hydroxyapatite scaffolds for bone tissue engineering. J Mater Sci Mater Med 2007; 18(2): 201-9.https://www.researchgate.net/publication/6483485
[http://dx.doi.org/10.1007/s10856-006-0682-9] [PMID: 17323151]

[97]   Prescott RS, Alsanea R, Fayad MI, *et al*. *In vivo* generation of dental pulp-like tissue by using dental pulp stem cells, a collagen scaffold, and dentin matrix protein 1 after subcutaneous transplantation in mice. J Endod 2008; 34(4): 421-6.
[http://dx.doi.org/10.1016/j.joen.2008.02.005] [PMID: 18358888]

[98]   Kim JY, Xin X, Moioli EK, *et al.* Regeneration of dental-pulp-like tissue by chemotaxis-induced cell homing. Tissue Eng Part A 2010; 16(10): 3023-31.
[http://dx.doi.org/10.1089/ten.tea.2010.0181] [PMID: 20486799]

[99]   Chan CP, Lan WH, Chang MC, *et al.* Effects of TGF-βs on the growth, collagen synthesis and collagen lattice contraction of human dental pulp fibroblasts in vitro. Arch Oral Biol 2005; 50(5): 469-79.
[http://dx.doi.org/10.1016/j.archoralbio.2004.10.005] [PMID: 15777529]

[100]   Jones GL, Motta A, Marshall MJ, El Haj AJ, Cartmell SH. Osteoblast: Osteoclast co-cultures on silk fibroin, chitosan and PLLA films. Biomaterials 2009; 30(29): 5376-84.
[http://dx.doi.org/10.1016/j.biomaterials.2009.07.028] [PMID: 19647869]

[101]   Zhang W, Ahluwalia IP, Literman R, Kaplan DL, Yelick PC. Human dental pulp progenitor cell behavior on aqueous and hexafluoroisopropanol based silk scaffolds. J Biomed Mater Res - Part A 2011 Jun 15; 97(A(4)): 414-22.

[102]   Mandal BB, Grinberg A, Gil ES, Panilaitis B, Kaplan DL. High-strength silk protein scaffolds for bone repair www.pnas.org/cgi/doi/10.1073/pnas.1119474109
[http://dx.doi.org/10.1073/pnas.1119474109]

[103]   Horan RL, Antle K, Collette AL, *et al.* In vitro degradation of silk fibroin. Biomaterials 2005; 26(17): 3385-93.
[http://dx.doi.org/10.1016/j.biomaterials.2004.09.020] [PMID: 15621227]

[104]   Kim KH, Jeong L, Park HN, *et al.* Biological efficacy of silk fibroin nanofiber membranes for guided bone regeneration. J Biotechnol 2005; 120(3): 327-39.
[http://dx.doi.org/10.1016/j.jbiotec.2005.06.033] [PMID: 16150508]

[105]   Panilaitis B, Altman GH, Chen J, Jin HJ, Karageorgiou V, Kaplan DL. Macrophage responses to silk. Biomaterials 2003; 24(18): 3079-85.
[http://dx.doi.org/10.1016/S0142-9612(03)00158-3] [PMID: 12895580]

[106]   Pérez-Rigueiro J, Elices M, Llorca J, Viney C. Tensile properties of silkworm silk obtained by forced silking. J Appl Polym Sci 2001; 82(8): 1928-35.
[http://dx.doi.org/10.1002/app.2038]

[107]   Celotti G, Landi E. From biomimetic apatite to biologically inspired composites 2005. https://www.researchgate.net/publication/8036945

[108]   Cao Y, Wang B. Biodegradation of silk biomaterials. Int J Mol Sci 2009; 10(4): 1514-24. www.mdpi.com/journal/ijms
[http://dx.doi.org/10.3390/ijms10041514] [PMID: 19468322]

[109]   Sell SA, Wolfe PS, Garg K, McCool JM, Rodriguez IA, Bowlin GL. The Use of Natural Polymers in Tissue Engineering: A Focus on Electrospun Extracellular Matrix Analogues. Polymers (Basel) 2010; 2(4): 522-53.www.mdpi.com/J./polymers [Internet].
[http://dx.doi.org/10.3390/polym2040522]

[110]   Huang GTJ, Yamaza T, Shea LD, Djouad F, Kuhn NZ, Tuan RS, *et al.* Stem/Progenitor cell-mediated de novo regeneration of dental pulp with newly deposited continuous layer of dentin in an *in vivo* model. Tissue Engineering - Part A. Mary Ann Liebert Inc. 2010; pp. 605-15.
[http://dx.doi.org/10.1089/ten.tea.2009.0518]

[111]   Xu WP, Zhang W, Asrican R, Kim HJ, Kaplan DL, Yelick PC. Accurately shaped tooth bud cell-derived mineralized tissue formation on silk scaffolds. Tissue Eng Part A 2008; 14(4): 549-57.
[http://dx.doi.org/10.1089/tea.2007.0227] [PMID: 18352829]

[112]   Huang Y, Onyeri S, Siewe M, Moshfeghian A, Madihally SV. In vitro characterization of chitosan–gelatin scaffolds for tissue engineering. Biomaterials 2005; 26(36): 7616-27.
[http://dx.doi.org/10.1016/j.biomaterials.2005.05.036] [PMID: 16005510]

[113] Schönwälder SMS, Bally F, Heinke L, *et al.* Interaction of human plasma proteins with thin gelatin-based hydrogel films: a QCM-D and ToF-SIMS study. Biomacromolecules 2014; 15(7): 2398-406.
[http://dx.doi.org/10.1021/bm500750v] [PMID: 24956040]

[114] Brovold M, Almeida JI. Pla-Palac\'\in I, Sainz-Arnal P, Sánchez-Romero N, Rivas JJ, *et al* Naturallyderived biomaterials for tissue engineering applications. Nov Biomater Regen Med 2018; pp. 421-49.

[115] Moussa DG, Aparicio C. Present and future of tissue engineering scaffolds for dentin-pulp complex regeneration. J Tissue Eng Regen Med 2019; 13(1): 58-75.
[PMID: 30376696]

[116] Vagropoulou G, Trentsiou M, Georgopoulou A, *et al.* Hybrid chitosan/gelatin/nanohydroxyapatite scaffolds promote odontogenic differentiation of dental pulp stem cells and in vitro biomineralization. Dent Mater 2021; 37(1): e23-36.
[http://dx.doi.org/10.1016/j.dental.2020.09.021] [PMID: 33208264]

[117] Ribeiro JS, Bordini EAF, Ferreira JA, Mei L, Dubey N, Fenno JC, *et al.* Injectable MMP-responsive nanotube-modified gelatin hydrogel for dental infection ablation. ACS Appl Mater \& interfaces. 2020; 12(14): 16006-7.

[118] Monteiro N, Thrivikraman G, Athirasala A, *et al.* Photopolymerization of cell-laden gelatin methacryloyl hydrogels using a dental curing light for regenerative dentistry. Dent Mater 2018; 34(3): 389-99.
[http://dx.doi.org/10.1016/j.dental.2017.11.020] [PMID: 29199008]

[119] Bakopoulou A, Georgopoulou A, Grivas I, *et al.* Dental pulp stem cells in chitosan/gelatin scaffolds for enhanced orofacial bone regeneration. Dent Mater 2019; 35(2): 310-27.
[http://dx.doi.org/10.1016/j.dental.2018.11.025] [PMID: 30527589]

[120] Jang JH, Moon JH, Kim SG, Kim SY. Pulp regeneration with hemostatic matrices as a scaffold in an immature tooth minipig model. Sci Rep 2020; 10(1): 12536.
[http://dx.doi.org/10.1038/s41598-020-69437-6] [PMID: 32719323]

[121] Alipour M, Firouzi N, Aghazadeh Z, *et al.* The osteogenic differentiation of human dental pulp stem cells in alginate-gelatin/Nano-hydroxyapatite microcapsules. BMC Biotechnol 2021; 21(1): 6.
[http://dx.doi.org/10.1186/s12896-020-00666-3] [PMID: 33430842]

[122] Wu S, Zhou Y, Yu Y, Zhou X, Du W, Wan M, *et al.* Evaluation of Chitosan Hydrogel for Sustained Delivery of VEGF for Odontogenic Differentiation of Dental Pulp Stem Cells Stem Cells Int 2019 2019.

[123] Xu X, Gu Z, Chen X, *et al.* An injectable and thermosensitive hydrogel: Promoting periodontal regeneration by controlled-release of aspirin and erythropoietin. Acta Biomater 2019; 86: 235-46.
[http://dx.doi.org/10.1016/j.actbio.2019.01.001] [PMID: 30611793]

[124] Bagheri B, Zarrintaj P, Samadi A, *et al.* Tissue engineering with electrospun electro-responsive chitosan-aniline oligomer/polyvinyl alcohol. Int J Biol Macromol 2020; 147: 160-9.
[http://dx.doi.org/10.1016/j.ijbiomac.2019.12.264] [PMID: 31904459]

[125] Wang H, Zhu D, Paul A, *et al.* Covalently adaptable elastin-like protein - hyaluronic acid (ELP - HA) hybrid hydrogels with secondary thermoresponsive crosslinking for injectable stem cell delivery. Adv Funct Mater 2017; 27(28): 1605609.
[http://dx.doi.org/10.1002/adfm.201605609] [PMID: 33041740]

[126] Silva CR, Babo PS, Gulino M, *et al.* Injectable and tunable hyaluronic acid hydrogels releasing chemotactic and angiogenic growth factors for endodontic regeneration. Acta Biomater 2018; 77: 155-71.
[http://dx.doi.org/10.1016/j.actbio.2018.07.035] [PMID: 30031163]

[127] Almeida LDF, Babo PS, Silva CR, *et al.* Hyaluronic acid hydrogels incorporating platelet lysate enhance human pulp cell proliferation and differentiation. J Mater Sci Mater Med 2018; 29(6): 88.

[http://dx.doi.org/10.1007/s10856-018-6088-7] [PMID: 29904797]

[128] Sancilio S, Gallorini M, Di Nisio C, Marsich E, Di Pietro R, Schweikl H. *et al.* Alginate/hydroxyapatite-based nanocomposite scaffolds for bone tissue engineering improve dental pulp biomineralization and differentiation. Stem Cells Int. 2018 2018.

[129] Devillard R, Rémy M, Kalisky J, *et al. In vitro* assessment of a collagen/alginate composite scaffold for regenerative endodontics. Int Endod J 2017; 50(1): 48-57.
[http://dx.doi.org/10.1111/iej.12591] [PMID: 26650723]

[130] Athirasala A, Lins F, Tahayeri A, *et al.* A Novel Strategy to Engineer Pre-Vascularized Full-Length Dental Pulp-like Tissue Constructs. Sci Rep 2017; 7(1): 3323.
[http://dx.doi.org/10.1038/s41598-017-02532-3] [PMID: 28607361]

[131] Sowmya S, Mony U, Jayachandran P, *et al.* Tri-Layered Nanocomposite Hydrogel Scaffold for the Concurrent Regeneration of Cementum, Periodontal Ligament, and Alveolar Bone. Adv Healthc Mater 2017; 6(7): 1601251.
[http://dx.doi.org/10.1002/adhm.201601251] [PMID: 28128898]

[132] Koch F, Meyer N, Valdec S, Jung RE, Mathes SH. Development and application of a 3D periodontal in vitro model for the evaluation of fibrillar biomaterials. BMC Oral Health 2020; 20(1): 148.
[http://dx.doi.org/10.1186/s12903-020-01124-4] [PMID: 32429904]

[133] Zhang W, Liu H, Yang W, *et al.* Hydroxyapatite/silk fibroin composite biomimetic scaffold for dental pulp repair. Bioinspired, Biomimetic and Nanobiomaterials 2019; 8(4): 231-8.
[http://dx.doi.org/10.1680/jbibn.18.00050]

[134] Jasiuk I, Abueidda DW, Kozuch C, Pang S, Su FY, McKittrick J. An Overview on Additive Manufacturing of Polymers. J Miner Met Mater Soc 2018; 70(3): 275-83.
[http://dx.doi.org/10.1007/s11837-017-2730-y]

[135] Baumgartner S, Gmeiner R, Schönherr JA, Stampfl J. Stereolithography-based additive manufacturing of lithium disilicate glass ceramic for dental applications. Mater Sci Eng C 2020; 116: 111180.
[http://dx.doi.org/10.1016/j.msec.2020.111180] [PMID: 32806296]

[136] Mederle N, Marin S, Marin MM, Danila E, Mederle O, Albu Kaya MG, *et al.* Innovative biomaterials based on collagen-hydroxyapatite and doxycycline for bone regeneration Adv Mater Sci Eng 2016 2016.

[137] Ngo TD, Kashani A, Imbalzano G, Nguyen KTQ, Hui D. Additive manufacturing (3D printing): A review of materials, methods, applications and challenges. Compos, Part B Eng 2018; 143: 172-96.
[http://dx.doi.org/10.1016/j.compositesb.2018.02.012]

[138] Zadpoor AA, Malda J. Additive Manufacturing of Biomaterials, Tissues, and Organs. Ann Biomed Eng 2017; 45(1): 1-11.https://link.springer.com/content/pdf/10.1007/s10439-016-1719-y.pdf
[http://dx.doi.org/10.1007/s10439-016-1719-y] [PMID: 27632024]

[139] Murphy SV, Atala A. 3D bioprinting of tissues and organs. Nat Biotechnol 2014; 32(8): 773-85.
[http://dx.doi.org/10.1038/nbt.2958] [PMID: 25093879]

[140] Xiongfa J, Hao Z, Liming Z, Jun X. Recent advances in 3D bioprinting for the regeneration of functional cartilage. Regenerative Medicine. Future Medicine Ltd. 2018; Vol. 13: pp. 73-87.

[141] Wang X, Ao Q, Tian X, *et al.* Correction: 3D Bioprinting Technologies for Hard Tissue and Organ Engineering. Materials 2016, 9, 802. Materials (Basel) 2016; 9(11): 911.
[http://dx.doi.org/10.3390/ma9110911] [PMID: 28774034]

[142] Hollister SJ. Porous scaffold design for tissue engineering. Nat Mater 2005; 4(7): 518-24.
[http://dx.doi.org/10.1038/nmat1421] [PMID: 16003400]

[143] Matai I, Kaur G, Seyedsalehi A, Biomaterials AM. 2020. https://www.sciencedirect.com/science/article/pii/S0142961219306350?casa_token=kTmUn3XUChcAAAAA:Pr4iHRKUWLcrl8s6HKevx6Vy-H92HiPPe29KWmtQyesel28AykvuTJBaKwLUyhlugHki0pILhOI

[144]   Sun W, Starly B, Daly A, Burdick J, *et al.* iopscience.iop.org2020.
        [http://dx.doi.org/10.1088/1758-5090/ab5158]

[145]   Roseti L, Parisi V, Petretta M, *et al.* CC-MS and 2017. https://www.sciencedirect.com/
        science/article/pii/S0928493117317228?casa_token= 8xoD7RNZpaEAAAAA:t2WMB8eQYazI6Yn1
        Hu_GVNSwXcTzI8-527IydDIvLTn4T06Bi-Z57d8NHB2-3zXpKY7HPcR0Oig

[146]   Wen Y, Xun S, Haoye M, *et al.* pubs.rsc.org https://pubs.rsc.org/no/content/articlehtml/2017/bm/
        c7bm00315c

[147]   Kim HD, Amirthalingam S, Kim SL, Lee SS, Rangasamy J, Hwang NS. Bone Tissue Engineering:
        Biomimetic Materials and Fabrication Approaches for Bone Tissue Engineering (Adv. Healthcare
        Mater. 23/2017). Adv Healthc Mater 2017; 6(23): 1770120.
        [http://dx.doi.org/10.1002/adhm.201770120] [PMID: 29171714]

[148]   Shah P, Chong BS. 3D imaging, 3D printing and 3D virtual planning in endodontics. Vol. 22, Clinical
        Oral Investigations. Springer Verlag; 2018. p. 641–54.

[149]   Yu H, Zhang X, Song W, *et al.* Effects of 3-dimensional bioprinting alginate/gelatin hydrogel scaffold
        extract on proliferation and differentiation of human dental pulp stem cells. J Endod 2019; 45(6): 706-
        15.
        [http://dx.doi.org/10.1016/j.joen.2019.03.004] [PMID: 31056297]

[150]   Athirasala A, Tahayeri A, Thrivikraman G, *et al.* A dentin-derived hydrogel bioink for 3D bioprinting
        of cell laden scaffolds for regenerative dentistry. Biofabrication 2018; 10(2): 024101.
        [http://dx.doi.org/10.1088/1758-5090/aa9b4e] [PMID: 29320372]

[151]   Dutta SD, Hexiu J, Patel DK, Ganguly K, Lim KT. 3D-printed bioactive and biodegradable hydrogel
        scaffolds of alginate/gelatin/cellulose nanocrystals for tissue engineering. Int J Biol Macromol 2021;
        167: 644-58.
        [http://dx.doi.org/10.1016/j.ijbiomac.2020.12.011] [PMID: 33285198]

[152]   Gao B, Yang Q, Zhao X, Jin G, Ma Y. https://www.sciencedirect.com/science/article/pii/S016777991
        6000664?casa_token=V_2x3MlGLgQAAAAA:hRmVIOzYXDPDeQ_Pf_yojZRU6wGpXYhnueqEdh
        RiwVW9S6x1voi9mslFou5J-KIdlrQ6sFLwqEM

[153]   Wan Z, Zhang P, Liu Y, Lv L. 2020. https://www.sciencedirect.com/science/article/pii/S174270
        6119307172

[154]   Tamay DG, Usal TD, Alagoz AS, Yucel D, Hasirci N, Hasirci V. 3D and 4D printing of polymers for
        tissue engineering applications. Frontiers in Bioengineering and Biotechnology. Frontiers Media S.A.
        2019; Vol. 7.

[155]   Sydney Gladman A, Matsumoto EA, Nuzzo RG, Mahadevan L, Lewis JA. Biomimetic 4D printing.
        Nat Mater 2016; 15(4): 413-8.
        [http://dx.doi.org/10.1038/nmat4544] [PMID: 26808461]

[156]   Shepherd J, Douglas I, Rimmer S, Swanson L, MacNeil S. Development of three-dimensional tissue-
        engineered models of bacterial infected human skin wounds. Tissue Eng Part C Methods 2009; 15(3):
        475-84.
        [http://dx.doi.org/10.1089/ten.tec.2008.0614] [PMID: 19292658]

CHAPTER 7

Scaffolds in Vascular Tissue Engineering Research

Jun W. Heng[1], Ubashini Vijakumaran[1], Rohaina C. Man[2] and **Nadiah Sulaiman[1,*]**

[1] *Centre for Tissue Engineering and Regenerative Medicine, Faculty of Medicine, Universiti Kebangsaan Malaysia, 56000, Cheras, Kuala Lumpur, Malaysia*

[2] *Department of Pathology, Faculty of Medicine, Universiti Kebangsaan Malaysia, 56000, Cheras, Kuala Lumpur, Malaysia*

Abstract: Scaffolds represent one of the key components in the tissue engineering triad. Construction of a vascular graft begins with the scaffold that acts as the base building material. Whether natural or synthetic, selecting the right scaffold material is essential to ensure the structural integrity of a graft. The structural integrity could further be strengthened with the addition of cells and regulatory signals that make up the whole tissue engineering triad. In this chapter, a selection of scaffold materials is discussed, and cell seeding strategies are later elaborated, covering the principle of the tissue engineering triad in vascular research.

Keywords: Blood vessel, Scaffold, Small diameter vascular graft, Tissue engineering triad, Vascular scaffold.

SCAFFOLDS IN VASCULAR TISSUE ENGINEERING RESEARCH

Tissue engineering is an interdisciplinary field that integrates the principles of engineering and biomedicine to produce biological materials that can integrate natively with the tissues of a patient to achieve the goal of restoring or enhancing physiological function [1]. A tissue-engineered vascular graft (TEVG) implanted with cells aims to produce a vessel that is capable of growing, remodeling, and repairing in vivo and represents a plausible solution for the advancement of vascular surgery, given the shortcomings of existing vascular bypass conduits [2]. The conventional tissue engineering framework consists of three components: a scaffold material, cellular grafting and tissue remodeling, and biological signals such as chemokines or growth factors to attract and promote cell assembly [1] (Fig. **1**). Biomaterials used as scaffolds for the production of TEVGs often mimic

---

* **Corresponding author Nadiah Sulaiman:** Centre for Tissue Engineering and Regenerative Medicine, Faculty of Medicine, Universiti Kebangsaan Malaysia, 56000, Cheras, Kuala Lumpur, Malaysia; E-mail: nadiahsulaiman@ukm.edu.my

Mohd Fauzi Mh Busra, Daniel Law Jia Xian, Yogeswaran Lokanathan and Ruszymah Haji Idrus (Eds.)

the properties of native extracellular matrices which allows them to direct cellular growth and tissue regeneration while the cellular component provides the capacity for physiological remodeling and biochemical signaling [3, 4]. As TEVGs will be integrated into the vasculature, the mechanical properties of the tissue-engineered vascular scaffolds cannot be overlooked and should be evaluated to ensure compatibility with native tissues [5]. It is essential for the TEVG to support unimpeded blood perfusion whilst withstanding and sustaining associated pressures without bursting or irreversibly deforming due to aneurysm formation [6, 7]. Vessel compliance is also a crucial factor to consider, as TEVGs need to be elastic enough to avoid high-stress areas developing around the anastomotic region [8, 9]. In addition, the TEVG should be devoid of cytotoxicity and immunogenicity to minimise or prevent adverse immune responses such as chronic inflammation when implanted [10].

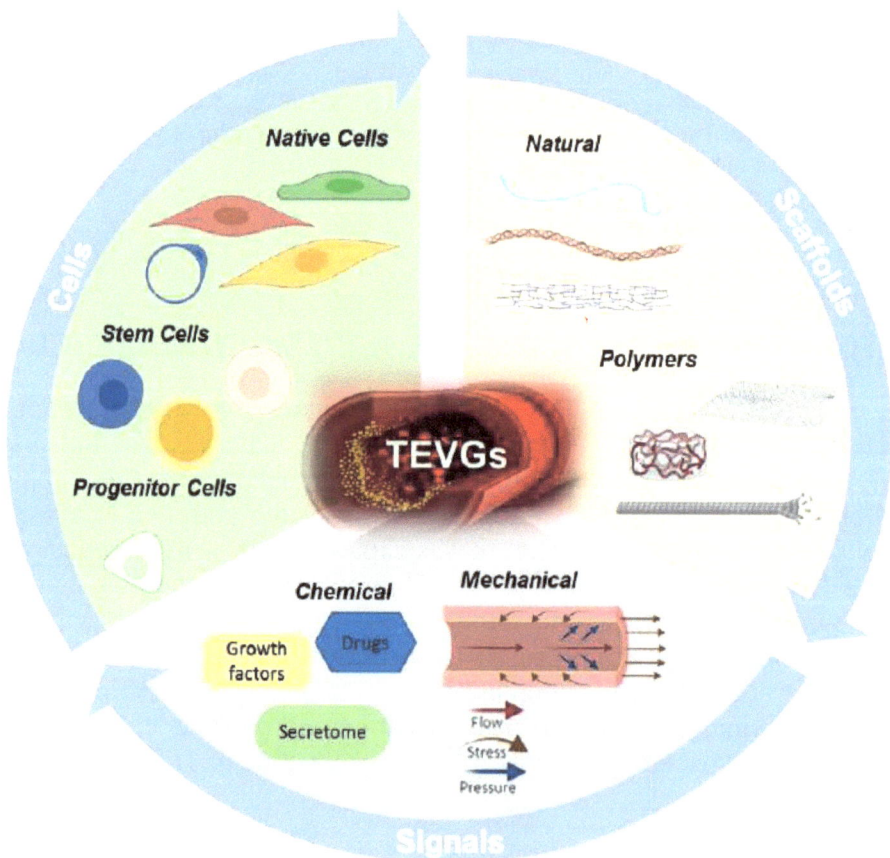

Fig. (1). Tissue-engineered vascular graft (TEVG) abides by the conventional tissue engineering triad, where the three components, including cells, scaffolding materials, and regulatory signals, are essential in fabricating a functional TEVG. Image created with Biorender.com.

Weinberg and Bell fabricated the first tissue-engineered vascular scaffold construct in 1986 through a combination of bovine ECs, smooth muscle cells (SMCs), and fibroblasts cultured in a collagen matrix to replicate the intimal, medial, and adventitial layers, respectively [11]. While they achieved tissue architectures resembling native blood vessels, the mechanical properties of the constructs proved to be extremely poor, with burst pressures below 10 mmHg, necessitating the introduction of a Dacron mesh for structural reinforcement [11]. Despite the addition of Dacron, burst pressures were still found to be within the range of maximal systolic blood pressure (burst pressure: 120-180 mmHg) [11. Despite this unfortunate failure, their ground-breaking research paved a new road for TEVG development, leading to a variety of different approaches to generate a clinically viable tissue-engineered vascular graft.

Scaffold

TEVGs can broadly be classified into two categories despite differences in structural components, manufacturing procedures, and cell sources: scaffold-based vascular grafts utilising natural or synthetic polymers and self-assembled vascular grafts. Natural polymers used for TEVG production can further be divided into two groups: ECM-based materials and decellularised natural matrices [2]. Scaffold-based techniques represent the most commonly employed process for TEVG design. This is attributed to the implementation of a physical, three-dimensional structure that can aid in directing cell migration and proliferation, allowing cells to organise into complex geometries [2, 5]. Synthetic polymers have seen extensively used in the fabrication of TEVGs to date due to the capacity and ease of reconfiguring characteristics (e.g., mechanical properties and degradation rate) of the resultant vascular graft to meet specific clinical requirements [12]. These modifications are carried out by altering the size, surface area, and composition of the materials incorporated into the TEVG.

Synthetic Polymers

Synthetic vascular grafts manufactured from non-biodegradable polymers such as polyethylene terephthalate (Dacron), expanded polytetrafluoroethylene (PTFE), and polyurethane (PU) have been developed as an alternative to autologous vessels to circumvent some of the limitations of using autologous vessels as bypass conduits [13, 14]. The aforementioned materials have been proven to be both mechanically and biologically compatible with native blood vessels and can be modified through processes such as heparin conjugation to instill anticoagulative functions which contribute to improving and maintaining satisfactory long-term patency when replacing large diameter (>8 mm) and middle diameter (6-8 mm) arteries [5, 14]. Unfortunately, studies have also shown that synthetic grafts exhibited increased thrombotic risk with increased probabilities for stenosis, ectopic calcification, and infection whilst lacking growth potential when replacing small diameter vessels, which include the coronary arteries [15, 16]. Autologous vessels remain the superior choice for these applications, with SV grafts exhibiting patency rates higher than 95% 1-year post-CABG compared to approximately 60% in PTFE grafts, with 2-year patency rates remaining above 90% in SV grafts and a critically low 32% in PTFE grafts [16, 17]. Endothelial cells (ECs) are crucial in the suppression of coagulation cascades activated by platelets in native blood vessels [8], hence, the presence of an adequate number of ECs on the luminal surface of a vascular graft can reduce the risk of thrombosis and extend graft patency [18]. Seeding of synthetic conduits with ECs has yielded improvements in patency. However, autologous vessels remain more effective [19]. As such, synthetic grafts can only be recommended as the bypass conduit for small-diameter vascular bypass procedures if compatible autologous vessels are absent [20]. The concept of tissue engineering was proposed by Langer and Vacanti as a potential solution to address the disadvantages associated with vascular bypass utilising autologous and synthetic grafts [1, 21].

Synthetic scaffolds that take longer to biodegrade can retain their mechanical strength and withstand blood pressures for longer periods, but this property could also be detrimental to the longevity of the graft as it may impede the formation of new tissue around the scaffold after implantation. Disequilibrium between scaffold degradation and tissue formation rates results in a mechanical mismatch and, consequently, graft failure [22]. In addition, these polymers are also limited by a lack of natural cell binding domains that are crucial for supporting cell adhesion and proliferation [23]. Polyglycolic acid (PGA), polylactic acid (PLA), poly(ε-caprolactone) (PCL), and poly(glycerol-sebacate) (PGS) represent some of the most commonly utilised synthetic polymers for the fabrication of TEVGs [24].

Polyglycolic Acid (PGA)

PGA is a non-immunogenic, biodegradable polyester that exhibits strong crystallinity and flexibility and is among the first polymers used for the fabrication TEVGs [24, 25]. As such, PGA grafts have been extensively studied and used in experiments with various animal models, including ovine, canine, porcine, and primate models [26, 27]. These grafts have a degradation rate of approximately 6 weeks, as evidenced by a previous study utilising a PGA TEVG as an inferior vena cava interposition graft [24, 28]. Unfortunately, this degradation rate is far too rapid for PGA to be used for clinical vascular applications as the scaffold degrades and loses mechanical integrity before sufficient numbers of neotissue form, leading to the development of aneurysms

[29]. Furthermore, the acidic by-products generated by the degradation of PGA scaffolds have been previously reported to cause luminal narrowing via the induction of SMC proliferation [30]. Fortunately, the mechanical integrity of PGA scaffolds can be enhanced via SMC seeding or by combining it with other polymers, such as PLA to form the poly (lactic-co-glycolic acid) (PGLA) copolymer [29, 31]. The mechanical properties of PGLA grafts are easily altered by modifying the ratio of lactic acid to glycolic acid in the polymer mixture [32].

In 1997, Niklason and Langer fabricated a small diameter TEVG using a PGA scaffold seeded with vascular SMCs cultured under pulsatile flow until maturation was achieved, and the burst pressure of their graft was determined to be promising being 2,150 mmHg [33, 34]. These results led to animal implantation studies which discovered that the TEVG retained maximum patency after 24 days in dogs and baboons, but its patency dropped to 88% 6 months post-implantation [35]. Melchiorri *et al.* fabricated a small-diameter TEVG by utilising a combination of PGLA with 10% and 15% poly (DL-caprolactone-co-lactic acid) (PCLLA) [36]. Their results showed that 10% PGLA-PCLLA was able to withstand 2.93 ± 0.26 MPa of pressure before tearing while 15% PGLA-PCLLA withstood 4.51 ± 0.97 MPa, both values higher than the ultimate tensile strength (UTS) of the human SV which can withstand 2.2 ± 0.2 MPa. The burst pressure of the Melchiorri *et al.*'s grafts was lower, however, at $1,002.17 \pm 181.98$ mmHg and $1,321.66 \pm 214.67$ mmHg in 10% and 15% PGLA-PCLLA respectively, as opposed to 1,680-2,273 mmHg in the SV [36, 37]. Another study conducted by Fukunishi *et al.* utilised a copolymer of 10 wt.% PGA and 5 wt.% poly (L-lactide-co-ε-caprolactone) (PLCL) in hexafluoro isopropanol to develop a scaffold through electrospinning and 3D printing [38]. Biomechanical testing of their TEVG showed no significant differences in burst pressure as compared to the native inferior vena cava (IVC), but the TEVG exhibited higher preoperative compliance compared to native IVC (4.0% ± 1.5% vs. 0.85%). Sufficient remodeling and scaffold degradation were detected 6 months post-implantation [38].

Polylactic Acid (PLA)

PLA represents another example of a widely used biodegradable and non-immunogenic polymer used to produce TEVGs. Due to the presence of an additional methyl group in the chemical structure of PLA when compared to PGA, scaffolds developed using PLA exhibit strong hydrophobic characteristics and, as a result, can retain their structural integrity and mechanical properties for a much longer period before degrading (6-12 months vs. 6 weeks) [29]. The hydrophobicity of PLA adversely affects cell adhesion and tissue remodeling, causing PLA grafts to tend toward early thrombogenicity, however [29, 39]. Additionally, PLA is a brittle polymer, easily sustaining fractures under impact loading [40]. To overcome this, PLA is commonly associated with other polymers, cells, or bioactive molecules to utilise and enhance its mechanical properties whilst reducing its thrombotic risk, resulting in increased graft patency [28, 39].

In 2007, Hashi *et al.* fabricated and implanted an electrospun nanofibrous poly (L-lactic acid) (PLLA) TEVG seeded with mesenchymal stem cells (MSCs) into the common carotid artery of rats using a bypass procedure [41]. Their results revealed that the use of nanofibrous PLLA scaffolds resulted in the induction of inflammatory responses leading to intimal hyperplasia, but the presence of MSCs on these TEVGs inhibited these inflammatory responses and consequently prevented intimal thickening. Their study also suggested that MSCs exhibit anti-thrombogenic properties as scanning electron microscopy of unseeded grafts revealed significant platelet aggregation, while MSC-seeded grafts had negligible amounts [41]. A 2017 study utilised electrospun scaffolds made from a mixture of PLLA and segmented polyurethane (PHD) functionalised via heparin immobilisation [42]. Contact angle measurements revealed that the heparin-modified PLLA/PHD scaffold exhibited hydrophilic properties, which proved advantageous for the adhesion and proliferation of human adipose-derived stem cells, as measured through the 3-(4,5-dimethylthiazol-2-yl)-2,5-diphenyl-tetrazolium bromide (MTT) assay. Most importantly, heparin-modified scaffolds were resistant to platelet adhesion and increased the migration, attachment, and development of ECs onto the TEVG [42].

Poly(E-Caprolactone) (PCL)

PCL is a low-cost, highly stable aliphatic polyester that represents the most commonly used synthetic polymer in vascular tissue engineering due to its astounding mechanical strength, hydrophobicity, and pliability at low temperatures, which consequently improves modifiability and ease of fabrication [43, 44]. A 2018 study conducted by Gao *et al.* illustrated that the mechanical strength of electrospun PCL grafts surpasses that of native vessels, with their fabricated vascular graft exhibiting a maximal tensile strength of 3 MPa with a maximal strain of 200% compared to the native femoral artery which exhibits a maximal tensile strength of 1-2 MPa with a maximal strain of 63-76% [3]. The findings from another study conducted by Asvar *et al.* further confirmed these results as they found that electrospun PCL grafts have a tensile strength of 3.6 MPa [45]. Chan *et al.* studied the characteristics of acellular electrospun PCL TEVGs implanted as a right common carotid artery interposition graft in mouse models and found that PCL grafts exhibited substantial endothelialisation 28 days post-implant but significant development of intimal hyperplasia, particularly near the anastomoses was also detected [46].

Due to the hydrophobicity and high crystallinity of the PCL polymer, scaffolds fabricated with this material have some of the longest degradation times (2-3 years or more) and can retain their mechanical properties for much longer periods compared to other synthetic polymers [47, 48]. However, this hydrophobicity can impede the adhesion and proliferation of cells, interfere with tissue remodeling, and increase the adhesion of platelet and plasma proteins, all of which leads to an increased risk of intimal hyperplasia, early thrombosis, and ultimately graft failure [18, 29, 49]. Therefore, PCL is commonly combined with other polymers or functionalized via surface modifications to improve the biological and mechanical properties of the graft [49]. Heparin and vascular endothelial growth factor (VEGF) are biomolecules utilised by Braghirolli *et al.* in 2017 to functionalise electrospun PCL scaffolds. Heparin-VEGF-modified grafts exhibited reduced thrombogenicity and increased MSC and endothelial progenitor cell (EPC) proliferation without affecting the structural integrity of the graft [8].

The combination of PLA and PCL results in the formation of the copolymer poly(l-lactic-co-ε-caprolactone) (PLCL), a synthetic elastic polymer with a slow degradation rate that overcomes some of the limitations of its constituting polymers, namely the brittle nature of PLA, the production of acidic by-products due to PLA degradation leading to acidification, and the low stiffness of PCL [50, 51]. Additionally, the mechanical properties and degradation rates of PLCL scaffolds can easily be adjusted to meet individual clinical requirements by adjusting PLA: PCL molar ratios during the production of the copolymer [29]. As with PCL, PLCL grafts can also undergo surface modification to enhance their mechanical and/or biological properties. He *et al.* constructed and investigated the properties of collagen type I-coated alkaline-modified PLCL (PLCL-COLI) scaffold using low-temperature deposition manufacturing 3D printing. Mechanical tests revealed that PLCL-COLI exhibits a lower Young's modulus than PLCL (0.21 ± 0.05 MPa vs. 0.32 ± 0.05 MPa), but significantly higher hydrophilicity than PLCL ($66.9 \pm 2.3\%$ vs. $52.0 \pm 2.7\%$). MTT assay showed increased cell proliferation in PLCL-COLI compared to PLCL [52].

Poly (Glycerol-Sebacate) (PGS)

PGS is an economical bioresorbable polyester elastomer composed of glycerol and sebacic acid. It exhibits thermoset elastomeric properties and has a short degradation and resorption time of approximately 4 weeks and 8 weeks, respectively, allowing for timely constructive remodeling of the vascular scaffold to a neoartery which is beneficial as it enhances graft-to-host integration efficiency, provides an anti-thrombogenic property to the lumen of the vascular graft, and improves the mechanical strength of the graft to matching with the native vessel [53]. Previous studies have shown that PGS has low thrombotic and inflammatory potential compared to poly(l-lactide-co-glycolide) (PLGA) and expanded PTFE [54]. As with other synthetic polymers, PGS grafts can easily be modified to achieve desired mechanical properties and degradation kinetics – Chen *et al.* fabricated a PGS using a 1:1 molar ratio of glycerol to sebacic acid at different three different temperatures (110°C, 120°C, 130°C) and found that Young's modulus and degradation times differed between each temperature [55].

Wu *et al.* interposition PCL-reinforced PGS TEVGs in the abdominal aortas of rats and discovered total endothelialisation of the luminal surface with cells staining positive for von Willebrand factor (vWF) with graft patency determined to be 80% 1-year post-implantation. SMC-like cells that stained for α-smooth muscle actin (α-SMA) and myosin heavy chain 11 (MHC-11) were also found inhabiting the middle layer of the neoartery, resembling the native arterial medial layer [53]. Another study utilising electrospun PGS reinforced with PCL as a mouse infrarenal aortic interposition disclosed that all grafts remained patent with a lack of thrombosis and stenosis during a 1-year post-operative examination [56].

Natural Polymers

Natural polymers such as collagen, elastin, and chitosan have been instrumental in the fabrication and refinement of TEVGs as they typically exhibit superior biological properties, are less likely to induce a foreign body reaction and are more biocompatible than synthetic polymers due to the presence of cell recognition and cell adhesion domains in their structure [12, 23]. Despite their advantages, natural polymers are subjected to higher degradation rates and suboptimal mechanical strength when compared to their synthetic counterparts, which is unfavourable as the probability of vessel rupture and aneurysm formation increases as a result. As such, natural polymers are usually combined with other materials, such as synthetic polymers, to form hybrid scaffolds, harnessing the superior mechanical properties of synthetic polymers while retaining the excellent biocompatibility of natural polymers to overcome the aforementioned limitations [23].

<u>*Collagen*</u>

Collagen is a protein that represents a primary structural constituent of the native ECM, and its usage in the fabrication of vascular scaffolds has seen a steady increase in recent years as a result of its strong biocompatibility and ability to facilitate cell adhesion coupled with its low antigenicity [4, 57]. However, collagen, as with other natural polymers, exhibits suboptimal mechanical properties and rapid biodegradation kinetics, which compromises graft performance, thus limiting their use in the production of TEVGs. This remains true regardless of the fabrication method utilised to create the collagen-based vascular graft, be it bioprinting, electrospinning, moulding, or freeze drying [58, 59].

The findings of a 2019 study conducted by Zhang *et al.* challenged this sentiment, however, Zhang's team fabricated a novel circular knitted collagen bilayer TEVG comprised of a circular knitted collagen filament outer layer and electrospun collagen inner layer produced from electrochemically aligned rat-derived collagen type I (ELAC). Burst pressure testing showed that the dry bilayer collagen graft withstood higher pressures prior to bursting compared to the ITA and SV but its burst pressure dropped massively when hydrated (2.11 ± 0.37 MPa vs 0.66 ± 0.09 MPa). Graft compliance was comparable to the SV but lower than the ITA. Human umbilical vein endothelial cell (HUVEC) adhesion and proliferation were also enhanced in the collagen graft when compared to the PLA control graft [60]. The same group of researchers fabricated a hybrid circular knitted vascular graft made from a combination of ELAC and PLA filaments plied into a hybrid multifilament yarn to incorporate the biological properties of collagen with the mechanical properties of PLA [61]. Biomechanical analyses of the resultant graft revealed a burst pressure of 1.89 ± 0.43 MPa with a suture retention strength of 10.86 ± 0.49 N, both of which are higher than the SV and ITA. Dynamic compliance was also superior in the hybrid graft as opposed to the coronary arteries. The hybrid graft also exhibited a 10-fold increase in HUVEC recruitment and a 3.2-fold higher cell proliferation compared to the PLA control graft at the end of 28 days [61].

Chitosan

Chitosan is a linear polysaccharide generated as a product of chitin deacetylation under highly basic conditions and is the second most frequently utilised natural polymer for the fabrication of TEVGs [5]. This is a consequence of chitosan's low toxicity and immunogenicity, strong mechanical strength alterable via pore size and orientation modifications, support for cellular colonisation and proliferation due to its interconnected porous structure, biodegradability with modifiable degradation rates, and natural antimicrobial properties [62]. In addition, chitosan has been reported in several studies to share structural similarities to glycosaminoglycans (GAGs), a major constituent of the native ECM. This is an important characteristic of vascular regeneration owing to its antithrombotic properties and its ability to control vascular SMC proliferation [63].

Fukunishi *et al.* utilised electrospun PCL and chitosan nanofibers for the fabrication of 1.0 and 5.0-mm hybrid vascular grafts. 1.0 mm TEVGs were implanted as infrarenal abdominal aortic interposition grafts in mice, while 5.0 mm TEVGs were implanted as carotid artery interposition grafts in sheep. Burst pressure of the hybrid graft pre-implantation was significantly lower than native carotid artery (0.39 ± 0.08 MPa vs. 1.46 ± 0.52 MPa), but no significant difference between the implanted graft and native carotid artery was detected after 6 months (1.37 ± 0.36 MPa vs. 1.46 ± 0.52 MPa). The inverse is true with regard to graft compliance, with no significant differences present when comparing the compliance of the pre-implanted graft to the native carotid artery ($14.04 \pm 1.50\%$ vs. $11.98 \pm 2.02\%$), while compliance of the TEVG 6 months post-implantation was significantly lower than the native carotid artery ($6.58\% \pm 1.76\%$ vs. $11.98 \pm 2.02\%$). The researchers found that after 6 months, all 1.0 mm grafts remained patent (n = 3) with an absence of aneurysms and calcification, but only 67% of 5.0 mm grafts remained patent (n = 6), concluding that cell migration and tissue remodeling was enhanced due to the rapid degradation kinetics of chitosan [64].

Fiqrianti and colleagues fabricated a hybrid scaffold TEVG through electrospinning a polymer mixture comprised of 10% PLLA, 1% collagen, and two different concentrations of chitosan, 0.5% and 0.6%, to evaluate its effects on the structural and biological properties of the TEVG. Samples used were as follows: A (100% PLLA; control sample), B (10% PLLA, 1% collagen, 0.5% chitosan), and C (10% PLLA, 1% collagen, 0.6% chitosan) [65]. Tensile strength testing showed that incorporating higher concentrations of chitosan resulted in higher graft UTS prior to failure, while burst pressure testing showed the opposite, with a downward trend seen in burst pressure with increasing concentrations of chitosan. Chitosan was shown to be non-toxic and capable of supporting cell growth, with the highest cell viability present in sample B. Overall, the hybrid scaffold TEVG made of 10% PLLA, 1% collagen, and 0.5% chitosan produced the best balance between biological performance and structural integrity.

Elastin

Elastin is a 67-kDa natural hydrophilic elastomeric protein that acts as the primary structural constituent of the extracellular matrix and is generally found in tissues frequently exposed to large elastic deformations such as the arteries; elastin encircles the arterial lumen to maintain the elasticity of arterial walls subjected to constant blood pressures [66]. In addition to contributing to the mechanical properties of arteries, the by-products of elastin degradation have been shown to impact critical cellular functions such as cell migration, adhesion, and proliferation, with previous studies showing the development of intimal hyperplasia as a consequence of excessive arterial SMC proliferation in elastin-deficient mice [67]. As such, the regulation of elastic fibre formation is crucial to regulate vascular wall thickness. In the context of vascular tissue engineering, elastin possesses several beneficial properties, namely its low thrombogenicity, resistance to degradation, ease of purification, and ability to positively affect vessel compliance 38, 100. Despite this, elastin remains highly insoluble and difficult to handle and suffers from poor UTS [59]. Hence, it is primarily utilised in the production of hybrid scaffolds, such as explained by Nyugen *et al.* who fabricated a bilayer scaffold incorporating soluble/insoluble elastin fibres within electrochemically aligned collagen fibres. Elastin incorporation was shown to reduce Young's modulus of the novel graft to a point comparable to native coronary arteries. α-SMA and calponin expression saw a substantial increase after 2 weeks of culturing rat aortic SMCs on the insoluble elastin graft, which suggests that a contractile phenotype has been adopted by the SMCs. These results highlight the potential of insoluble elastin in vascular tissue engineering [68].

Decellularised Scaffolds

The discrepancies between the biological and mechanical properties of existing synthetic and natural polymer tissue-engineered vascular grafts led to the development of decellularised natural matrices with comparable structures and mechanical strength to native vessels. Focused removal of cellular and nuclear contents from existing allogeneic or xenogeneic tissues with minimal disruption to its extracellular matrix constituents enables the retention of existing ECM structure and function whilst reducing the immunogenicity of the decellularised scaffold to prevent adverse immunological responses upon implantation [47] (Fig. **2**). Though inadequate cell removal risks immune activation, aggressive decellularisation adversely affects the structural integrity of the scaffold, consequently increasing the chances of graft failure [69]. Hence, the optimisation of the decellularisation protocol is essential to meet the delicate balance required for the benefits of decellularised scaffolds. Decellularisation agents typically consist of detergents and alcohols, which include examples such as sodium dodecyl sulphate (SDS), 3-[(3-cholamidopropyl)dimethylammonio--1-propanesulfonate (CHAPS), glycerol and isopropanol, and enzymes such as dispase and thermolysin in combination with mechanical abrasion for effective cell removal [47]. Several studies have shown the capabilities of decellularised vascular scaffolds in enabling EC and SMC migration, adhesion, and proliferation, making decellularisation a promising approach for the fabrication of TEVGs [70, 71].

Rosenberg *et al.* pioneered the first decellularised vascular graft with the enzymatic digestion of bovine carotid arteries in 1966, but advancements in vascular tissue engineering techniques since then have led to the decellularisation of a vast number of tissues, with some scaffolds derived from bovine origins made commercially available [2, 72]. Despite this, decellularised vascular scaffolds have not been implemented outside of clinical trials due to thrombotic risk along with possible aneurysmal dilatation and infection, which several studies have proven occur as a consequence of the absence of a viable endothelial layer on the lumen of decellularised scaffolds [73, 74]. Seeding decellularised scaffolds with cells, as illustrated by a study conducted by Lin *et al.,* and coating or treating these scaffolds with bioactive molecules such as heparin, vascular endothelial growth factor, and fibronectin are methods frequently used to improve the endothelialisation efficiency, and hence, biocompatibility, mechanical properties, and ultimately, the feasibility of decellularised scaffolds as fully functional TEVGs [74].

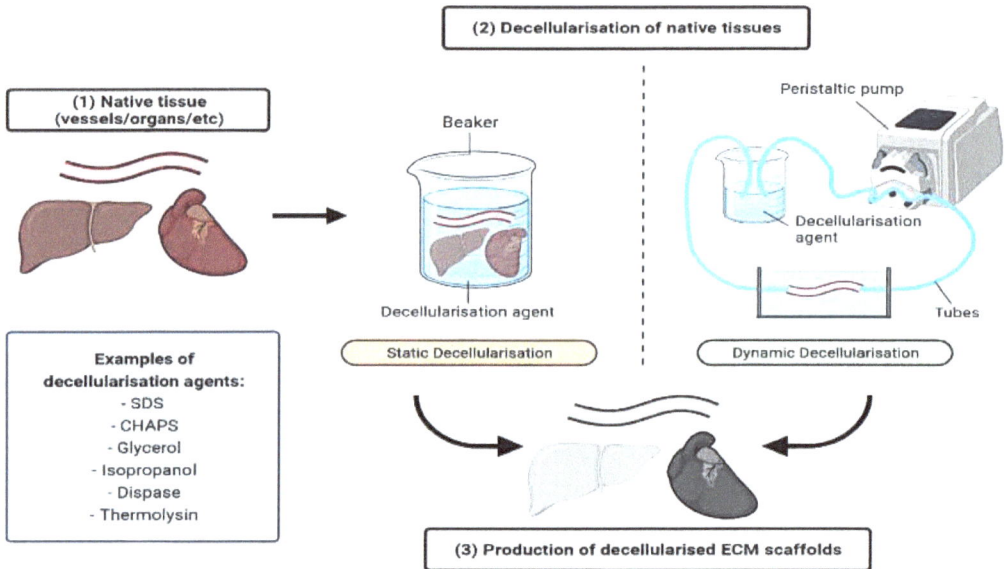

Fig. (2). (1) Existing native tissues (e.g., blood vessels, organs) can undergo static decellularisation, whereby decellularisation agents are added directly onto the native tissue, or dynamic decellularisation whereby decellularisation agents are circulated through the target tissue via a perfusion bioreactor as shown in (2). Some examples of chemical-based decellularisation agents include sodium dodecyl sulphate (SDS), 3-[(--cholamidopropyl)dimethylammonio]-1-propanesulfonate (CHAPS), glycerol, and isopropanol, while dispase and thermolysin represent enzyme-based decellularisation agents. Successful decellularisation of native tissues will result in the production of extracellular matrix-based scaffolds that can be used for the production of tissue-engineered vascular grafts [3].

Scaffold Cell Seeding Strategies

Intimal hyperplasia develops as a vascular response to endothelial injury due to interventional and surgical procedures that are done to treat advanced stages of atherosclerosis. Excessive and uncontrolled proliferation of smooth muscle cells (SMC) to remodel the injured vascular bed causes subsequent atherosclerosis at the area of intervention e.g., stented vessel and vascular graft [75].

Atherosclerosis due to plaque formation and intimal hyperplasia shares a common initial point which is endothelial dysfunction and subsequent pathologic events. In fabricating a functional TEVG, the body's response to materials needs to be anticipated.

Cell seeding techniques are being developed for the small diameter of vascular grafts. For *in vitro* cell seeding, various strategies, including dynamic, static, magnetic, and electrostatic cell seeding, are employed depending on the application.

Static Cell Seeding

Gravitational or static cell seeding is the most conventional and simplest technique used in TEVG seeding. Cells are seeded directly on the lumen of the vascular scaffold (Fig. **3**). However, this technique usually requires pre-coating with cell adhesion molecules, such as fibronectins, laminin, and ECM proteins. Fibronectin was used by Foxall and friends (1986) to coat small-caliber PTFE and PET/Dacron vascular grafts to enhance ECs attachment and migration on the implanted graft [76]. Similarly, ECM molecules such as fibrin, collagen, and gelatine-coated lumen of PTFE and PET/Dacron grafts also increase EC proliferation and migration in *vitro* models [77]. One of the drawbacks of static cell seeding is the inconsistency of seeding density, poor efficiency, longer culture maintenance (typically 2 weeks), and risk of contamination [78]. Moreover, coating the lumen with adhesion molecules attracts free platelets in the blood. Therefore, it is necessary to protect the graft with anti-thrombotic drugs after the establishment of cells in the lumen.

Dynamic Cell Seeding

Dynamic cell seeding employs shear stress, vacuum pressure, and centrifugal force to increase the seeding efficiency Fig. (**3**). Pores in the graft plays an essential key role in efficient cell seeding. Nevertheless, synthetic grafts such as PTFE and PET/Dacron required pre-coating to cover the pores in the graft. This pre-coating is a challenging method since pre-coated surfaces tend to be rough and could trigger platelet adhesion and activation, which eventually results in intimal hyperplasia. Therefore, patients are required to be on anti-coagulants and anti-thrombotic drugs before implantation procedures [79].

A recent study by Daum *et al.* (2020) has shown that the coated electrospun synthetic vascular grafts with fibronectin successfully attracted endothelial progenitor cells and increased the endothelialisation process in dynamic *in vitro* culture [80]. With the emergence of bioreactor designs, various kinds of physiological conditions can be mimicked, and the desired condition can be controlled. For instance, the dynamic physiological pulse can be recreated using perfusion bioreactors to promote endothelialisation of vascular grafts. A novel two-phase shear conditioning technique with a computer-controlled perfusion circuit was developed, where axial rotation is used to seed the ECs monolayer into the luminal surface of decellularized umbilical cord [70].

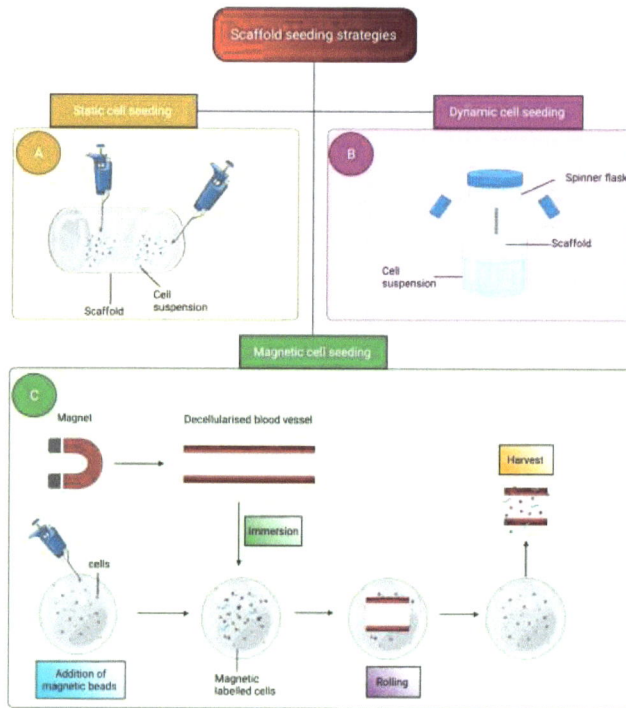

Fig. (3). (A) Static cell seeding: Cells are seeded directly on the lumen of the vascular scaffold; (B) Dynamic cell seeding: Scaffold fixed to a needle placed in a spinner flask with cell suspension. The rotation of the medium will attract cells into the scaffold; (C) Magnetic seeding: Scaffold immersed and rolled into magnetic labeled cells suspension to evenly distribute cells.

Magnetic and Electrostatic Cell Seeding

Magnetic cell seeding is a novel strategy employed to achieve more efficient cell seeding via the use of magnetic beads for cell labeling and regulating cellular distribution. It has great potential to produce rapid and reproducible results, which are essential for clinical translation [81]. Fayol and colleagues have successfully designed a tubular scaffold with magnetically labeled cells, where the endothelialisation process is monitored via magnetic resonance imaging (MRI) scanner before transplantation procedures [82]. Furthermore, carboxy dextran-coated superparamagnetic nanoparticles (Resovist®) were also used to label human umbilical vein endothelial cells (HUVECs) in TEVG fabrication [82].

Cell attachment and migration are very dependent on the material used for grafting. For instance, the surface of platelets and ECs are negatively charged, similar to synthetic grafts like ePTFE [18]. Thus, the different approaches in cell seeding must overcome the repulsive force that is present between the material and cell interface. Electrostatic cell seeding regulates the electrical charge of the graft for a short duration to promote cell attachment. For example, if a graft is dielectric when it is attached to a capacitor, the oppositely charged nuclei are attracted toward the surface graft. Hence, these temporary positive charges can enhance ECs proliferation [83].

CONCLUSION

The biomaterial utilised for the production of vascular scaffolds remains a crucial consideration as it can dictate both the structural and mechanical properties of the resulting scaffold. However, scaffold composition alone is not sufficient for the production of a fully functional tissue-engineered vascular graft, as evidenced by some studies showing the development of intimal hyperplasia, thrombosis, and premature graft failure. Seeding of endothelial or endothelial progenitor cells using some of the cell seeding methods discussed in this chapter has proven to be effective in reducing the occurrence of the aforementioned limitations. As such, the combination of incorporating an appropriate scaffolding material and an appropriate cell seeding method is essential for the successful production of fully functional tissue-engineered vascular grafts.

CONFLICT OF INTEREST

The authors declare that the research was conducted in the absence of any commercial or financial relationships that could be construed as a potential conflict of interest.

ACKNOWLEDGEMENTS

All authors would like to thank the Faculty of Medicine, UKM, for the resources used to complete this book chapter.

REFERENCES

[1]   Langer R, Vacanti JP. Tissue Engineering. Science 1993; 260(5110): 920-6.
        [http://dx.doi.org/10.1126/science.8493529] [PMID: 8493529]

[2]   Pashneh-Tala S, MacNeil S, Claeyssens F. The Tissue-Engineered Vascular Graft—Past, Present, and Future. Tissue Eng Part B Rev 2016; 22(1): 68-100.
        [http://dx.doi.org/10.1089/ten.teb.2015.0100] [PMID: 26447530]

[3]   Gao J, Jiang L, Liang Q, *et al.* The grafts modified by heparinization and catalytic nitric oxide generation used for vascular implantation in rats. Regen Biomater 2018; 5(2): 105-14.
        [http://dx.doi.org/10.1093/rb/rby003] [PMID: 29644092]

[4]   Jia W, Li M, Weng H, Gu G, Chen Z. Design and comprehensive assessment of a biomimetic tri-layer tubular scaffold via biodegradable polymers for vascular tissue engineering applications. Mater Sci Eng C 2020; 110: 110717.
[http://dx.doi.org/10.1016/j.msec.2020.110717] [PMID: 32204029]

[5]   Leal BBJ, Wakabayashi N, Oyama K, Kamiya H, Braghirolli DI, Pranke P. Vascular Tissue Engineering: Polymers and Methodologies for Small Caliber Vascular Grafts. Front Cardiovasc Med 2021; 7: 592361.
[http://dx.doi.org/10.3389/fcvm.2020.592361] [PMID: 33585576]

[6]   Sarkar S, Salacinski HJ, Hamilton G, Seifalian AM. The mechanical properties of infrainguinal vascular bypass grafts: their role in influencing patency. Eur J Vasc Endovasc Surg 2006; 31(6): 627-36.
[http://dx.doi.org/10.1016/j.ejvs.2006.01.006] [PMID: 16513376]

[7]   Haruguchi H, Teraoka S. Intimal hyperplasia and hemodynamic factors in arterial bypass and arteriovenous grafts: a review. J Artif Organs 2003; 6(4): 227-35.
[http://dx.doi.org/10.1007/s10047-003-0232-x] [PMID: 14691664]

[8]   Braghirolli DI, Helfer VE, Chagastelles PC, Dalberto TP, Gamba D, Pranke P. Electrospun scaffolds functionalized with heparin and vascular endothelial growth factor increase the proliferation of endothelial progenitor cells. Biomed Mater 2017; 12(2): 025003.
[http://dx.doi.org/10.1088/1748-605X/aa5bbc] [PMID: 28140340]

[9]   Ballyk PD, Walsh C, Butany J, Ojha M. Compliance mismatch may promote graft–artery intimal hyperplasia by altering suture-line stresses. J Biomech 1997; 31(3): 229-37.
[http://dx.doi.org/10.1016/S0197-3975(97)00111-5] [PMID: 9645537]

[10]   G N, Tan A, Gundogan B, *et al.* Tissue engineering vascular grafts a fortiori: looking back and going forward. Expert Opin Biol Ther 2015; 15(2): 231-44.
[http://dx.doi.org/10.1517/14712598.2015.980234] [PMID: 25427995]

[11]   Weinberg CB, Bell E. A blood vessel model constructed from collagen and cultured vascular cells. Science 1986; 231(4736): 397-400.
[http://dx.doi.org/10.1126/science.2934816] [PMID: 2934816]

[12]   Ercolani E, Del Gaudio C, Bianco A. Vascular tissue engineering of small-diameter blood vessels: reviewing the electrospinning approach. J Tissue Eng Regen Med 2015; 9(8): 861-88.
[http://dx.doi.org/10.1002/term.1697] [PMID: 23365048]

[13]   van der Slegt J, Steunenberg SL, Donker JMW, *et al.* The current position of precuffed expanded polytetrafluoroethylene bypass grafts in peripheral vascular surgery. J Vasc Surg 2014; 60(1): 120-8.
[http://dx.doi.org/10.1016/j.jvs.2014.01.062] [PMID: 24629990]

[14]   Chlupáč J, Filová E, Bačáková L. Blood vessel replacement: 50 years of development and tissue engineering paradigms in vascular surgery. Physiol Res 2009; 58 (Suppl. 2): S119-40.
[http://dx.doi.org/10.33549/physiolres.931918] [PMID: 20131930]

[15]   Drews JD, Miyachi H, Shinoka T. Tissue-engineered vascular grafts for congenital cardiac disease: Clinical experience and current status. Trends Cardiovasc Med 2017; 27(8): 521-31.
[http://dx.doi.org/10.1016/j.tcm.2017.06.013] [PMID: 28754230]

[16]   Hadinata IE, Hayward PAR, Hare DL, *et al.* Choice of conduit for the right coronary system: 8-year analysis of Radial Artery Patency and Clinical Outcomes trial. Ann Thorac Surg 2009; 88(5): 1404-9.
[http://dx.doi.org/10.1016/j.athoracsur.2009.06.010] [PMID: 19853082]

[17]   Shah PJ, Bui K, Blackmore S, *et al.* Has the in situ right internal thoracic artery been overlooked? An angiographic study of the radial artery, internal thoracic arteries and saphenous vein graft patencies in symptomatic patients. Eur J Cardiothorac Surg 2005; 27(5): 870-5.
[http://dx.doi.org/10.1016/j.ejcts.2005.01.027] [PMID: 15848328]

[18]   Sarkar S, Sales KM, Hamilton G, Seifalian AM. Addressing thrombogenicity in vascular graft

construction. J Biomed Mater Res B Appl Biomater 2007; 82B(1): 100-8.
[http://dx.doi.org/10.1002/jbm.b.30710] [PMID: 17078085]

[19]   Deutsch M, Meinhart J, Zilla P, *et al.* Long-term experience in autologous in vitro endothelialization of infrainguinal ePTFE grafts. J Vasc Surg 2009; 49(2): 352-62.
[http://dx.doi.org/10.1016/j.jvs.2008.08.101] [PMID: 19110397]

[20]   Hehrlein FW, Schlepper M, Loskot F, Scheld HH, Walter P, Mulch J. The use of expanded polytetrafluoroethylene (PTFE) grafts for myocardial revascularization. J Cardiovasc Surg (Torino) 1984; 25(6): 549-53.
[PMID: 6334688]

[21]   Vacanti JP. Beyond Transplantation. Arch Surg 1988; 123(5): 545-9.
[http://dx.doi.org/10.1001/archsurg.1988.01400290027003] [PMID: 3282491]

[22]   Seifu DG, Purnama A, Mequanint K, Mantovani D. Small-diameter vascular tissue engineering. Nat Rev Cardiol 2013; 10(7): 410-21.
[http://dx.doi.org/10.1038/nrcardio.2013.77] [PMID: 23689702]

[23]   Carrabba M, Madeddu P. Current Strategies for the Manufacture of Small Size Tissue Engineering Vascular Grafts. Front Bioeng Biotechnol 2018; 6: 41.
[http://dx.doi.org/10.3389/fbioe.2018.00041] [PMID: 29721495]

[24]   Matsuzaki Y, John K, Shoji T, Shinoka T. The Evolution of Tissue Engineered Vascular Graft Technologies: From Preclinical Trials to Advancing Patient Care. Appl Sci (Basel) 2019; 9(7): 1274.
[http://dx.doi.org/10.3390/app9071274] [PMID: 31890320]

[25]   Maurmann N, Sperling LE, Pranke P. Electrospun and Electrosprayed Scaffolds for Tissue Engineering. Adv Exp Med Biol 2018; 1078: 79-100.
[http://dx.doi.org/10.1007/978-981-13-0950-2_5] [PMID: 30357619]

[26]   Brennan MP, Dardik A, Hibino N, *et al.* Tissue-engineered vascular grafts demonstrate evidence of growth and development when implanted in a juvenile animal model. Ann Surg 2008; 248(3): 370-7.
[http://dx.doi.org/10.1097/SLA.0b013e318184dcbd] [PMID: 18791357]

[27]   Cummings I, George S, Kelm J, *et al.* Tissue-engineered vascular graft remodeling in a growing lamb model: expression of matrix metalloproteinases. Eur J Cardiothorac Surg 2011.
[http://dx.doi.org/10.1016/j.ejcts.2011.02.077] [PMID: 21530291]

[28]   Xue L, Greisler HP. Biomaterials in the development and future of vascular grafts. J Vasc Surg 2003; 37(2): 472-80.
[http://dx.doi.org/10.1067/mva.2003.88] [PMID: 12563226]

[29]   Tara S, Rocco KA, Hibino N, *et al.* Vessel Bioengineering. Circ J 2014; 78(1): 12-9.
[http://dx.doi.org/10.1253/circj.CJ-13-1440] [PMID: 24334558]

[30]   Higgins SP, Solan AK, Niklason LE. Effects of polyglycolic acid on porcine smooth muscle cell growth and differentiation. J Biomed Mater Res 2003; 67A(1): 295-302.
[http://dx.doi.org/10.1002/jbm.a.10599] [PMID: 14517889]

[31]   O'Brien FJ. Biomaterials & scaffolds for tissue engineering. Mater Today 2011; 14(3): 88-95.
[http://dx.doi.org/10.1016/S1369-7021(11)70058-X]

[32]   Hajiali H, Shahgasempour S, Naimi-Jamal MR, Peirovi H. Electrospun PGA/gelatin nanofibrous scaffolds and their potential application in vascular tissue engineering. Int J Nanomedicine 2011; 6: 2133-41.
[http://dx.doi.org/10.2147/IJN.S24312] [PMID: 22114477]

[33]   Niklason LE, Langer RS. Advances in tissue engineering of blood vessels and other tissues. Transpl Immunol 1997; 5(4): 303-6.
[http://dx.doi.org/10.1016/S0966-3274(97)80013-5] [PMID: 9504152]

[34]   Niklason LE, Gao J, Abbott WM, *et al.* Functional arteries grown in vitro. Science 1999; 284(5413):

489-93.
[http://dx.doi.org/10.1126/science.284.5413.489] [PMID: 10205057]

[35]   Dahl SLM, Kypson AP, Lawson JH, *et al.* Readily available tissue-engineered vascular grafts. Sci Transl Med 2011; 3(68): 68ra9.
[http://dx.doi.org/10.1126/scitranslmed.3001426] [PMID: 21289273]

[36]   Melchiorri AJ, Hibino N, Brandes ZR, Jonas RA, Fisher JP. Development and assessment of a biodegradable solvent cast polyester fabric small-diameter vascular graft. J Biomed Mater Res A 2014; 102(6): 1972-81.
[http://dx.doi.org/10.1002/jbm.a.34872] [PMID: 23852776]

[37]   Falco EE, Coates EE, Li E, Roth JS, Fisher JP. Fabrication and characterization of porous EH scaffolds and EH-PEG bilayers. J Biomed Mater Res A 2011; 97A(3): 264-71.
[http://dx.doi.org/10.1002/jbm.a.33052] [PMID: 21442727]

[38]   Fukunishi T, Best CA, Sugiura T, *et al.* Preclinical study of patient-specific cell-free nanofiber tissue-engineered vascular grafts using 3-dimensional printing in a sheep model. J Thorac Cardiovasc Surg 2017; 153(4): 924-32.
[http://dx.doi.org/10.1016/j.jtcvs.2016.10.066] [PMID: 27938900]

[39]   Lin C, Liu C, Zhang L, *et al.* Interaction of iPSC-derived neural stem cells on poly(L-lactic acid) nanofibrous scaffolds for possible use in neural tissue engineering. Int J Mol Med 2017.
[http://dx.doi.org/10.3892/ijmm.2017.3299] [PMID: 29207038]

[40]   Vilay V, Mariatti M, Ahmad Z, Pasomsouk K, Todo M. Characterization of the mechanical and thermal properties and morphological behavior of biodegradable poly(L-lactide)/poly(ε-caprolactone) and poly(L-lactide)/poly(butylene succinate- *co* -L-lactate) polymeric blends. J Appl Polym Sci 2009; 114(3): 1784-92.
[http://dx.doi.org/10.1002/app.30683]

[41]   Hashi CK, Zhu Y, Yang GY, *et al.* Antithrombogenic property of bone marrow mesenchymal stem cells in nanofibrous vascular grafts. Proc Natl Acad Sci USA 2007; 104(29): 11915-20.
[http://dx.doi.org/10.1073/pnas.0704581104] [PMID: 17615237]

[42]   Caracciolo PC, Rial-Hermida MI, Montini-Ballarin F, Abraham GA, Concheiro A, Alvarez-Lorenzo C. Surface-modified bioresorbable electrospun scaffolds for improving hemocompatibility of vascular grafts. Mater Sci Eng C 2017; 75: 1115-27.
[http://dx.doi.org/10.1016/j.msec.2017.02.151] [PMID: 28415397]

[43]   Bertram U, Steiner D, Poppitz B, *et al.* Vascular Tissue Engineering: Effects of Integrating Collagen into a PCL Based Nanofiber Material. BioMed Res Int 2017; 2017: 1-11.
[http://dx.doi.org/10.1155/2017/9616939] [PMID: 28932749]

[44]   Sugiura T, Matsumura G, Miyamoto S, Miyachi H, Breuer CK, Shinoka T. Tissue-engineered Vascular Grafts in Children With Congenital Heart Disease: Intermediate Term Follow-up. Semin Thorac Cardiovasc Surg 2018; 30(2): 175-9.
[http://dx.doi.org/10.1053/j.semtcvs.2018.02.002] [PMID: 29427773]

[45]   Asvar Z, Mirzaei E, Azarpira N, Geramizadeh B, Fadaie M. Evaluation of electrospinning parameters on the tensile strength and suture retention strength of polycaprolactone nanofibrous scaffolds through surface response methodology. J Mech Behav Biomed Mater 2017; 75: 369-78.
[http://dx.doi.org/10.1016/j.jmbbm.2017.08.004] [PMID: 28802205]

[46]   Chan A, Tan R, Michael P, *et al.* A Novel Mouse Carotid Grafting Model for Evaluation of Synthetic Vascular Grafts. Heart Lung Circ 2017; 26: S309.
[http://dx.doi.org/10.1016/j.hlc.2017.06.616]

[47]   Crapo PM, Gilbert TW, Badylak SF. An overview of tissue and whole organ decellularization processes. Biomaterials 2011; 32(12): 3233-43.
[http://dx.doi.org/10.1016/j.biomaterials.2011.01.057] [PMID: 21296410]

[48]   Woodard LN, Grunlan MA. Hydrolytic Degradation and Erosion of Polyester Biomaterials. ACS Macro Lett 2018; 7(8): 976-82.
[http://dx.doi.org/10.1021/acsmacrolett.8b00424] [PMID: 30705783]

[49]   Nagiah N, Johnson R, Anderson R, Elliott W, Tan W. Highly Compliant Vascular Grafts with Gelatin-Sheathed Coaxially Structured Nanofibers. Langmuir 2015; 31(47): 12993-3002.
[http://dx.doi.org/10.1021/acs.langmuir.5b03177] [PMID: 26529143]

[50]   Laurent CP, Vaquette C, Liu X, Schmitt JF, Rahouadj R. Suitability of a PLCL fibrous scaffold for soft tissue engineering applications: A combined biological and mechanical characterisation. J Biomater Appl 2018; 32(9): 1276-88.
[http://dx.doi.org/10.1177/0885328218757064] [PMID: 29409376]

[51]   Park S, Kim J, Lee MK, *et al.* Fabrication of strong, bioactive vascular grafts with PCL/collagen and PCL/silica bilayers for small-diameter vascular applications. Mater Des 2019; 181: 108079.
[http://dx.doi.org/10.1016/j.matdes.2019.108079]

[52]   He Y, Liu W, Guan L, *et al.* A 3D-Printed PLCL Scaffold Coated with Collagen Type I and Its Biocompatibility. BioMed Res Int 2018; 2018: 1-10.
[http://dx.doi.org/10.1155/2018/5147156] [PMID: 29850530]

[53]   Wu W, Allen RA, Wang Y. Fast-degrading elastomer enables rapid remodeling of a cell-free synthetic graft into a neoartery. Nat Med 2012; 18(7): 1148-53.
[http://dx.doi.org/10.1038/nm.2821] [PMID: 22729285]

[54]   Motlagh D, Yang J, Lui KY, Webb AR, Ameer GA. Hemocompatibility evaluation of poly(glycerol-sebacate) in vitro for vascular tissue engineering. Biomaterials 2006; 27(24): 4315-24.
[http://dx.doi.org/10.1016/j.biomaterials.2006.04.010] [PMID: 16675010]

[55]   Chen QZ, Bismarck A, Hansen U, *et al.* Characterisation of a soft elastomer poly(glycerol sebacate) designed to match the mechanical properties of myocardial tissue. Biomaterials 2008; 29(1): 47-57.
[http://dx.doi.org/10.1016/j.biomaterials.2007.09.010] [PMID: 17915309]

[56]   Khosravi R, Best CA, Allen RA, *et al.* Long-Term Functional Efficacy of a Novel Electrospun Poly(Glycerol Sebacate)-Based Arterial Graft in Mice. Ann Biomed Eng 2016; 44(8): 2402-16.
[http://dx.doi.org/10.1007/s10439-015-1545-7] [PMID: 26795977]

[57]   Duan N, Geng X, Ye L, *et al.* A vascular tissue engineering scaffold with core–shell structured nano-fibers formed by coaxial electrospinning and its biocompatibility evaluation. Biomed Mater 2016; 11(3): 035007.
[http://dx.doi.org/10.1088/1748-6041/11/3/035007] [PMID: 27206161]

[58]   Koens MJW, Faraj KA, Wismans RG, *et al.* Controlled fabrication of triple layered and molecularly defined collagen/elastin vascular grafts resembling the native blood vessel. Acta Biomater 2010; 6(12): 4666-74.
[http://dx.doi.org/10.1016/j.actbio.2010.06.038] [PMID: 20619367]

[59]   Kumar VA, Caves JM, Haller CA, *et al.* Acellular vascular grafts generated from collagen and elastin analogs. Acta Biomater 2013; 9(9): 8067-74.
[http://dx.doi.org/10.1016/j.actbio.2013.05.024] [PMID: 23743129]

[60]   Zhang F, Xie Y, Celik H, Akkus O, Bernacki SH, King MW. Engineering small-caliber vascular grafts from collagen filaments and nanofibers with comparable mechanical properties to native vessels. Biofabrication 2019; 11(3): 035020.
[http://dx.doi.org/10.1088/1758-5090/ab15ce] [PMID: 30943452]

[61]   Zhang F, Bambharoliya T, Xie Y, *et al.* A hybrid vascular graft harnessing the superior mechanical properties of synthetic fibers and the biological performance of collagen filaments. Mater Sci Eng C 2021; 118: 111418.
[http://dx.doi.org/10.1016/j.msec.2020.111418] [PMID: 33255019]

[62]   Kim IY, Seo SJ, Moon HS, *et al.* Chitosan and its derivatives for tissue engineering applications.

Biotechnol Adv 2008; 26(1): 1-21.
[http://dx.doi.org/10.1016/j.biotechadv.2007.07.009] [PMID: 17884325]

[63] Ranganathan S, Balagangadharan K, Selvamurugan N. Chitosan and gelatin-based electrospun fibers for bone tissue engineering. Int J Biol Macromol 2019; 133: 354-64.
[http://dx.doi.org/10.1016/j.ijbiomac.2019.04.115] [PMID: 31002907]

[64] Fukunishi T, Best CA, Sugiura T, *et al.* Tissue-Engineered Small Diameter Arterial Vascular Grafts from Cell-Free Nanofiber PCL/Chitosan Scaffolds in a Sheep Model. PLoS One 2016; 11(7): e0158555.
[http://dx.doi.org/10.1371/journal.pone.0158555] [PMID: 27467821]

[65] Fiqrianti I, Widiyanti P, Manaf M, Savira C, Cahyani N, Bella F. Poly-L-lactic Acid (PLLA)-Chitosan-Collagen Electrospun Tube for Vascular Graft Application. J Funct Biomater 2018; 9(2): 32.
[http://dx.doi.org/10.3390/jfb9020032] [PMID: 29710843]

[66] Gonzalez de Torre I, Alonso M, Rodriguez-Cabello JC. Elastin-Based Materials: Promising Candidates for Cardiac Tissue Regeneration. Front Bioeng Biotechnol 2020; 8: 657.
[http://dx.doi.org/10.3389/fbioe.2020.00657] [PMID: 32695756]

[67] Rodgers UR, Weiss AS. Cellular interactions with elastin. Pathol Biol (Paris) 2005; 53(7): 390-8.
[http://dx.doi.org/10.1016/j.patbio.2004.12.022] [PMID: 16085115]

[68] Nguyen TU, Bashur CA, Kishore V. Impact of elastin incorporation into electrochemically aligned collagen fibers on mechanical properties and smooth muscle cell phenotype. Biomed Mater 2016; 11(2): 025008.
[http://dx.doi.org/10.1088/1748-6041/11/2/025008] [PMID: 26987364]

[69] Keane TJ, Londono R, Turner NJ, Badylak SF. Consequences of ineffective decellularization of biologic scaffolds on the host response. Biomaterials 2012; 33(6): 1771-81.
[http://dx.doi.org/10.1016/j.biomaterials.2011.10.054] [PMID: 22137126]

[70] Uzarski JS, Cores J, McFetridge PS. Physiologically Modeled Pulse Dynamics to Improve Function in *In Vitro* -Endothelialized Small-Diameter Vascular Grafts. Tissue Eng Part C Methods 2015; 21(11): 1125-34.
[http://dx.doi.org/10.1089/ten.tec.2015.0110] [PMID: 25996580]

[71] Rosario-Quinones F, Magid MS, Yau J, Pawale A, Nguyen K. Tissue reaction to porcine intestinal Submucosa (CorMatrix) implants in pediatric cardiac patients: a single-center experience. Ann Thorac Surg 2015; 99(4): 1373-7.
[http://dx.doi.org/10.1016/j.athoracsur.2014.11.064] [PMID: 25707584]

[72] Rosenbehc N, Mahtinez A, Sawyer PN, Wesolowski SA, Postlethwait RW, Dillon ML Jr. Tanned collagen arterial prosthesis of bovine carotid origin in man. Preliminary studies of enzyme-treated heterografts. Ann Surg 1966; 164(2): 247-56.
[http://dx.doi.org/10.1097/00000658-196608000-00010] [PMID: 5950359]

[73] Niklason L. Bioengineered Human Acellular Vessels as Dialysis Access Grafts. FASEB J 2020; 34(S1): 1-1.
[http://dx.doi.org/10.1096/fasebj.2020.34.s1.00352]

[74] Lin CH, Hsia K, Tsai CH, Ma H, Lu JH, Tsay RY. Decellularized porcine coronary artery with adipose stem cells for vascular tissue engineering. Biomed Mater 2019; 14(4): 045014.
[http://dx.doi.org/10.1088/1748-605X/ab2329] [PMID: 31108479]

[75] Porter KE, Varty K, Jones L, Bell PRF, London NJM. Human saphenous vein organ culture: A useful model of intimal hyperplasia? Eur J Vasc Endovasc Surg 1996; 11(1): 48-58.
[http://dx.doi.org/10.1016/S1078-5884(96)80134-1] [PMID: 8564487]

[76] Foxall TL, Auger KR, Callow AD, Libby P. Adult human endothelial cell coverage of small-caliber dacron and polytetrafluoroethylene vascular prostheses in vitro. J Surg Res 1986; 41(2): 158-72.
[http://dx.doi.org/10.1016/0022-4804(86)90021-1] [PMID: 2945052]

[77]   Anderson JS, Price TM, Hanson SR, Harker LA. In vitro endothelialization of small-caliber vascular grafts. Surgery 1987; 101(5): 577-86.
[PMID: 2953082]

[78]   Roh JD, Nelson GN, Udelsman BV, *et al.* Centrifugal seeding increases seeding efficiency and cellular distribution of bone marrow stromal cells in porous biodegradable scaffolds. Tissue Eng 2007; 13(11): 2743-9.
[http://dx.doi.org/10.1089/ten.2007.0171] [PMID: 17880269]

[79]   Yates SG, BARROS D'SA AAB, Berger K, *et al.* The preclotting of porous arterial prostheses. Ann Surg 1978; 188(5): 611-22.
[http://dx.doi.org/10.1097/00000658-197811000-00005] [PMID: 152614]

[80]   Daum R, Visser D, Wild C, *et al.* Fibronectin Adsorption on Electrospun Synthetic Vascular Grafts Attracts Endothelial Progenitor Cells and Promotes Endothelialization in Dynamic In Vitro Culture. Cells 2020; 9(3): 778.
[http://dx.doi.org/10.3390/cells9030778] [PMID: 32210018]

[81]   Villalona GA, Udelsman B, Duncan DR, *et al.* Cell-seeding techniques in vascular tissue engineering. Tissue Eng Part B Rev 2010; 16(3): 341-50.
[http://dx.doi.org/10.1089/ten.teb.2009.0527] [PMID: 20085439]

[82]   Fayol D, Le Visage C, Ino J, Gazeau F, Letourneur D, Wilhelm C. Design of biomimetic vascular grafts with magnetic endothelial patterning. Cell Transplant 2013; 22(11): 2105-18.
[http://dx.doi.org/10.3727/096368912X661300] [PMID: 23295155]

[83]   Bowlin GL, Rittgers SE. Electrostatic endothelial cell transplantation within small-diameter (<6 mm) vascular prostheses: a prototype apparatus and procedure. Cell Transplant 1997; 6(6): 631-7.
[http://dx.doi.org/10.1177/096368979700600614] [PMID: 9440873]

CHAPTER 8

Recent Bio-Based Material Strategies to Regenerate Periodontal Tissue in Clinical Setting

Osa Amila Hafiyyah[1], Anton Kusumo Widagdo[2], Ahmad Syaify[1] and Retno Ardhani[3,4,*]

[1] *Department of Periodontology, Faculty of Dentistry, Universitas Gadjah Mada, Yogyakarta, Indonesia*

[2] *Indramayu Bhayangkara Hospital, Indonesian National Police, 45285, Indonesia*

[3] *Department of Dental Biomedical Sciences, Faculty of Dentistry, Universitas Gadjah Yogyakarta, Indonesia*

[4] *Centre for Tissue Engineering and Regenerative Medicine, Faculty of Medicine, Universiti Kebangsaan Malaysia, 56000, Cheras, Kuala Lumpur, Malaysia*

Abstract: Periodontitis draws much attention because of its escalating burden on the healthcare economy in both developed and developing countries. For decades, periodontitis has been acknowledged as the most common oral disease worldwide and mostly found in the productive age. The inflammation in periodontal tissue destructs periodontal complex structures: periodontal ligament, cementum, and alveolar bone. Hence, its therapy is directed to interrupt disease progression and restore damaged tissue. The regenerative approach has been recognized by the periodontal association, and it has been integrated in their clinical practice guidelines for treating periodontitis. Various regenerative therapies have been introduced to dental clinics, which provide a wide range of treatment services. The regenerative approach is selected based on the consideration involving the interest of patients and clinicians. However, in its development, regulatory, public, and manufacturer concerns must also be taken into account. This paper exclusively discusses bio-functional materials used in dental clinics to regenerate periodontal defects. The brief evaluation describes recent periodontal regenerative materials available in clinics and clinician's expectations of future therapies.

Keywords: Guided-tissue regeneration, Membrane barrier, Periodontitis, Periodontal regeneration.

---

* **Corresponding author Retno Ardhani:** Department of Dental Biomedical Sciences, Faculty of Dentistry, Universitas Gadjah Yogyakarta, Indonesia; E-mail: retnoardhani@mail.ugm.ac.id

Mohd Fauzi Mh Busra, Daniel Law Jia Xian, Yogeswaran Lokanathan and Ruszymah Haji Idrus (Eds.)

CHANCES AND CHALLENGES IN PERIODONTITIS THERAPY

There has been a global concern about the aging population worldwide [1], especially when it comes to the challenge of maintaining good health of the elderly population, including their oral health status. The Oral Health-Related Quality of Life (OHRQOL) is reflected by people's ability to comfortably eat, sleep, communicate, and socialize [2]. A study showed that poor OHRQOL is closely related to the impairment of nutritional status [3]. Thus, complete dentition and disease-free oral tissue are expected to be maintained for a lifetime.

Normal human teeth are supported by the periodontium, which is a complex of the gingiva, periodontal ligament, cementum, and alveolar bone. The last three mentioned form a tooth-anchoring structure called the attachment apparatus [4]. Pathogenic destruction of the attachment apparatus, especially the periodontal ligament, and alveolar bone, is the hallmark of periodontitis [5,6]. Clinically, periodontitis is diagnosed by the identification of attachment loss and the radiographic indication of bone defect with or without tooth mobility [6].

Periodontitis is not classified as a lethal disease but a debilitating one. It causes discomfort and eating problems because of tooth migration, mobility, or even loss, bad oral odor, and an increase in susceptibility to systemic disease [6, 7]. Epidemiologic evidence indicates periodontitis is associated with other systemic inflammation-related conditions, such as cardio-metabolic, neurodegenerative, and autoimmune diseases, also cancer [8]. A multicenter case-control study was performed on 568 COVID-19 patients in Qatar. A study denoted the possibility of a correlation between periodontitis and more severe symptoms of COVID-19 [9].

Global Burden Diseases 2017 study estimated that the number of prevalent cases of periodontitis amounted to 796 million worldwide [10]. Further analysis denotes the prevalence of periodontitis among adolescents, adults, and the older population, with a high prevalence among the elderly [11]. Demographic trends, alteration of risk factors, and prolonged tooth retention are estimated to increase the socio-economic burden of periodontitis. Thus, the public, policymakers, educators, and professional organizations are encouraged to contribute to the prevention, detection, and care of periodontitis [7]. Such contribution involves the participation of experts in regenerative medicine to develop an effective and efficient therapy for periodontitis treatments.

Periodontitis therapies aim to terminate disease progression and achieve a healthy state of tissue stability and thus avoiding tooth loss. In periodontitis, destructive inflammation progresses as a response not only to microorganism infection but also to the host's own immune response to the periodontium. In order to control the progress of the disease, careful cleaning of contaminated root surfaces from microorganisms and their product is mandatory [12, 13]. Both systemic and local antimicrobial agents are available as adjunctive therapy for mechanical debridement [4]. At the same time, efforts to regenerate the periodontium to prevent early loss of the teeth are highly recommended. The ultimate goal of periodontal regenerative therapy is to restore the gingiva, periodontal ligament, cementum, and alveolar bone. However, it should be considered that clinicians constantly encounter challenges in daily practices that may exceed the subject criteria in controlled clinical studies. Consequently, treatment outcomes of periodontal regenerative surgery are unpredictable [13].

One of the contributions of biomedical engineers is the development of biomaterials to improve the results of periodontitis therapies. Biomaterials are designed to play a part in eliminating infection, controlling inflammation, and regenerating periodontal tissue [14]. Readily marketed biomaterials are available for use in clinical settings. However, new approaches are explored to provide the procedure with the most predictable result. Simultaneously, the biomaterials must satisfy the concerns of regulators, public, patients, clinicians, and manufacturers. The regulator mandates the safety and efficacy of proposed periodontitis therapy modalities, while patients consider its cost-effectiveness and medical risks. From the clinician's side, the biomaterial must be easy to sterilize, manipulate, and store. Clinicians prefer a simple method of applying biomaterials with minimal adjustment to reduce surgery durations. Sustainability, reproducibility, and ease of storage, transportation, and distribution are important for manufacturers. Public acceptance is also a crucial aspect to consider. For example, in the case of Indonesia, porcine-containing products are avoided, and halal certification is substantial. Fig. (1) summarizes the collective concerns in the development of biomaterials for regenerative periodontal therapy.

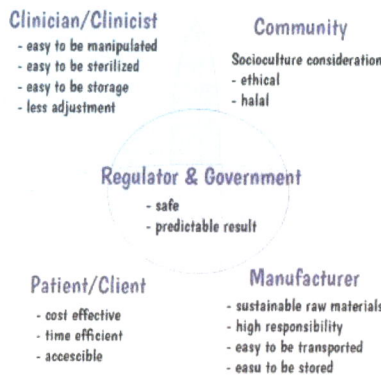

Fig. (1). Considerations in developing periodontal regenerative materials.

MEMBRANES IN PERIODONTAL REGENERATIVE THERAPY

Apart from the total removal of contaminated and necrotic tissue of the periodontium, the use of an adjunctive regenerative approach is suggested to completely restore the tissue deformation. In 2020, the European Federation of Periodontology issued clinical practice guidelines for treating periodontitis. They strongly recommend periodontal regenerative surgery as one of the interventions to treat dentition with clinical attachment loss that does not adequately respond to non-surgical therapy. The periodontal regenerative approach involves the application of pro-regenerative factors and biomaterials [16]. The approaches are decided based on the morphology of defects. For example, the use of pro-regeneration factors is preferred for a narrow intrabony defect with ≥3 mm depth. In a wider defect, single bone graft use or its combination with regenerative factors is selected [17].

The applied biomaterials generally include ceramics, polymers, or their combination. Ceramics are used for osteogenic, osteoconductive, and osteoinductive properties. Polymer is applied when a physical barrier is needed for space provision [18]. Periodontal regenerative materials are readily available in the market. The products offered a single ceramic or polymer preparation and a combination of ceramic-ceramic, polymer-polymer, or ceramic-polymer. The material is derived from natural or synthetic sources and prepared as powder, bulk, injectable gel, or sheet.

The anatomical architecture of the periodontium is a challenge in performing total debridement. Different types of defects are inflicted by periodontitis, as shown in Fig. (**2**). Surgical procedure is required to expand the field of view and allow a thorough cleaning, which leaves an empty space. The dominant cell to occupy the void determines the fate of periodontal tissue. If the population of epithelial cells is larger, the periodontium is repaired by the down growth of a long epithelial junction. The repair by bone or connective tissue adhesion on the root surface, with or without root resorption, progresses if bone cells or connective tissue predominantly proliferate into the void [19]. The repair tissues halt the formation of the true attachment apparatus. Periodontal regenerative therapy is mostly subjected to intrabony, infrabony, or bifurcation defects Fig. (**2**). Table **1** describe the types of periodontal defects due to periodontitis.

The idea to employ a physical barrier around the periodontal defect was proposed to prevent repair by means of epithelial, connective, or bone tissue formation and allow true periodontal tissue regeneration into the defective area. This strategy is an inseparable part of the Guided Tissue Regeneration (GTR) approach, whose development is also driven by biomaterials evolution. There are three generations of membrane barriers for GTR. First-generation membranes are non-degradable, second-generation are degradable, and third-generation membranes are designed with an additional function as a delivery system [20]. All three generations remain clinical options, as depicted in (Table **2**).

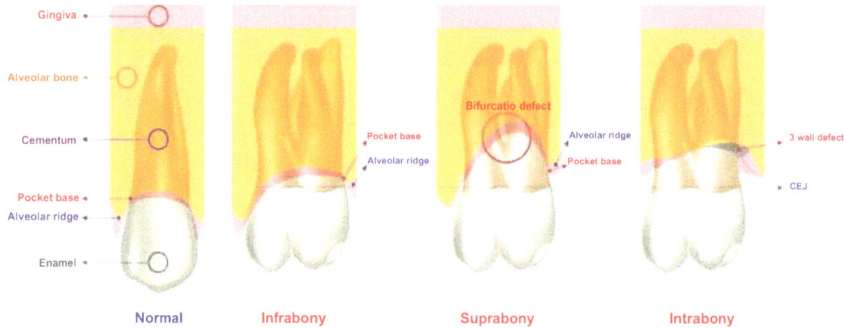

Fig. (2). Periodontitis promotes types of defects. Regenerative therapy studies are mostly dedicated but not limited to treat infrabony, intrabony, and bifurcatio defects.

Table 1. Types of Defects of Periodontal Tissue.

Periodontal Tissue Condition/ Defect	Periodontal Tissue	Alveolar Bone Tissue
Normal periodontium	Periodontal tissue is intact; the base of the periodontal tissue is called the "sulcus base".	Alveolar bone tissue is on the normal level, around 2-3 mm below the sulcus base.
Infrabony defects	"Infra-bony" literally means the pocket is under the bone. The deepest pocket base is positioned deeper (more apically) than the alveolar crest.	Alveolar bone usually has narrow yet deep defects; radiographically, it will be shown as vertical defects.
Suprabony defects	"Supra-bony" literally means the pocket is above the bone. The deepest pocket base is positioned higher than the alveolar crest.	Alveolar bone usually has broader defects; radiographically, it will be shown as horizontal defects.
Intrabony defects	"Intra-bony" literally means the pocket is located inside or trapped on the alveolar bone structure. The pocket structure is mainly similar to the infrabony defects.	The defect is characterized as "three-wall defect", which means that defects are confined to bone tissue surrounding.

Non-degradable polymers and metals with superior mechanical strength and biocompatibility are utilized to prepare the first generations of GTR membranes. Poly-tetrafluoroethylene (PTFE) or titanium-based materials are used in mesh or dense film form. The first non-absorbable membrane for dental purposes was made of expandable-PTFE (e-PTFE), with or without titanium reinforcement [21]. The e-PTFE porosity increases the possibility of an early infection because of microbial colonization on the membrane. Thus, a non-expandable or high-density

PTFE is introduced [21, 22]. Titanium mesh is the only whole metal GTR membrane [23]. A study demonstrated that the clinical parameters of periodontal regeneration in the use of titanium mesh are equal to e-PTFE [24]. Titanium mesh is chosen for its high stiffness, low density, corrosion resistance, and good biocompatibility. However, titanium mesh is hardly adapted to periodontal lesions due to its stiffness and the fact that its sharp edges may harm the tissue [23].

Table 2. Commercial Guided Tissue Regeneration Barrier.

	Products	Ingredient	Form
	Non-biodegradable		
1.	Gore-tex® (W.L. Gore & Associates, Flagstaff, AZ, USA)	Expanded- polytetrafluoroethylene	Sheet
	Biodegradable		
1.	Bio-Gide® (Geistlich Pharma, Wolhusen, Switzerland)	Type 1 collagen from porcine	Sheet
2.	BioMend (Zimmer Biomet Holdings, Inc., USA)	Type 1 collagen from bovine	Sheet
3.	Epi-Guide (Curasan, Inc., USA)	Polylactic acid	Sheet
4.	Resolute XT (WL Gore & Associates Ltd., Flagstaff, AZ, USA)	Polylactic acid, polyglycolic acid	Sheet
5.	Tissue Guide	Atelocollagen from bovine	Sheet
6.	BioMesh-S™ (Samyang corp., Korea)	polyglycolide, poly (d,l-lactide-co glycolide), poly (L-lactide) copolymer	Sheet
7.	Atrisorb® barrier FreeFlow™	Poly-DL-lactide (PLA) in N-Methyl-2-pyrrolidone	Injectable (syringe)

First-generation GTR membranes provide good mechanical support, but the need for second surgery to remove the film encourages the use of biodegradable materials. A randomized clinical trial on 23 patients with 29 pairs of the damaged periodontal site is performed to compare non-biodegradable (e-PTFE) and biodegradable material (polyglactin) as GTR membrane. A study highlighted that clinical and radiographic parameters are not different, but the biodegradable membrane is recommended to avoid surgical re-entry [25].

Biodegradable materials as the second-generation membrane are derived from natural and synthetic sources. The natural polymer used for GTR membrane is mostly collagen type 1 from porcine or bovine, whereas the commercially available synthetic GTR membranes are made of poly-lactic acid (PLA), poly-glycolic acid (PGA), and poly-lactic glycolic acid (PLGA) (Table **2**). Natural membranes offer excellent biocompatibility but lack of mechanical strength. On the other hand, synthetic membranes provide controllable degradation and mechanical properties [15].

It is recommended to use filler material to support the barrier membranes, as illustrated in Fig. (3). Various bone grafts are suggested. Bone grafts not only assist in the maintenance of the space but accelerate regeneration, especially bone tissue [26]. We list the commercially available bone grafts used in dental clinics for periodontal regenerative purposes in Table 3. Hydroxyapatite (HA), tricalcium phosphate (TCP), and bioglass (BG), with or without collagen, are provided in granule or block forms.

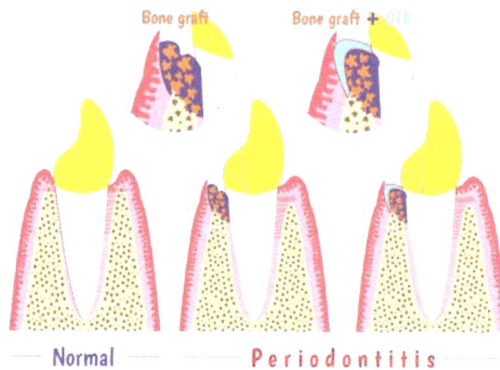

Fig. (3). The application of bone graft only or in combination with a guided tissue regeneration membrane to treat a periodontal defect due to periodontitis.

Table 3. Commercial Bone graft used for periodontal therapy materials without active agent.

	Products	**Ingredient**	**Form**
	Synthetic Sources		
1.	Bonelike® (Medmat Innovation, Porto, Portugal)	Hydroxyapatite, tricalcium phosphate, bioactive glass	granules
2.	Biograft-HT® (IFGL Bioceramics Limited, Calcutta)	biphasic calcium phosphate consisting of hydroxyapatite, beta-tricalcium phosphate	granules
3.	Osteon™ II (Dentium, USA)	Hydroxyapatite scaffold with beta-tricalcium phosphate	granules
4.	PerioGlas®, (NovaBone Products, USA)	calcium phospho-silicate bioactive glass	granules
	Natural Sources		
	Bio-Oss® (Geistlich Pharma, Wolhusen, Switzerland)	bovine-derived bone tissue	Granules
	Bio-Oss® Collagen (Geistlich Pharma, Wolhusen, Switzerland)	Bone apatite, porcine collagen	Block
	OsteBiol® Gen-Os® (Tecnoss, Giaveno, Italy)	Hydroxyapatite, type 1 collagen from porcine	Block

In periodontitis therapy, a bone graft is expected to have a regenerative effect on the attachment apparatus. A systematic review in 2002 concluded that the use of bone graft enhanced the clinical regenerative outcomes of GTR membrane application to treat furcation defects, but not in intrabony defects [27]. Periodontal defect, which extends to the furcation area, occupies a greater area of defect, morphologically, demanding better scaffolding properties in order to restore the periodontal complex structure surgically. Another systematic review in 2013 further compared the effectiveness of GTR in treating furcation involvement of periodontal defects. It concluded that the application of bone graft in GTR generates superior results clinically compared to GTR only [28].

Bioactive molecules, in addition to the combination of bone graft and GTR membrane, are expected to enhance the regenerative potential. Bioactive molecules, including enamel matrix derivative (EMD), platelet concentrates, and growth factors, are commonly used for treating patients. A clinical trial was performed on the bioactive molecule alone or bioactive molecule-bone graft or bioactive molecules-bone graft-GTR. The results were varied, and thus, more controlled, well-designed clinical trials are needed to be done.

The EMD is an acidic extract of enamel extracellular matrix protein and contains 90% amelogenin [29]. A study showed that the application of recombinant human amelogenin protein-induced regeneration process mimics the normal pattern of periodontal development *in vivo*. It is initiated with cementum formation and followed by ligament periodontal and alveolar bone establishment [29]. In patients with intrabony defects, EMD induced comparable periodontal regeneration with GTR [30]. Clinical advantages were found in the use of EMD in combination with bovine porous bone mineral as bone graft and collagen/poly-lactic acid membrane as a GTR barrier [31].

Platelet-rich plasma (PRP) is one of the most accessible growth factor sources for periodontal regenerative surgery. It usually prepares from a patient's own blood and contains 3-5 times higher platelets and growth factors than the whole blood [32]. A systematic review evaluated the benefits of adding PRP to the GTR/ GBR therapy. The study could not conclude the effectiveness of PRP in gaining better clinical parameters. Although some of the RCTs revealed the contribution of PRP to improving the clinical parameters, other research also provided contrary results [33]. One clinical trial also found evidence that PRP failed to improve the regeneration effect of bone graft and GTR membrane combination in deep and narrow periodontal defects [34]. On the contrary, another study revealed that PRP increased the clinical parameters more significantly than using bone graft only [35].

Within a shorter time and more cost-effective preparation method than PRP, the process could produce platelet-rich fibrin (PRF) from autologous blood. The PRF contains a three-dimensional matrix of fibrin, cytokines, and growth factors [32]. A split-mouth design clinical study was performed on 16 patients with intrabony defects, in addition to the PRF enhanced of the periodontal regenerative potential of a collagen membrane [36]. The positive effects of PRF on the periodontal regeneration process were reported, either as a single therapeutic agent or in combination with other modalities. However, no standard procedures for PRF preparation and handling are available [37].

The advancement in regenerative medicine also inspired the development of a new approach to periodontal therapy. This development includes the use of cell therapy. In a single-centered randomized clinical trial, an autologous Periodontal Ligament Stem Cell (PDLSC) sheet is used to enhance the therapeutic effect of bone tissue xenograft and collagen type 1 membrane. The study failed to prove the advantage of cell therapy as an adjunctive to GBR and GTR combination. Significant alveolar bone height gain ($p < 0.001$) was identified in patients who received GBR and GTR with or without PDLSC sheet. However, the increase in alveolar bone height and clinical attachment level (CAL), as well as the reduction of pocket depth (PD) and gingival recession (GR) ($p > 0.05$), was not statistically different [38].

Advanced technologies in modifying and manipulating biomaterials agents, for example, using cell therapy, have increased the expectation of clinical results. Clinically, the result is contradictory to the previous statement. Additional technology applied in clinical practice means an additional invasive cost. From this perspective, further research is expected to be more effective, more economical, and faster, considering the clinical benefit in using minimal manipulation of "technology" [39].

The third generation of GTR membranes is developed based on the idea of improving its function. The membrane is not only dedicated as a physical barrier but also actively influences and directs the regeneration process. The researcher incorporates antimicrobial, anti-inflammation, or pro-regeneration molecules into the membrane polymers. This strategy could be effective *in vitro* and *in vivo* evaluation without examining the risk of re-infection in a clinical setting.

BIOACTIVE MEMBRANE BARRIER

The highly advanced strategy is developing membranes from a polymer that owns an innate capacity to stimulate tissue regeneration. Advances in materials science encourage the creation of a membrane barrier with the ability to activate cellular functions. This bioactive/biofunctional membrane serves as a scaffold while retaining its primary function of maintaining the periodontal space [40]. Biomaterials from natural sources are commonly used for this purpose. Chitosan is well-known for its antimicrobial and anti-inflammatory properties. Chitosan particles inhibit periodontitis-related bacteria, *Aggregatibacter actinomycetemcomitans* (Aa), and *Porphyromonas gingivalis* (Pg) growth. It simultaneously suppresses prostaglandin E production in human gingival fibroblasts after the stimulation of Interleukin [41].

The incorporation of antimicrobials into a GTR membrane has been made applicable for patients, as shown in (Table **4**). Local application of antimicrobial agents is more effective than systemic use in preventing GTR membrane contamination [42]. The idea to prepare an antimicrobial-containing GTR membrane is considered to provide a controlled-release system for local application. For example, a gelatin-carbonated apatite hydrogel was prepared as a periodontal regenerative membrane with the ability to act as a metronidazole delivery system [43]. A meta-analysis of randomized controlled clinical trials from 2008 to 2012 recommended the use of local antibiotics in moderate and severe periodontitis cases to control inflammation. However, there is no consensus about the products and dosages [44], and the issue of resistance put us to reconsider the use of antibiotic agents. The alternatives of antibiotics are explored, such as, employing ZnO in a polycaprolactone (PCL) membrane. The ZnO-impregnated PCL membrane showed antibacterial activity against Pg and biocompatibility with human dental pulp stem cells [45].

Table 4. Commercial Active Agent Impregnated Periodontal Regenerative Material as Local Adjuvant Periodontitis Treatment.

	Products	Carrier	Active Agent	Preparations
		Drugs		
1.	ATRIDOX (TOLMAR Inc, USA)	Poly-(DL-lactide)	Doxycycline-Hyclate	Two-syringe gel
2.	Arestin (Bausch Health Companies Inc., USA)	Poly (glycolide-co--l-lactide) or PGLA	Minocycline hydrochloride	Gel in cartridge
3.	Periochip (Dexcel Pharma/AmediusTec, Israel)	Hydrolyzed gelatine (porcine) cross-linked with glutaraldehyde	Chlorhexidine gluconate	Film
4.	PerioCol-CG (EUCARE PHARMACEUTICALS (P) LTD., India)	Type 1 collagen derived from fish sources	Chlorhexidine gluconate	Chip
5.	Periodontal Plus AB (Advanced Biotech Product (P) Ltd., India)	Collagen type-1	Tetracycline hydrochloride	Fibres

(Table 4) cont.....

	Products	Carrier	Active Agent	Preparations
6.	CHLO-SITE (Zantomed, Germany)	Xanthan gum	Chlorhexidine dihydrochloride, chlorhexidine digluconate	Xanthan-based gel
	Growth Factor			
1	GEM 21S® (Lynch Biologics, LLC., USA)	ß-TCP	rhPDGF-BB	granule

There are several developments in the synthesis of bioactive/ biofunctional membranes for GTR. These researches mainly focused on fabricating a new formula of alloplast membranes with tunability, antibacterial, and cell occlusion [46 - 48]. Hence, these studies were only performed at the cellular level and animal model. More studies are obligatory to be further developed into clinical settings through clinical trials.

Limited clinical trials were performed to evaluate allograft bioactive membrane barrier, and amnion chorion membrane, as a treatment for intrabony defect in comparison to bone allograft materials. Both groups showed significant improvement in clinical parameters with no statistical difference [49]. Another clinical trial was performed to evaluate the classic naturally derived material, chitosan. A clinical trial for chronic periodontitis patients proved that the treatment group using chitosan gel had better clinical improvement than the control group [50]. Despite the fact that there are only limited clinical trials regarding the use of chitosan for periodontal defects, the potential of chitosan as natural bioactive material is worth to be considered.

ENGINEERED BIO-FUNCTIONAL BARRIER TO DIRECT PERIODONTAL TISSUE REGENERATION

In addition to efficacy, developed products that are oriented toward clinical application problems receive special attention. For example, the new membrane may offer simplification of application procedures to reduce the working time. Membrane barrier adaptation into periodontal defect areas is intricate. In this situation, a high precision barrier may be considered.

In 2015, Rasperini *et al.* presented a clinical case of individual-designed membranes in combination with recombinant human platelet-derived growth factor-BB (rhPDGF-BB) [51]. They employed a computed-tomography scan and selective laser sintering to provide a membrane barrier from polycaprolactone powder containing 4% hydroxyapatite. The approach afforded a three-dimensional (3D) matrix with perforation for fixation, an internal port for delivering rhPDGF-BB, and pegs oriented perpendicularly to the root for periodontal ligament formation. This illustrates the feasibility of the precise barrier application in periodontal regenerative therapy.

Biomaterial aspects must be considered in designing a precise matrix. First, appropriate medical-grade materials must meet the needs of controllable degradability. Second, the geometry must be able to allow the regenerating tissue to form 3D morphology of the natural structure of the periodontal ligament, cementum, and alveolar bone. Third, it is suggested to explore the modification of topography that is able to direct the regeneration of periodontal ligament and cementum [52].

It is widely accepted that the topography of materials defines a periodontal tissue cell's behaviour. *In vitro*, a microporous surface (50-400 μm) facilitates better adhesion and fiber elongation of mouse periodontal ligament cells than a smoothened one. The periodontal extracellular matrix marker, including tropoelastin, tenascin, periostin, and fibronectin, is elevated [53]. The aforementioned situation highlights the importance of topography design to direct cell's regeneration. Cell's behaviours correspond to the surface, mechanical, electrical, and morphological characteristics of the scaffold [40].

CONCLUSION

Recent biomaterials developed for periodontal regenerative therapy urge to be assessed further to investigate the best design and composition that meet users' needs and are in line with government and industry expectations. The complexity of the periodontal tissue structures and varied defect morphologies challenge both clinicians and biomaterial scientists. The development of strategies to improve the predictability of treatment outcomes, as well as accessibility and good economic value, is encouraged . Aligned expectation is key for auspicious and predictable treatment results.

REFERENCES

[1]   World Health Organization. Global strategy and action plan on ageing and health. Geneva, World Health Organization. 2017; 1-56.

[2]   Bennadi D, Reddy C. Oral health related quality of life. JInt Soc Prevent Communit Dent. 2013; 3(1): 1-6.

[3]   Rosli TI, Chan YM, Kadir RA et al. Association between oral health-related quality of life and nutritional status among older adults in district of Kuala Pilah, Malaysia. BMC Public Health. 2019; 19(Suppl 4)): 547-54.

[4]   Fiorellini JD, Kim D, Chang YC. Anatomy, structure, and function of the periodontium. In: Newman MG, Takei HH, Klokkevold PR, Carranza FA, Eds. Newman and Carranza's Clinical Periodontology 13th ed. St. Louis, Elsevier Saunders, 2019; 19-49.

[5]   Slots J. Periodontitis: facts, fallacies, and the future. Periodontol 2000 2017; 75(1): 7-23.

[6]   Papapanou PN, Susin C. Periodontitis epidemiology: is periodontitis under-recognized, over-diagnosed, or both. Periodontol 2000 2017; 75(1): 45-51.

[7]   Tonetti MS, Jepsen S, Jin L, Otomo-Corgel J. Impact of the global burden of periodontal diseases on health, nutrition and wellbeing of mankind: A call for global action. J Clin Periodontol 2017; 44(5): 456-62.
[http://dx.doi.org/10.1111/jcpe.12732] [PMID: 28419559]

[8]   Hajishengallis G, Chavakis T. Local and systemic mechanisms linking periodontal disease and inflammatory comorbidities. Nat Rev Immunol 2021; 21(7): 426-40.
[http://dx.doi.org/10.1038/s41577-020-00488-6] [PMID: 33510490]

[9]   Marouf N, Cai W, Said KN, *et al.* Association between periodontitis and severity of Covid-19 infection: a case-control study. J Clin Periodontol 00: 1-9.
[http://dx.doi.org/10.1111/jcpe.13435] [PMID: 33527378]

[10]   Bernabe E, Marcenes W, Hernandez CR, *et al.* GBD 2017 Oral Disorders Collaborators. Global, regional, and national levels and trends in burden of oral conditions from 1990 to 2017: a systematic analysis for the global burden of disease 2017 study. J Dent Res 2020; 99(4): 362-73.
[http://dx.doi.org/10.1177/0022034520908533] [PMID: 32122215]

[11]   Nazir M, Al-Ansari A, Al-Khalifa K, Alhareky M, Gaffar B, Almas K. Global prevalence of periodontal disease and lack of its surveillance. ScientificWorldJournal 2020; 2020: 1-8.
[http://dx.doi.org/10.1155/2020/2146160] [PMID: 32549797]

[12]   Hienz SA, Paliwal S, Ivanovski S. Mechanisms of Bone Resorption in Periodontitis. J Immunol Res 2015; 2015: 1-10.
[http://dx.doi.org/10.1155/2015/615486] [PMID: 26065002]

[13]   Bosshardt DD, Sculean A. Does periodontal tissue regeneration really work? Periodontol 2000 2009; 51(1): 208-19.
[http://dx.doi.org/10.1111/j.1600-0757.2009.00317.x] [PMID: 19878476]

[14]   Herrera D, Matesanz P, Bascones-Martínez A, Sanz M. Local and systemic antimicrobial therapy in periodontics. J Evid Based Dent Pract 2012; 12(3) (Suppl.): 50-60.
[http://dx.doi.org/10.1016/S1532-3382(12)70013-1] [PMID: 23040339]

[15]   Liang Y, Luan X, Liu X. Recent advances in periodontal regeneration: A biomaterial perspective. Bioact Mater 2020; 5(2): 297-308.
[http://dx.doi.org/10.1016/j.bioactmat.2020.02.012] [PMID: 32154444]

[16]   Sanz M, Herrera D, Kebschull M, *et al.* Treatment of stage I–III periodontitis—The EFP S3 level clinical practice guideline. J Clin Periodontol 2020; 47(S22) (Suppl. 22): 4-60.
[http://dx.doi.org/10.1111/jcpe.13290] [PMID: 32383274]

[17]   Hägi TT, Laugisch O, Ivanovic A, Sculean A. Regenerative periodontal therapy. Quintessence Int 2014; 45(3): 185-92.
[PMID: 24570985]

[18]   Shue L, Yufeng Z, Mony U. Biomaterials for periodontal regeneration. Biomatter 2012; 2(4): 271-7.
[http://dx.doi.org/10.4161/biom.22948] [PMID: 23507891]

[19]   Kao RT, Takei HH, Cochran DL. Periodontal regeneration and reconstructive surgery. In: Newman MG, Takei HH, Klokkevold PR, Carranza FA, Eds. Newman and Carranza's Clinical Periodontology. 13th ed. St. Louis: Elsevier Saunders 2019; pp. 642-52.

[20]   Sam G, Pillai BRM. Evolution of barrier membranes in periodontal regeneration - are the third generation membranes really here? J Clin Diagn Res 2014; 8(12): ZE14-7.
[http://dx.doi.org/10.7860/JCDR/2014/9957.5272] [PMID: 25654055]

[21]   Barboza EP, Stutz B, Ferreira VF, Carvalho W. Guided bone regeneration using nonexpanded

polytetrafluoroethylene membranes in preparation for dental implant placements--a report of 420 cases. Implant Dent 2010; 19(1): 2-7.
[http://dx.doi.org/10.1097/ID.0b013e3181cda72c] [PMID: 20147810]

[22]   Carbonell JM, Martín IS, Santos A, Pujol A, Sanz-Moliner JD, Nart J. High-density polytetrafluoroethylene membranes in guided bone and tissue regeneration procedures: a literature review. Int J Oral Maxillofac Surg 2014; 43(1): 75-84.
[http://dx.doi.org/10.1016/j.ijom.2013.05.017] [PMID: 23810680]

[23]   Xie Y, Li S, Zhang T, Wang C, Cai X. Titanium mesh for bone augmentation in oral implantology: current application and progress. Int J Oral Sci 2020; 12(1): 37.
[http://dx.doi.org/10.1038/s41368-020-00107-z] [PMID: 33380722]

[24]   Toygar HU, Guzeldemir E, Cilasun U, Akkor D, Arpak N. Long□term clinical evaluation and SEM analysis of the e□PTFE and titanium membranes in guided tissue regeneration. J Biomed Mater Res B Appl Biomater 2009; 91B(2): 772-9.
[http://dx.doi.org/10.1002/jbm.b.31454] [PMID: 19572297]

[25]   Eickholz P, Kim TS, Holle R. Regenerative periodontal surgery with non-resorbable and biodegradable barriers: results after 24 months. J Clin Periodontol 1998; 25(8): 666-76.
[http://dx.doi.org/10.1111/j.1600-051X.1998.tb02504.x] [PMID: 9722272]

[26]   Schenk RK, Buser D, Hardwick WR, Dahlin C. Healing pattern of bone regeneration in membrane-protected defects: a histologic study in the canine mandible. Int J Oral Maxillofac Implants 1994; 9(1): 13-29.
[PMID: 8150509]

[27]   Murphy KG, Gunsolley JC. Guided tissue regeneration for the treatment of periodontal intrabony and furcation defects. A systematic review. Ann Periodontol 2003; 8(1): 266-302.
[http://dx.doi.org/10.1902/annals.2003.8.1.266] [PMID: 14971257]

[28]   Chen TH, Tu YK, Yen CC, Lu H-K. A systematic review and meta-analysis of guided tissue regeneration/osseous grafting for the treatment of Class II furcation defects. J Dent Sci 2013; 8(3): 209-24.
[http://dx.doi.org/10.1016/j.jds.2013.06.006]

[29]   Haze A, Taylor AL, Haegewald S, *et al.* Regeneration of bone and periodontal ligament induced by recombinant amelogenin after periodontitis. J Cell Mol Med 2009; 13(6): 1110-24.
[http://dx.doi.org/10.1111/j.1582-4934.2009.00700.x] [PMID: 19228267]

[30]   Esposito M, Grusovin MG, Papanikolaou N, Coulthard P, Worthington HV. Enamel matrix derivative (Emdogain®) for periodontal tissue regeneration in intrabony defects. Cochrane Libr 2009; 2009(4): CD003875.
[http://dx.doi.org/10.1002/14651858.CD003875.pub3] [PMID: 19821315]

[31]   Lekovic V, Camargo PM, Weinlaender M, Kenney EB, Vasilic N. Combination use of bovine porous bone mineral, enamel matrix proteins, and a bioabsorbable membrane in intrabony periodontal defects in humans. J Periodontol 2001; 72(5): 583-9.
[http://dx.doi.org/10.1902/jop.2001.72.5.583] [PMID: 11394392]

[32]   Mijiritsky E, Assaf HD, Peleg O, Shacham M, Cerroni L, Mangani L. Use of PRP, PRF, and CGF in periodontal regeneration and facial rejuvenation-a narrative review. Biology (Basel) 2021; 10(4): 317.
[http://dx.doi.org/10.3390/biology10040317] [PMID: 33920204]

[33]   Saleem M, Pisani F, Zadid FM, *et al.* Adjunctive Platelet-Rich Plasma (PRP) in infrabony regenerative treatment: A systematic review and rct's meta-analysis. Stem Cell Int 2018; pp. 1-10.

[34]   Döri F, Huszár T, Nikolidakis D, Arweiler NB, Gera I, Sculean A. Effect of platelet-rich plasma on the healing of intra-bony defects treated with a natural bone mineral and a collagen membrane. J Clin Periodontol 2007; 34(3): 254-61.
[http://dx.doi.org/10.1111/j.1600-051X.2006.01044.x] [PMID: 17257158]

[35]   Kaushick BT, Jayakumar ND. Padmalatha et al. Treatment of human periodontal infrabony defects with hydroxyapatite + β tricalcium phosphate bone graft alone and in combination with platelet rich plasma: A randomized clinical trial. IJDR 2011; 22(4): 505-10.

[36]   Panda S, Sankari M, Satpathy A, *et al.* Adjunctive effect of autologous platelet-rich fibrin to barrier membrane in the treatment of periodontal intrabony defects. J Craniofac Surg 2016; 27(3): 691-6.
[http://dx.doi.org/10.1097/SCS.0000000000002524] [PMID: 27046472]

[37]   Castro AB, Meschi N, Temmerman A, *et al.* Regenerative potential of leucocyte- and platelet-rich fibrin. Part A: intra-bony defects, furcation defects and periodontal plastic surgery. A systematic review and meta-analysis. J Clin Periodontol 2017; 44(1): 67-82.
[http://dx.doi.org/10.1111/jcpe.12643] [PMID: 27783851]

[38]   Chen FM, Gao LN, Tian BM, *et al.* Treatment of periodontal intrabony defects using autologous periodontal ligament stem cells: a randomized clinical trial. Stem Cell Res Ther 2016; 7(1): 33.
[http://dx.doi.org/10.1186/s13287-016-0288-1] [PMID: 26895633]

[39]   Moreno Sancho F, Leira Y, Orlandi M, Buti J, Giannobile WV, D'Aiuto F. Cell-based therapies for alveolar bone and periodontal regeneration: concise review. Stem Cells Transl Med 2019; 8(12): 1286-95.
[http://dx.doi.org/10.1002/sctm.19-0183] [PMID: 31692298]

[40]   Shimauchi H, Nemoto E, Ishihata H, Shimomura M. Possible functional scaffolds for periodontal regeneration. Jpn Dent Sci Rev 2013; 49(4): 118-30.
[http://dx.doi.org/10.1016/j.jdsr.2013.05.001]

[41]   Arancibia R, Maturana C, Silva D, *et al.* Effects of chitosan particles in periodontal pathogens and gingival fibroblasts. J Dent Res 2013; 92(8): 740-5.
[http://dx.doi.org/10.1177/0022034513494816] [PMID: 23788611]

[42]   Zucchelli G, Sforza NM, Clauser C, Cesari C, Sanctis MD. Topical and systemic antimicrobial therapy in guided tissue regeneration. J Periodontol 1999; 70(3): 239-47.
[http://dx.doi.org/10.1902/jop.1999.70.3.239] [PMID: 10225539]

[43]   Ardhani R. Setyaningsih, Hafiyyah OA et al. Preparation o carbonate apatite membrane as metronidazole delivery system for periodontal application. KEM 2016; 696: 250-8.

[44]   Herrera D, Matesanz P, Bascones-Martínez A, Sanz M. Local and systemic antimicrobial therapy in periodontics. J Evid Based Dent Pract 2012; 12(3) (Suppl.): 50-60.
[http://dx.doi.org/10.1016/S1532-3382(12)70013-1] [PMID: 23040339]

[45]   Münchow EA, Albuquerque MTP, Zero B, *et al.* Development and characterization of novel ZnO-loaded electrospun membranes for periodontal regeneration. Dent Mater 2015; 31(9): 1038-51.
[http://dx.doi.org/10.1016/j.dental.2015.06.004] [PMID: 26116414]

[46]   Khorsand B, Elangovan S, Hong L, Kormann MSD, Salem AK. A bioactive collagen membrane that enhances bone regeneration. J Biomed Mater Res B Appl Biomater 2019; 107(6): 1824-32.
[http://dx.doi.org/10.1002/jbm.b.34275] [PMID: 30466196]

[47]   Dubey N, Ferreira JA, Daghrery A, *et al.* Highly tunable bioactive fiber-reinforced hydrogel for guided bone regeneration. Acta Biomater 2020; 113: 164-76.
[http://dx.doi.org/10.1016/j.actbio.2020.06.011] [PMID: 32540497]

[48]   Abdelaziz D, Hefnawy A, Al-Wakeel E, El-Fallal A, El-Sherbiny IM. New biodegradable nanoparticles-in-nanofibers based membranes for guided periodontal tissue and bone regeneration with enhanced antibacterial activity. J Adv Res 2021; 28: 51-62.
[http://dx.doi.org/10.1016/j.jare.2020.06.014] [PMID: 33364045]

[49]   Temraz A, Ghallab NA, Hamdy R, El-Dahab OA. Clinical and radiographic evaluation of amnion chorion membrane and demineralized bone matrix putty allograft for management of periodontal intrabony defects: a randomized clinical trial. Cell Tissue Bank 2019; 20(1): 117-28.
[http://dx.doi.org/10.1007/s10561-018-09743-6] [PMID: 30631986]

[50]   Akıncıbay H, Şenel S, Yetkin Ay Z. Application of chitosan gel in the treatment of chronic periodontitis. J Biomed Mater Res B Appl Biomater 2007; 80B(2): 290-6.
[http://dx.doi.org/10.1002/jbm.b.30596] [PMID: 16767723]

[51]   Rasperini G, Pilipchuk SP, Flanagan CL, *et al.* 3D-printed bioresorbable scaffold for periodontal repair. J Dent Res 2015; 94(9_suppl) (Suppl.): 153S-7S.
[http://dx.doi.org/10.1177/0022034515588303] [PMID: 26124215]

[52]   Park C, Kim KH, Lee YM, Seol YJ. Advanced Engineering Strategies for Periodontal Complex Regeneration. Materials (Basel) 2016; 9(1): 57.
[http://dx.doi.org/10.3390/ma9010057] [PMID: 28787856]

[53]   Dangaria SJ, Ito Y, Yin L, *et al.* Apatite Microtopographies Instruct Signaling Tapestries For Progenitor-Driven New Attachment of Teeth Tissue Eng Part A 2011; 17(3 and 4): 279-90.

CHAPTER 9

Tissue Engineering Approach for Corneal Regeneration

Mohamed Salih[1] and **Bakiah Shaharuddin**[1,*]

[1] *Regenerative Medicine Cluster, Advanced Medical and Dental Institute, Universiti Sains Malaysia, Bertam, 13200 Kepala Batas, Pulau Pinang, Malaysia*

Abstract: There is an inadequate supply of tissues and organs for transplantation due to limitations in organ donors and challenges surrounding the use of autografts. The search for biodegradable and compatible tissue constructs as a platform for cellular, gene, and immune therapies, as well as drug deliveries, warrant intensive investigations. Biologically compatible materials with unique properties are needed as substrates or scaffolds for many types of cellular and gene therapies, which include treatment for ocular surface regeneration. Although the cornea is one of the most successful organ transplantations because it is considered an immune-privileged site, there are limitations like the risk of graft rejection, the transmission of diseases, and the scarcity of donors. Based on a clear understanding of the anatomy and physiology of the cornea, types of biomaterials, fabrication, and adjunct use of biologics are among the regenerative strategies employed in the tissue engineering approach for corneal regeneration. This chapter highlights the indications for cornea replacement, common biomaterials, and biologics used in this field.

Keywords: Cornea regenerative medicine, Tissue engineering, Ocular surface regeneration.

INTRODUCTION

The main purpose of corneal epithelial regenerative strategies is to achieve successful tissue transplantation with a minimum risk of immune system rejection. Many tissue engineering techniques and strategies are utilized to reach this goal. Tissue engineering methods aim to repair damaged tissues and organs by biological substitutes. The main principle of tissue engineering is the use of cells, scaffolds, and biologically active molecules to restore the normal functions of tissues or organs (Fig. **1**). Scaffold materials, fabrication, and the method of scaffold manufacturing are among the important factors involved in this field. The

* **Corresponding author Bakiah Shaharuddin:** Regenerative Medicine Cluster, Advanced Medical and Dental Institute, Universiti Sains Malaysia, Bertam, 13200 Kepala Batas, Pulau Pinang, Malaysia; E-mail: bakiah@usm.my

Mohd Fauzi Mh Busra, Daniel Law Jia Xian, Yogeswaran Lokanathan and Ruszymah Haji Idrus (Eds.)

implementation of tissue engineering methods for corneal regeneration weighs heavily on a good understanding of corneal anatomy and physiological functions in the design of the tissue-engineered construct.

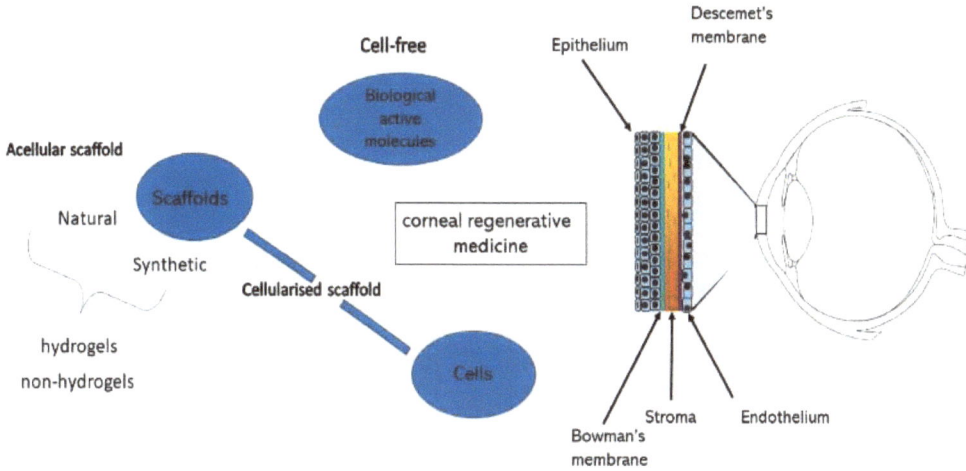

Fig. (1).   Corneal regenerative medicine encompasses three major approaches; cellular component, biomaterials fabrication into tissue scaffolds, and use of biologically active molecules (cell-free approach). Regenerative strategies are employed to treat corneal conditions arising from the epithelium, stroma, or endothelial layers. Among commonly used biomaterials are hydrogel or non-hydrogel-based polymers, either natural or synthetic. A Cellularised scaffold is also an option to regenerate a damaged site. The cellular component includes cells from ocular source or non-ocular sources.

The Burden of Corneal Blindness

Approximately 6 million people globally are experiencing blindness or visual impairment caused by corneal diseases [1]. A cataract is the main cause of blindness worldwide; glaucoma comes in second and corneal blindness is the third cause on the list [2]. Corneal blindness is one of the serious conditions affecting millions of people annually worldwide. Among the common causes of corneal blindness are inflammatory conditions and infections and corneal scarring due to keratoconus. Corneal regenerative medicine is one of the therapeutic strategies to improve visual acuity.

Anatomical Considerations for Corneal Tissue Engineering

The cornea is essential for clarity of vision as it provides 40 - 44 Diopter; approximately two-thirds of the refractive power of the eye [3]. The cornea is flat at the periphery and steep at the center. This variation in thickness is due to the high amount of collagen in the peripheral stroma. Corneal components are divided into cellular and non-cellular components. Cellular components are epithelial, endothelial, and keratocytes or corneal fibroblasts, which are the major cells of the corneal stroma.

Non-cellular components are collagen and glycosaminoglycan. Keratin sulphate is the primary glycosaminoglycan comprising about 65% of the glycosaminoglycan content. There are five layers of the human cornea: corneal epithelium, Bowman's layer, corneal stroma, Descemet's membrane, and corneal endothelium (Doughty and Jonuscheit, 2019). Cornea is an avascular anterior most structure of the eye which acts as a physical barrier and protection to the eye [6]. Cornea is responsible for focusing the light that enters the eye onto the retina (Sridhar, 2017).

Corneal Epithelium

This is the outermost layer of the cornea with five to six layers of non-keratinized stratified squamous epithelium, and it is a layer of highly regenerative cells. It plays a role in heat and gas exchange [7]. Corneal epithelium comprises approximately 10% of the general corneal thickness, and its function is to protect the eye and absorb oxygen and nutrients. The corneal epithelium serves as a barrier between the cornea and the outside environment [8]. The posterior most layer of the corneal epithelium includes basal epithelial cells.

To re-populate the cornea, pre-limbal basal epithelial cells first differentiate and then migrate anteriorly. During this process, the surface microvilli started to appear in a gradual manner. Hemidesmosomes adhere to the basement membrane and stroma by the utilization of basal cells. The link between the intracellular skeleton of basal cells and stroma is through the anchoring complex. This complex is composed of the hemidesmosome, anchoring fibril, and anchoring filament complex [9].

The life span of the corneal epithelial cells is 7 to 10 days; after that, it starts apoptosis and desquamation, which is subsequently followed by the replacement process by the limbal stem cells [10]. Epithelial basement membrane is an extracellular matrix that anchors epithelial cells to the stroma, and it serves as a scaffold for the purpose of embryonic development. It is composed of collagen, laminin, heparan sulphate proteoglycans, nidogens, thrombospondin-1 (THBS1), matrilin-2 (MATN2), and matrilin-4 (MATN4) and fibronectin. Vinculin is located in focal adhesion sites together with integrin $\beta1$ subunits, and this is essential for cellular adhesion, and vinculin is a major factor in corneal wound healing as well [11]. F-actin, which always binds to phalloidin, is found in the corneal epithelial cells, mainly in the lateral cell membrane [12].

Bowman's Layer and Stroma

The second corneal layer which is an acellular non-regenerating layer presenting as unorganized fibril composed mainly of collagen [13]. Stroma layer contributes to 80-85% corneal thickness, measuring around 500 μm in humans, and it contains collagen fibers type I and type IV. The extracellular matrix contains glycoproteins, water, proteoglycans like lumican and keratocan, and salts [14]. Collagen fibers are arranged in packs called fibrils; fibrils are also packed to form lamellae [200-250 in the human eye] [15].

Major cells of the stroma are keratocytes, which are the source of the production of collagen, matrix metalloproteinases, and glycosaminoglycans [8]. The stromal fibers and extracellular matrix are perfectly organized, and that make the stroma quite unique in comparison to other collagenous structures; the stroma is unique in its transparency [16]. The passage of light through this organized network of fibrils allow the light to pass without scattering. Keratocytes differentiation is crucial to stromal clarity. In response to TGF-β1 and PDGF, myofibroblasts which are derived from keratocytes, form corneal haze and promote corneal opacification [17]. The descemet membrane is a layer located just under the stroma, composed of collagen-like fibrils [7]. It is the corneal endothelium basement membrane. The descemet membrane, the basement membrane of corneal epithelium, assists in corneal dehydration maintenance.

Corneal Endothelium

The endothelium plays a role in the transport of necessary substances from intraocular fluid to the cornea [7]. Located in the posterior end of the cornea, it is composed of a layer of flat polygonal cells 20 μm in diameter. It maintains the stroma dehydrated through an ionic pump located in the plasma membrane. It contains Actin filaments which are located as dense peripheral bands, and its function is to facilitate the cell migration process [18]. Corneal endothelial also contains gap junction and play a role in stromal dehydration; this process depends on the tight junction of corneal endothelial cells together with Na^+/K^+-ATPase and bicarbonate-dependent Mg^{2+}-ATPase [19].

Corneal Wound Healing

Corneal cells contain stratified squamous epithelium cells, which are self-renewing, and these cells are maintained by stem cells. These stem cells are located at corneal periphery, in the limbus area, and not present in the central cornea, specifically in the stromal invaginations named Palisades of Vogt [20]. The cells start to divide when they are activated; they divide asymmetrically into two cells; one will be stored in the stem cell pool, and the other one will continue to differentiate and migrate to replace the cells shed from the ocular surface due to aging or injury. If the limbal stem cell depleted, such as in the case of limbal stem cell deficiency, the corneal area will be re-epithelized by conjunctival cells, which lead to impaired vision or blindness, and eye pain.

REQUIREMENTS FOR CORNEAL REGENERATIVE STRATEGIES

Various strategies are employed in corneal regenerative medicine, which include the use of biologics, growth factors/small molecules, scaffold-free methods, and biomaterials for scaffold fabrication.

Biologically Active Molecules

Cornea tissue engineering also exploits active biological molecules, including some growth factors and cytokines. These bio-signals commonly work as receptor-ligand interactions, acting on complex mechanisms or cross-talk between cells.

Exosome

First found in the supernatant of the sheep blood cells cultured in the laboratory [21], exosomes are rich with many components like proteins, miRNAs, lipids, and IncRNAs. Exosomes can be found in many sources like the supernatant of cell culture, sweat, milk, blood, and tears. Exosomes proved to be an important factor in the treatment of ocular diseases, and it has been used in many eye diseases like retinopathy, autoimmune diseases, and corneal conditions [22]. Exosomes derived from human MSC are a potential agent for corneal wound healing [23].

Small Molecules

Using the newly discovered human induced pluripotent stem cells (hiPSC) is a very useful addition to the tissue engineering cell-based therapy field [24]. Protocols that demonstrate iPSC differentiation are drawn from our understanding of the ectodermal development of the eye. Combination of specific growth mediums, supplements, and small molecules is used to improve and enhance the yield of differentiated cells. Selective TGF-inhibitors, SB-505124, and its analogue, the SB-431542 were coupled with IWP-2, Wnt inhibitor, to induce neural commitment. Several studies showed combination of SB-505124 along with IWP-2 and bFGF has led to corneal epithelial cell fate due to the activation of FGF signaling [25, 26]. A similar growth factor cocktail resulted in corneal epithelial commitment with raised corneal differentiation markers, such as PAX6 and its transcription factor Wnt7A. Garcia *et al.* have reported that the combination of IWP-2 and SB with Rho-kinase (ROCK) inhibitor favours corneal epithelial fate [27].

ROCK Inhibitor

Human corneal endothelial cells form a layer of flat hexagonal shape responsible for the corneal dehydration, which results in maintaining corneal transparency.

This mechanism is possible by altering Na^+/K^+-ATPase pumps and barrier function facilitated by tight junctions. Rho-associated kinase (ROCK) inhibitors have been extensively investigated for corneal endothelial regenerative strategies *in vitro* and *in vivo* [28 - 35]. Corneal endothelium is challenged by the limited regenerative capacity of the native cells and the specialised barrier functions of the endothelial cells to maintain homeostasis. ROCK inhibitors were demonstrated to enhance proliferative capacity, promotes adhesion and suppress apoptosis. In the form of eye drops, the effects of a selective ROCK inhibitor Y-27632 is the potential to be developed for translational strategies in managing cornea endothelial diseases [27, 28, 31]. Combined use of Y-27632 and MSC-conditioned media also showed remarkable cellular proliferation and suppression of senescence [29].

Cellular Components

Cell therapies for cornea regeneration may involve a 2D cell sheet or 3D arrangement of cultivated cells. It may be used concurrently with biomaterials, in which case, it is usually labelled as 'cellularised scaffolds'. The source of cells can be derived from cornea native cells or from the extra-ocular source of cells such as buccal mucosa, and embryonic or adult stem cells.

Corneal Stem Cells

Corneal stem cells that are located in the limbus are identified as limbal stem cells (LSC), which are responsible for the regeneration of corneal stroma [36] and epithelium [37]. LSCs were cultivated for the treatment of limbal stem cell deficiency (LSCD). Nakamura *et al.* collected autologous serum (AS) from the patients and used it in a feeder-free culture of corneal epithelial cells on AM as the biological scaffold. Removal of 3 mm limbal biopsy was initially performed, followed by cultivated tissue transplantation on the ocular surface [38].

Extra-ocular Cells

Autologous transplantation is usually the best option to avoid the disadvantages related to allogenic transplantation. In the case of bilateral LSCD, the best option will be using stem cells from a non-ocular source, such as conjunctival epithelial cells obtained from biopsies [39]; however, this is hindered by an opaque media. Another strategy is cultivated oral mucosal epithelial transplantation (COMET). It has been used for treating patients with persistent epithelial defect (PET) and LSCD. In a study by Sotozono and colleagues, they achieved a complete and full reepithelization and managed to stabilize the ocular surface in patients with PET. They extracted oral mucosal epithelial cells from the patients (autologous) and cocultured them on the amniotic membrane with 3T3 feeder cells which are mitomycin-C inactivated and transplanted into the patients [40].

Mesenchymal Stem Cells (MSC)

MSC is a non-clonal and heterogenous mixture of multipotent stem cells, differentiated cells together with committed progenitors, and due to this, the proposed proper name for these cells is Mesenchymal Stromal Cells [41]. Many sources of MSCs have been identified, such as from the amniotic fluid, skin, umbilical cord [42], cord blood [43], peri vasculature [44], Wharton's Jelly connective tissues [45] as well as cord vein subendothelial layer [46].

MSCs are widely used in tissue engineering and regenerative medicine because they can be easily obtained due to their high differentiation ability. The risk of graft rejection of MSCs is less because these cells do not express the major histocompatibility proteins [47]. In 1970, A.J. Friedenstein managed to develop a fibroblast colony in monolayer cultures of Guinea Pig bone marrow and spleen. His work suggested that the stromal cells are the precursors of bone marrow and spleen fibroblasts [48]. Friedenstein also found these fibroblast precursors in normal and irradiated mouse hematopoietic organs. It is now also clear that the bone marrow contains cells that can differentiate into other cells. He found that the morphology is like fibroblasts, and the cells are adherent and able to differentiate [48].

Scaffold-free Cell Delivery

This method is attractive to researchers without the need for biodegradable scaffolds. The technique entails the preparation of 2D or 3D cell sheets for transplantation [49 - 51]. A thin layer of thermosensitive polymer, poly(N-isopropylacrylamide) (PIPAAm) was used as tissue culture coating [52], which facilitates cell harvesting with a reduction of temperature. Transplantable endothelial cell sheet with an abundant extracellular matrix containing collagen type IV and fibronectin was observed after cell sheet harvesting from the dishes [53].

Biomaterials for Corneal Tissue Regeneration

Tissue-engineered corneal replacement often require biomaterial scaffold system. The choice of scaffolds is matched to the properties of the tissue substitutes. For corneal stem cell transplantation, a scaffold which can support cells and act as the extracellular matrix would have to be permeable, thin, and flexible. The scaffold should also be degradable, and when it degrades, it should not release any cytotoxic or inflammatory materials. Thicker 3D scaffold is preferred, as opposed to 2D cell sheet for epithelium and endothelial layers, which are needed for corneal stroma replacement [54].

Cellularised Scaffolds

It is important to consider whether to integrate the cellular component into the scaffold or implant acellular scaffold [55]. The latter is commonly adopted to deliver certain biomolecules to inhibit inflammation, scarring, and overt vascularisation [55]. The choice of cellular source will be discussed in the cellular component section. The chemical and physical properties of the scaffold, such as stiffness, will influence cell adhesion, migration, proliferation, and production of the extracellular matrix [54]. Expression of the proliferation markers phospho-extracellular responsive kinase (pERK) and nuclear protein Ki67 is higher in the stiffer substrate than the softer one. Cells on the stiffer substrate also have higher expression of the cytokeratin gene (*CK3*), a marker for mature epithelial cells. Therefore, tuning the stiffness of the scaffold by either polymer/crosslinker concentration or crosslinking time is a likely modification.

Polymers in Corneal Tissue Engineering

Polymers show a good performance in tissue engineering as the cells can perform well on the polymer surface. Cells can adhere, migrate, proliferate, and differentiate very well with many polymers [56]. Polymers used in this field are either naturally occurring or synthetic polymers. Naturally occurring polymers are well known as good biocompatible materials and are categorized into protein, hyaluronic acid products, polynucleotides, and polysaccharides. Polymers are favoured in tissue engineering due to the ease of synthesis and manipulation of different properties of their monomers to suit the type of applications.

Natural Scaffolds

The traditional use of natural biological scaffolds such as human amniotic membrane (AM) has undergone intense scrutiny. A human AM is usually harvested from donors during elective lower-segment caesarean section, subjected to costly infectious screening, and presents donor-to-donor variability. Although enriched with growth factors with anti-inflammatory and anti-angiogenic properties, human AM cell carriers are challenged with membrane thickness, mechanical strength, and translucency [57].

Fibrin Cell Carrier

Limbal stem cells cultivated on fibrin cell carriers with the use of a lethally inactivated 3T3-J2 feeder layer had demonstrated a successful outcome in treating eyes with limbal stem cell deficiency (LSCD) [58]. Holoclar emerged as the first commercially available advanced therapy medicinal product for LSCD in 2015 [59]. However, it was reserved for autologous treatment following chemical or thermal burns. Fibrin carriers were also associated with xenogenic culture protocols and feeder cells [58].

Collagen Hydrogels

Hydrogels are widely used in tissue regeneration because of their high water content, three-dimensional (3D) structure, adjustable properties, and ample mass transfer. Real Architecture for 3D tissues (RAFT) is a technology used to treat corneal disorders [60]. The initial type I collagen hydrogel 3D model was fundamentally weak due to the high proportion of water content, which was subsequently improved by blending it with other polymers to form a composite [61]. RAFT development introduced an optimum biomimetic endothelial and epithelial tissues for transplantation and worked as a model to study *in vitro* interaction between cells [60]. RAFT demonstrates successful co-culture of human limbal epithelial cells and corneal stromal stem cells with a minimal need for animal feeder cells [36].

Chitosan and Alginate Hydrogels

Chitosan has been used as well in the corneal epithelium regeneration as a scaffold. A study modified a chitosan membrane by crosslinking the membrane with [62]. One of the most widely investigated biopolymer hydrogels is calcium alginate which has a long history of supporting wound healing and biocompatibility [63]. Alginate is readily acceptable since it is quite similar to the epithelial extracellular matrix, which favours the adhesion, spread, and growth of cultivated corneal epithelia. Alginate microspheres have been encapsulated with collagen hydrogels as a composite for the development of drug delivery in the eye or as a corneal substitute [64].

Synthetic Polymers

Poor mechanical properties and high degradation rates are among some of the challenges with natural or biological scaffolds. The higher mechanical strength of non-hydrogel-based scaffolds made them a favourable choice in regenerative medicine.

Poly D,L-lactide-co-glycolide (PLGA)

PLGA has been used successfully in cornea tissue engineering. It is a biodegradable membrane of lactide and glycolide (50:50), which can be fabricated by electrospinning technique. PLGA has the ability to degrade *ex vivo* after one to one and a half month [65]. The use of electro-spun scaffold poly (lactide-c--glycoside)- PLGA was studied as a candidate to replace AM due to low cost and biodegradability, and prior serological screening was not essential [66]. Electrospinning technique allows firm control of the fiber diameter and the thickness of the polymer. PLGA was successfully tested on the rabbit cornea model, showing good expression of differentiated epithelia and corneal stem cells [65].

Polyhydroxyalkanoate (PHA)

Tissue-engineered nanofibrous scaffolds prepared by the electrospinning technique stimulate protein fibers in the extracellular matrix. One of the common polymers used in the synthesis of electrospun nanofibers scaffolds is PHA which has been used as a cell carrier for corneal transplant cells. Blending PHAs with natural and synthetic polymers is done by the electrospinning method to enhance the mechanical properties and reduce the crystallinity of the polymer, and this is often carried out as a strategy in regenerative medicine [67]. The *in vivo* studies showed the high rate of biocompatibility of the PHAs and could be tolerated in an excellent way inside the body [68].

Comparison between PHA to other polymers like Polylactic acid (PLA) demonstrated that *in vivo* degradation of PHA is slower than PLGA and PLA [69]. It is now common to improve and adjust the degradation rates, biocompatibility, mechanical properties, and biodegradability based on the purpose of the functional applications, which is possible by alteration of the monomeric structure of the PHAs [70]. The biodegradation of PHAs varies between different types, and the rate is governed by many factors like molecular weight, surface area, crystallinity, and the composition of the polymer as well as external factors like pH, temperature, and humidity.

PHAs have been used in many ocular applications, such as poly(3-hydroxybutyrate-co-3-hydroxyvalerate); which has been investigated for subretinal retinal pigment epithelium cell transplantation [71]. As a solution to avoid fibrosis following glaucoma drainage surgery [72]. In eyelid reconstruction, poly(3-hydroxybutyrate-co-3-hydroxyhexanoate) (PHBHHx) has been tested to substitute the tarsal plate repair [73]. Electrospun nanofibrous scaffold of PHBV/gelatin is another application for the expansion of limbal stem cells [74]. PCL and PHBV electrospun scaffolds have also been investigated as cellularised scaffolds for corneal keratocytes [75].

CONCLUSION

Regenerative strategies in the cornea evolve to find solutions for the limitations in corneal transplantation, such as graft rejection risks, scarcity of tissue donors, and disease transmission. The choice of biomaterials, biologics, or small molecules, with or without cellular components, weighs heavily on the knowledge and understanding of the anatomy and physiology of the ocular. Future directions in this area include induced pluripotent stem cells (iPSC) technology to answer the scarcity of cells and tissues and bioprinting to generate 3D corneal structures. Acellular carriers or scaffolds are emerging as a safer method in corneal regeneration with reduced cell-mediated or immune-related complications.

ACKNOWLEDGEMENTS

The authors acknowledge USM Research University (Individual) to grant funding to Bakiah Shaharuddin (1001/CIPPT/8012263) and the National University of Sudan for an academic grant to Mohamed Salih; We also thank Advanced Medical and Dental Institute librarians and Professor Sudesh Kumar of the Ecobiomaterial Research Laboratory, School of Biological Sciences, Universiti Sains Malaysia, for their assistance and collaboration.

REFERENCES

[1]   Shalom-Feuerstein R, Serror L, De La Forest Divonne S, *et al.* Pluripotent stem cell model reveals essential roles for miR-450b-5p and miR-184 in embryonic corneal lineage specification. Stem Cells 2012; 30(5): 898-909.
[http://dx.doi.org/10.1002/stem.1068] [PMID: 22367714]

[2]   Resnikoff S, Pascolini D, Etya'ale D, *et al.* Global data on visual impairment in the year 2002. Bull World Health Organ 2004; 82(11): 844-51.
[PMID: 15640920]

[3]   Meek KM, Knupp C. Corneal structure and transparency. Prog Retin Eye Res 2015; 49: 1-16.
[http://dx.doi.org/10.1016/j.preteyeres.2015.07.001] [PMID: 26145225]

[4]   Doughty MJ, Jonuscheit S. Corneal structure, transparency, thickness and optical density (densitometry), especially as relevant to contact lens wear—a review. Cont Lens Anterior Eye 2019; 42(3): 238-45.
[http://dx.doi.org/10.1016/j.clae.2018.11.014] [PMID: 30502960]

[5]   Dua HS, Faraj LA, Said DG, Gray T, Lowe J. Human corneal anatomy redefined: a novel pre-Descemet's layer (Dua's layer). Ophthalmology 2013; 120(9): 1778-85.
[http://dx.doi.org/10.1016/j.ophtha.2013.01.018] [PMID: 23714320]

[6]   Espana EM, Birk DE. Composition, structure and function of the corneal stroma. Exp Eye Res 2020; 198: 108137.
[http://dx.doi.org/10.1016/j.exer.2020.108137] [PMID: 32663498]

[7]   Mglinets VA. [Molecular genetics of development of cornea]. Genetika 2015; 51(1): 5-13.
[PMID: 25857188]

[8]   DelMonte DW, Kim T. Anatomy and physiology of the cornea. J Cataract Refract Surg 2011; 37(3): 588-98.

[http://dx.doi.org/10.1016/j.jcrs.2010.12.037] [PMID: 21333881]

[9]   Gipson IK, Spurr-Michaud SJ, Tisdale AS. Anchoring fibrils form a complex network in human and rabbit cornea. Invest Ophthalmol Vis Sci 1987; 28(2): 212-20.
[PMID: 8591898]

[10]   Hanna C, Bicknell DS, O'Brien JE. Cell turnover in the adult human eye. Arch Ophthalmol 1961; 65(5): 695-8.
[http://dx.doi.org/10.1001/archopht.1961.01840020697016] [PMID: 13711260]

[11]   Trinkaus-Randall V, Newton AW, Franzblau C. The synthesis and role of integrin in corneal epithelial cells in culture. Invest Ophthalmol Vis Sci 1990; 31(3): 440-7.
[PMID: 2108096]

[12]   Wu XY, Svoboda KKH, Trinkaus-Randall V. Distribution of F-actin, vinculin and integrin subunits (alpha6 and beta4) in response to corneal substrata. Exp Eye Res 1995; 60(4): 445-58.
[http://dx.doi.org/10.1016/S0014-4835(05)80101-0] [PMID: 7789424]

[13]   Jacobsen I, Jensen OA, Prause JU. Structure and composition of Bowman's membrane. Study by frozen resin cracking. Acta Ophthalmol 1984; 62(1): 39-53.
[http://dx.doi.org/10.1111/j.1755-3768.1984.tb06755.x] [PMID: 6720276]

[14]   Torricelli AAM, Wilson SE. Cellular and extracellular matrix modulation of corneal stromal opacity. Exp Eye Res 2014; 129: 151-60.
[http://dx.doi.org/10.1016/j.exer.2014.09.013] [PMID: 25281830]

[15]   Ambati BK, Nozaki M, Singh N, *et al.* Corneal avascularity is due to soluble VEGF receptor-1. Nature 2006; 443(7114): 993-7.
[http://dx.doi.org/10.1038/nature05249] [PMID: 17051153]

[16]   Boote C, Dennis S, Newton RH, Puri H, Meek KM. Collagen fibrils appear more closely packed in the prepupillary cornea: optical and biomechanical implications. Invest Ophthalmol Vis Sci 2003; 44(7): 2941-8.
[http://dx.doi.org/10.1167/iovs.03-0131] [PMID: 12824235]

[17]   Kamil S, Mohan RR. Corneal stromal wound healing: Major regulators and therapeutic targets. Ocul Surf 2021; 19: 290-306.
[http://dx.doi.org/10.1016/j.jtos.2020.10.006] [PMID: 33127599]

[18]   Olsen EG, Davanger M, Moen T. The role of microfilaments in the healing of the corneal endothelium. Acta Ophthalmol 1985; 63(1): 104-8.
[http://dx.doi.org/10.1111/j.1755-3768.1985.tb05226.x] [PMID: 4039518]

[19]   Eghrari AO, Riazuddin SA, Gottsch JD. Overview of the Cornea: Structure, Function, and Development. 1st ed. Elsevier Inc. 2015; Vol. 134.
[http://dx.doi.org/10.1016/bs.pmbts.2015.04.001]

[20]   Liu W, Lagutin OV, Mende M, Streit A, Oliver G. Six3 activation of Pax6 expression is essential for mammalian lens induction and specification. EMBO J 2006; 25(22): 5383-95.
[http://dx.doi.org/10.1038/sj.emboj.7601398] [PMID: 17066077]

[21]   Mathivanan S, Ji H, Simpson RJ. Exosomes: Extracellular organelles important in intercellular communication. J Proteomics 2010; 73(10): 1907-20.
[http://dx.doi.org/10.1016/j.jprot.2010.06.006] [PMID: 20601276]

[22]   Li SF, Han Y, Wang F, Su Y. Progress in exosomes and their potential use in ocular diseases. Int J Ophthalmol 2020; 13(9): 1493-8.
[http://dx.doi.org/10.18240/ijo.2020.09.23] [PMID: 32953591]

[23]   Samaeekia R, Rabiee B, Putra I, *et al.* Effect of human corneal mesenchymal stromal cell-derived exosomes on corneal epithelial wound healing. Invest Ophthalmol Vis Sci 2018; 59(12): 5194-200.
[http://dx.doi.org/10.1167/iovs.18-24803] [PMID: 30372747]

[24] Takahashi K, Yamanaka S. Induction of pluripotent stem cells from mouse embryonic and adult fibroblast cultures by defined factors. Cell 2006; 126(4): 663-76.
[http://dx.doi.org/10.1016/j.cell.2006.07.024] [PMID: 16904174]

[25] Mikhailova A, Ilmarinen T, Uusitalo H, Skottman H. Small-molecule induction promotes corneal epithelial cell differentiation from human induced pluripotent stem cells. Stem Cell Reports 2014; 2(2): 219-31.
[http://dx.doi.org/10.1016/j.stemcr.2013.12.014] [PMID: 24527395]

[26] Hongisto H, Ilmarinen T, Vattulainen M, Mikhailova A, Skottman H. Xeno- and feeder-free differentiation of human pluripotent stem cells to two distinct ocular epithelial cell types using simple modifications of one method. Stem Cell Res Ther 2017; 8(1): 291.
[http://dx.doi.org/10.1186/s13287-017-0738-4] [PMID: 29284513]

[27] Martínez García de la Torre RA, Nieto-Nicolau N, Morales-Pastor A, Casaroli-Marano RP. Determination of the Culture Time Point to Induce Corneal Epithelial Differentiation in Induced Pluripotent Stem Cells. Transplant Proc 2017; 49(10): 2292-5.
[http://dx.doi.org/10.1016/j.transproceed.2017.09.047] [PMID: 29198663]

[28] Koizumi N, Okumura N, Ueno M, Kinoshita S. New therapeutic modality for corneal endothelial disease using Rho-associated kinase inhibitor eye drops. Cornea 2014; 33(11) (Suppl. 11): S25-31.
[http://dx.doi.org/10.1097/ICO.0000000000000240] [PMID: 25289721]

[29] Jung B, Lee H, Kim S, Tchah H, Hwang C. Effect of Rho-Associated Kinase Inhibitor and Mesenchymal Stem Cell-Derived Conditioned Medium on Corneal Endothelial Cell Senescence and Proliferation. Cells 2021; 10(6): 1463.
[http://dx.doi.org/10.3390/cells10061463] [PMID: 34207965]

[30] Okumura N, Kakutani K, Inoue R, et al. Generation and feasibility assessment of a new vehicle for cell-based therapy for treating corneal endothelial dysfunction. PLoS One 2016; 11(6): e0158427.
[http://dx.doi.org/10.1371/journal.pone.0158427] [PMID: 27355373]

[31] Koizumi N, Okumura N, Kinoshita S. Development of new therapeutic modalities for corneal endothelial disease focused on the proliferation of corneal endothelial cells using animal models. Exp Eye Res 2012; 95(1): 60-7.
[http://dx.doi.org/10.1016/j.exer.2011.10.014] [PMID: 22067130]

[32] Miyagi H, Kim S, Li J, Murphy CJ, Thomasy SM. Topical rho-associated kinase inhibitor, Y27632, accelerates corneal endothelial regeneration in a canine cryoinjury model. Cornea 2019; 38(3): 352-9.
[http://dx.doi.org/10.1097/ICO.0000000000001823] [PMID: 30516555]

[33] Okumura N, Sakamoto Y, Fujii K, et al. Rho kinase inhibitor enables cell-based therapy for corneal endothelial dysfunction. Sci Rep 2016; 6(1): 26113.
[http://dx.doi.org/10.1038/srep26113] [PMID: 27189516]

[34] Meekins LC, Rosado-Adames N, Maddala R, Zhao JJ, Rao PV, Afshari NA. Corneal endothelial cell migration and proliferation enhanced by rho kinase (ROCK) inhibitors in *in vitro* and *in vivo* models. Invest Ophthalmol Vis Sci 2016; 57(15): 6731-8.
[http://dx.doi.org/10.1167/iovs.16-20414] [PMID: 27951595]

[35] Schlötzer-Schrehardt U, Zenkel M, Strunz M, et al. Potential Functional Restoration of Corneal Endothelial Cells in Fuchs Endothelial Corneal Dystrophy by ROCK Inhibitor (Ripasudil). Am J Ophthalmol 2021; 224: 185-99.
[http://dx.doi.org/10.1016/j.ajo.2020.12.006] [PMID: 33316261]

[36] Kureshi AK, Dziasko M, Funderburgh JL, Daniels JT. Human corneal stromal stem cells support limbal epithelial cells cultured on RAFT tissue equivalents. Sci Rep 2015; 5(1): 16186.
[http://dx.doi.org/10.1038/srep16186] [PMID: 26531048]

[37] Kruse FE. Stem cells and corneal epithelial regeneration. Eye (Lond) 1994; 8(2): 170-83.
[http://dx.doi.org/10.1038/eye.1994.42] [PMID: 7958018]

[38]   Mobaraki M, Abbasi R, Omidian Vandchali S, Ghaffari M, Moztarzadeh F, Mozafari M. Corneal repair and regeneration: Current concepts and future directions. Front Bioeng Biotechnol 2019; 7: 135.
[http://dx.doi.org/10.3389/fbioe.2019.00135] [PMID: 31245365]

[39]   Di Girolamo N, Bosch M, Zamora K, Coroneo MT, Wakefield D, Watson SL. A contact lens-based technique for expansion and transplantation of autologous epithelial progenitors for ocular surface reconstruction. Transplantation 2009; 87(10): 1571-8.
[http://dx.doi.org/10.1097/TP.0b013e3181a4bbf2] [PMID: 19461496]

[40]   Sotozono C, Inatomi T, Nakamura T, *et al.* Cultivated oral mucosal epithelial transplantation for persistent epithelial defect in severe ocular surface diseases with acute inflammatory activity. Acta Ophthalmol 2014; 92(6): e447-53.
[http://dx.doi.org/10.1111/aos.12397] [PMID: 24835597]

[41]   Squillaro T, Peluso G, Galderisi U. Clinical trials with mesenchymal stem cells: An update. Cell Transplant 2016; 25(5): 829-48.
[http://dx.doi.org/10.3727/096368915X689622] [PMID: 26423725]

[42]   Baksh D, Yao R, Tuan RS. Comparison of proliferative and multilineage differentiation potential of human mesenchymal stem cells derived from umbilical cord and bone marrow. Stem Cells 2007; 25(6): 1384-92.
[http://dx.doi.org/10.1634/stemcells.2006-0709] [PMID: 17332507]

[43]   Kögler G, Sensken S, Airey JA, *et al.* A new human somatic stem cell from placental cord blood with intrinsic pluripotent differentiation potential. J Exp Med 2004; 200(2): 123-35.
[http://dx.doi.org/10.1084/jem.20040440] [PMID: 15263023]

[44]   Sarugaser R, Lickorish D, Baksh D, Hosseini MM, Davies JE. Human umbilical cord perivascular (HUCPV) cells: a source of mesenchymal progenitors. Stem Cells 2005; 23(2): 220-9.
[http://dx.doi.org/10.1634/stemcells.2004-0166] [PMID: 15671145]

[45]   Wang HS, Hung SC, Peng ST, *et al.* Mesenchymal stem cells in the Wharton's jelly of the human umbilical cord. Stem Cells 2004; 22(7): 1330-7.
[http://dx.doi.org/10.1634/stemcells.2004-0013] [PMID: 15579650]

[46]   Covas DT, Siufi JLC, Silva ARL, Orellana MD. Isolation and culture of umbilical vein mesenchymal stem cells. Braz J Med Biol Res 2003; 36(9): 1179-83.
[http://dx.doi.org/10.1590/S0100-879X2003000900006] [PMID: 12937783]

[47]   Han Y, Li X, Zhang Y, Han Y, Chang F, Ding J. Mesenchymal Stem Cells for Regenerative Medicine. Cells 2019; 8(8): 886.
[http://dx.doi.org/10.3390/cells8080886] [PMID: 31412678]

[48]   Friedenstein AJ, Chailakhjan RK, Lalykin KS. The development of fibroblast colonies in marrow and spleen cells. Cell Tissue Kinet 1970; 3: 393-403.
[PMID: 5523063]

[49]   Ang SL, Sivashankari R, Shaharuddin B, Chuah JA, Tsuge T, Abe H, *et al.* Potential Applications of Polyhydroxyalkanoates as a Biomaterial for the Aging Population. Polym Degrad Stab 2020; p. 181.

[50]   Casaroli-Marano RP, Nieto-Nicolau N, Martínez-Conesa EM, Edel M, B Álvarez-Palomo A. Potential Role of Induced Pluripotent Stem Cells (IPSCs) for Cell-Based Therapy of the Ocular Surface. J Clin Med 2015; 4(2): 318-42.
[http://dx.doi.org/10.3390/jcm4020318] [PMID: 26239129]

[51]   Casaroli-Marano RP, Nieto-Nicolau N, Martínez-Conesa EM. Progenitor cells for ocular surface regenerative therapy. Ophthalmic Res 2013; 49(3): 115-21.
[http://dx.doi.org/10.1159/000345257] [PMID: 23257987]

[52]   Alexander A, Ajazuddin , Khan J, Saraf S, Saraf S. Polyethylene glycol (PEG)–Poly(N-isopropylacrylamide) (PNIPAAm) based thermosensitive injectable hydrogels for biomedical applications. Eur J Pharm Biopharm 2014; 88(3): 575-85.

[http://dx.doi.org/10.1016/j.ejpb.2014.07.005] [PMID: 25092423]

[53] Ide T, Nishida K, Yamato M, *et al.* Structural characterization of bioengineered human corneal endothelial cell sheets fabricated on temperature-responsive culture dishes. Biomaterials 2006; 27(4): 607-14.
[http://dx.doi.org/10.1016/j.biomaterials.2005.06.005] [PMID: 16099037]

[54] Ahearne M, Fernández-Pérez J, Masterton S, Madden PW, Bhattacharjee P. Designing Scaffolds for Corneal Regeneration. Adv Funct Mater 2020; 30.

[55] Liu J, Sheha H, Fu Y, Liang L, Tseng SCG. Update on amniotic membrane transplantation. Expert Rev Ophthalmol 2010; 5(5): 645-61.
[http://dx.doi.org/10.1586/eop.10.63] [PMID: 21436959]

[56] Saad B, Neuenschwander P, Uhlschmid GK, Suter UW. New versatile, elastomeric, degradable polymeric materials for medicine. Int J Biol Macromol 1999; 25(1-3): 293-301.
[http://dx.doi.org/10.1016/S0141-8130(99)00044-6] [PMID: 10416677]

[57] Pauklin M, Fuchsluger TA, Westekemper H, Steuhl KP, Meller D. Midterm results of cultivated autologous and allogeneic limbal epithelial transplantation in limbal stem cell deficiency. Dev Ophthalmol 2010; 45: 57-70.
[http://dx.doi.org/10.1159/000315020] [PMID: 20502027]

[58] Rama P, Matuska S, Paganoni G, Spinelli A, De Luca M, Pellegrini G. Limbal stem-cell therapy and long-term corneal regeneration. N Engl J Med 2010; 363(2): 147-55.
[http://dx.doi.org/10.1056/NEJMoa0905955] [PMID: 20573916]

[59] Pellegrini G, Lambiase A, Macaluso C, *et al.* From discovery to approval of an advanced therapy medicinal product-containing stem cells, in the EU. Regen Med 2016; 11(4): 407-20.
[http://dx.doi.org/10.2217/rme-2015-0051] [PMID: 27091398]

[60] Levis H, Kureshi A, Massie I, Morgan L, Vernon A, Daniels J. Tissue Engineering the Cornea: The Evolution of RAFT. J Funct Biomater 2015; 6(1): 50-65.
[http://dx.doi.org/10.3390/jfb6010050] [PMID: 25809689]

[61] Liu W, Deng C, McLaughlin CR, *et al.* Collagen–phosphorylcholine interpenetrating network hydrogels as corneal substitutes. Biomaterials 2009; 30(8): 1551-9.
[http://dx.doi.org/10.1016/j.biomaterials.2008.11.022] [PMID: 19097643]

[62] Li YH, Cheng CY, Wang NK, *et al.* Characterization of the modified chitosan membrane cross-linked with genipin for the cultured corneal epithelial cells. Colloids Surf B Biointerfaces 2015; 126: 237-44.
[http://dx.doi.org/10.1016/j.colsurfb.2014.12.029] [PMID: 25576808]

[63] Hunt NC, Grover LM. Encapsulation and culture of mammalian cells including corneal cells in alginate hydrogels. Methods Mol Biol 2013; 1014: 201-10.
[http://dx.doi.org/10.1007/978-1-62703-432-6_14] [PMID: 23690015]

[64] Majid QA, Fricker ATR, Gregory DA, *et al.* Natural Biomaterials for Cardiac Tissue Engineering: A Highly Biocompatible Solution. Front Cardiovasc Med 2020; 7: 554597.
[http://dx.doi.org/10.3389/fcvm.2020.554597] [PMID: 33195451]

[65] Deshpande P, Ramachandran C, Sefat F, *et al.* Simplifying corneal surface regeneration using a biodegradable synthetic membrane and limbal tissue explants. Biomaterials 2013; 34(21): 5088-106.
[http://dx.doi.org/10.1016/j.biomaterials.2013.03.064] [PMID: 23591389]

[66] Deshpande P, Ramachandran C, Sangwan VS, MacNeil S. Cultivation of limbal epithelial cells on electrospun poly (lactide-co-glycolide) scaffolds for delivery to the cornea. Methods Mol Biol 2013; 1014: 179-85.
[http://dx.doi.org/10.1007/978-1-62703-432-6_12] [PMID: 23690013]

[67] Sanhueza C, Acevedo F, Rocha S, Villegas P, Seeger M, Navia R. Polyhydroxyalkanoates as biomaterial for electrospun scaffolds. Int J Biol Macromol 2019; 124: 102-10.
[http://dx.doi.org/10.1016/j.ijbiomac.2018.11.068] [PMID: 30445089]

[68] Nelson T, Kaufman E, Kline J, Sokoloff L. The extraneural distribution of γ-hydroxybutyrate. J Neurochem 1981; 37(5): 1345-8.
[http://dx.doi.org/10.1111/j.1471-4159.1981.tb04689.x] [PMID: 7299403]

[69] Gogolewski S, Jovanovic M, Perren SM, Dillon JG, Hughes MK. Tissue response andin vivo degradation of selected polyhydroxyacids: Polylactides (PLA), poly(3-hydroxybutyrate) (PHB), and poly(3-hydroxybutyrate-co-3-hydroxyvalerate) (PHB/VA). J Biomed Mater Res 1993; 27(9): 1135-48.
[http://dx.doi.org/10.1002/jbm.820270904] [PMID: 8126012]

[70] Valappil SP, Misra SK, Boccaccini AR, Roy I. Biomedical applications of polyhydroxyalkanoates, an overview of animal testing and *in vivo* responses. Expert Rev Med Devices 2006; 3(6): 853-68.
[http://dx.doi.org/10.1586/17434440.3.6.853] [PMID: 17280548]

[71] Tezcaner A, Bugra K, Hasırcı V. Retinal pigment epithelium cell culture on surface modified poly(hydroxybutyrate-co-hydroxyvalerate) thin films. Biomaterials 2003; 24(25): 4573-83.
[http://dx.doi.org/10.1016/S0142-9612(03)00302-8] [PMID: 12951000]

[72] Löbler M, Sternberg K, Stachs O, Allemann R, Grabow N, Roock A, *et al.* et al. Polymers and drugs suitable for the development of a drug delivery drainage system in glaucoma surgery. J Biomed Mater Res - Part B Appl Biomater 2011; 97(B): 388-95.

[73] Zhou J, Peng SW, Wang YY, Zheng SB, Wang Y, Chen GQ. The use of poly(3-hydroxybutyrate-c--3-hydroxyhexanoate) scaffolds for tarsal repair in eyelid reconstruction in the rat. Biomaterials 2010; 31(29): 7512-8.
[http://dx.doi.org/10.1016/j.biomaterials.2010.06.044] [PMID: 20663550]

[74] Baradaran-Rafii A, Biazar E, Heidari-Keshel S. Cellular response of limbal stem cells on PHBV/gelatin nanofibrous scaffold for ocular epithelial regeneration. Int J Polym Mater 2015; 64(17): 879-87.
[http://dx.doi.org/10.1080/00914037.2015.1030658]

[75] Azari P, Luan NS, Gan SN, *et al.* Electrospun Biopolyesters as Drug Screening Platforms for Corneal Keratocytes. Int J Polym Mater 2015; 64(15): 785-91.
[http://dx.doi.org/10.1080/00914037.2015.1030648]

CHAPTER 10

Biomaterials and Their Applications for Bone Regeneration

Norazlina Mohamed[1,*]

[1] *Department of Pharmacology, Faculty of Medicine, Universiti Kebangsaan Malaysia, Cheras, Kuala Lumpur, 56000, Malaysia*

Abstract: Bones are the hardest tissue in the human body, but they may also sustain injuries when stressed. The most common injury that can occur to bone is fractures. Bones are unique in that they can heal themselves. However, failure of healing may occur if the bone defect is large. The healing process that occurred may not be perfect; nonunion and scar formation may occur, which eventually impair the function of the bone. The elderly is prone to the incidence of falling, which may cause bone fractures. This age group of individuals, especially women who are experiencing menopause, will face delays in fracture healing. This will ultimately affect the quality of life of these individuals. This situation has led researchers to venture into bone engineering or bone regeneration in order to facilitate bone healing and induce new bone formation which can restore bone function. Bone regeneration involves the usage of the bone scaffold as a starting point for new bone formation. The scaffolds must have specific characteristics to allow new bone growth without causing adverse effects on the surrounding tissue. This chapter discusses the biomaterials that can be used in developing scaffolds for use in bone regeneration. Their characteristics (advantages and disadvantages) and modifications of the scaffold to enhance their performance are also highlighted. Their usage as a drug delivery system is also described.

Keywords: Biomaterials, Bone engineering, Bone regeneration, Drug delivery, Scaffolds.

INTRODUCTION

Bone is a specialized tissue that is able to regenerate and heal itself upon injury. The most common bone injury that may occur is a bone fracture. The healing of bone fracture involves three major phases: reactive phase, reparative phase, and the remodeling phase [1]. The bone healing process usually occurs within a few months; however, remodeling phase may last until a few years [2]. However, the capacity of bone to regenerate is often limited by the size of the injury, which re-

---

* **Corresponding author Norazlina Mohamed:** Department of Pharmacology, Faculty of Medicine, Universiti Kebangsaan Malaysia, Cheras, Kuala Lumpur, 56000, Malaysia; E-mail: azlina@ppukm.ukm.edu.my

Mohd Fauzi Mh Busra, Daniel Law Jia Xian, Yogeswaran Lokanathan and Ruszymah Haji Idrus (Eds.)

sults in nonunion and the formation of scar tissue. This will eventually affect the strength and function of the bone.

Autologous bone graft (bone acquired from the same individual) is considered the gold standard for enhancing bone regeneration. The most common site for bone harvest is the iliac crest. However, several complications have been associated with autologous bone grafts, such as pain, sensory disturbances, infection, and hematoma [3]. As an alternative to autologous bone graft, allograft, *i.e.*, tissue graft from a donor of the same species as the recipient but not genetically identical, is also practiced. Despite the safety and availability of a large amount of bone with allograft, it still poses several complications, such as nonunion, fracture of the allograft, and infection [4]. Another alternative to bone graft is xenograft, bone obtained from a donor of different species such as coral, bovine or porcine. The risk of transmission of zoonotic diseases is the major setback of xenograft as well as loss of osteogenic and osteoinductive characteristics during the processing [5]. Due to the many complications which result from the autologous bone graft, bone allograft, and bone xenograft, the tissue engineering technique is being extensively studied for bone regeneration.

There are three key components that make up the triad of tissue engineering: i) Progenitor or stem cells for tissue formation, ii) Biomaterial scaffolds, either natural or synthetic, as a platform for tissue growth and development, and iii) Signaling molecules (proteins and growth factors) which will drive the growth and differentiation of cells within the scaffold [6]. This chapter will discuss one of the elements in tissue engineering *i.e.* the scaffolds, particularly for bone regeneration.

TYPES OF BIOMATERIALS FOR BONE SCAFFOLD

Biomaterial used as bone scaffold is responsible for providing structural and mechanical support for the regeneration and proliferation of cells, differentiation to suitable cell types, and, eventually, the synthesis of a mineralized new bone matrix that will replace the scaffold itself. Thus, in designing a scaffold for bone application, several criteria must be met, as depicted in Fig. (**1**).

The scaffold must have a suitable geometrical shape to be able to fill into the defective bone and acts as a guide for new bone formation. It must have bioactivity, biocompatibility, and biological properties that stimulate tissue attachment, avoid the formation of scars, support normal cellular activity without causing toxic effects, promote angiogenesis, and stimulate cell differentiation. The materials that make up the scaffold should be stable, have mechanical competence to support the load of new tissue, and have the ability to degrade gradually and eventually be replaced by natural host tissue. The porous structure of the scaffold is essential to allow cell penetration and tissue in-growth and facilitate vascularization and nutrient transport. The fabrication of the scaffold should be easily tailored to fit the size and shape of the defective bone area. It also must be easily reproducible for commercialization [7].

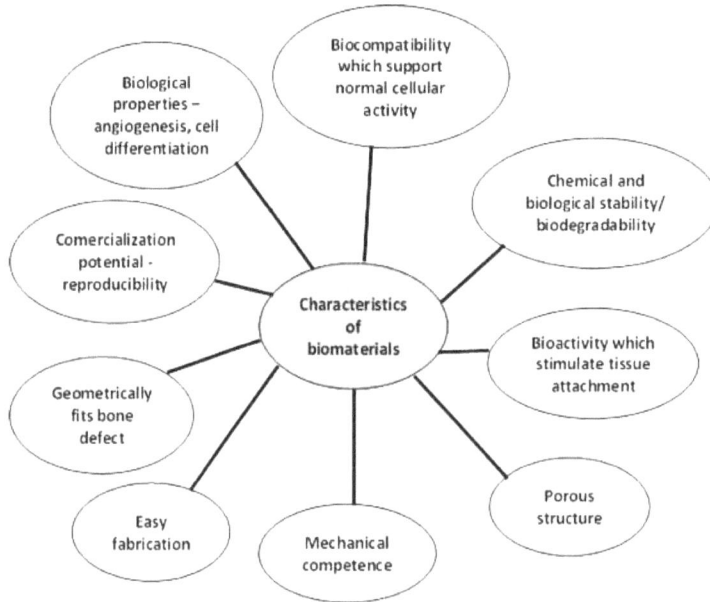

Fig. (1). Characteristics of biomaterials for bone regeneration.

In order to design a scaffold with the above characteristics, biomaterials that are used should also possess certain characteristics such as biocompatibility, biodegradability, specific porosity, and the ability to stimulate cellular proliferation and osteogenic differentiation at the healing site [8]. Good biomaterials should have a pore size ranging from 100 to 500 μm, the ability to allow the exchange of nutrients, and be able to promote vascularization and bone ingrowth [9]. Pore size is an important factor that can affect the number of nutrients being transported and the extent of cell penetration and ingrowth. The size must be large enough for cell migration but small enough for the binding of cells to the scaffold [10]. The scaffold will eventually degrade; however, the degradation rate must be in a controlled manner so that the newly generated bone is strong enough and able to provide support [11]. Scaffolds that are developed for bone regeneration should also be able to retain their shape, strength, and biological integrity throughout the regeneration process [12]. There are a few biomaterials that are suitable to be used as a bone substitute for bone repair, such as ceramics, metals, naturally derived polymers, and synthetic polymers.

Metallic Biomaterials

The available metallic biomaterials which are used for bone regeneration are silver, magnesium, cobalt, niobium, strontium, and titanium, with titanium being the most commonly used [13]. Metal ions influence the equilibrium between osteoblasts, osteoclasts, and osteocytes and thus may enhance or inhibit bone regeneration. For instance, magnesium (Mg^{2+}) enhances osteogenic differentiation, osteoblast proliferation, bone formation, and bone mineralization, while ferrous iron (Fe^{2+}) inhibits these processes [14].

As mentioned above, titanium is the metal most commonly used for bone regeneration. A study in rabbits has shown that titanium implants allow bone formation, which depends on porosity and pore sizes; with increased porosity and pore sizes, the bone formation will be enhanced [15]. Properties of titanium and titanium-based alloys, such as their biocompatibility, resistance to corrosion and wear, and high strength, are suitable for biomedical applications [16]. Titanium can react with other metal elements such as silver, aluminium, vanadium, and zinc to form alloys that improve their properties such as an increase in strength and a decrease in weight [17]. Pure titanium has sufficient mechanical and biocompatibility properties, which is favorable for use in dental implants [18]. For bone applications, such as hip and knee implants, which require better mechanical properties, the titanium-based alloy is commonly used [19]. However, studies have reported that pure titanium had similar properties as titanium-based alloy [20, 21].

It is difficult to manufacture titanium and its alloy using traditional manufacturing methods; thus, additive manufacturing is the solution that improves the end product that can be customized to patient's needs with high accuracy [22]. The two additive manufacturing processes that are suitable for bone implant applications are selective laser melting and electron beam melting. Titanium alloy scaffolds manufactured by selective laser melting displayed greater hardness and strength [23], good biocompatibility [24], and enhanced osteogenesis as well as osteointegration [25]. Similarly, the electron beam melting technique also improved the properties of titanium alloy as scaffolds for bone defects [26, 27].

Other alloys have also been reported to be beneficial as bone scaffolds. In an *in vivo* study, a combination of zinc and manganese was tested in a rat model of femoral condyle defect. Manganese was added to overcome the low strength and brittleness of pure zinc. It was observed that the addition of manganese improved the cytocompatibility and osteogenic properties of pure Zn. In addition, the porous Zn-Mn alloy scaffolds were able to induce new bone formation, indicating their potential for bone repair in the clinical setting [28]. Magnesium alloy has been shown to be superior to titanium-based alloy in terms of bone strength and osseointegration [29].

Metallic biomaterials are limited with several disadvantages, such as high elastic modulus, the release of metallic ions that cause adverse effects on tissue, the release of debris that cause toxicity to tissue, no bioactivity [30], and the risk of infection [31]. Surface modifications can be employed to the metal biomaterials to overcome the disadvantages. Modifications such as rapid electrochemical anodization treatment can enhance the bio-corrosion resistance, and bone cell responses [32], sand-blasted and acid-etched modified implants can produce higher bone contact and stability [33], atomic layer deposition can improve surface wettability [34] and nanohydroxyapatite coatings with nanosilver and nano copper can enhance antibacterial efficiency [35].

Ceramic Materials

Ceramic materials such as ceramic, glass, and glass-ceramic can be used as bone substitutes. Clinically, ceramic materials are used as solid pieces (in the reconstruction of middle ear ossicles or as load-bearing components of joint prostheses), as bone filling in powder or granule form, coatings on metal joint prostheses, as bone cement and porous scaffolds [7]. These materials are grouped under bioceramics which can be classified into i) Bioinert ceramics, ii) Bioactive ceramics, glasses, and glass-ceramics, and iii) Bioresorbable ceramics (Table **1**). Alumina and zirconia composites were shown to have biological compatibility for arthroplasty applications without any deleterious effects both *in vivo* and in vitro [36]. They are considered inert and thus have high biological safety. Their hard structure also makes them suitable as biomaterials in joint replacement [37].

Table 1. Classification of bioceramics [38].

Bioinert ceramics	Bioactive ceramics, glasses, and glass-ceramics	Bioresorbable ceramics
• Carbon • Alumina • Zirconia ceramics	• Hydroxyapatite • Bioglass • A-W glass-ceramic	• Tricalcium phosphate • Calcium sulphate

Calcium phosphate-based materials are the most studied and being used to elicit a biological response that is beneficial for bone repair [39]. In another report, it was observed that for the past ten years, hydroxyapatite (HA) was the most cited ceramic in studies related to bone regeneration, followed by calcium phosphate (CaP) and glass [13]. The advantages of ceramic materials are their hardness, good wettability, thus decreased adhesive wear, inert wear debris, thus no toxic effects, and high compressive strength. Their disadvantages include high brittleness, which lead to unexpected fractures, limitation in component fixation, high elastic modulus, and no bioactivity [40].

The most common ceramic materials used in bone regeneration are composed of calcium phosphate and tricalcium phosphate. These materials have a composition that is similar to human bone minerals and display bioactivity as well as osteoconductivity, which are suitable for bone regeneration [41]. In a previous study that compared hydroxyapatite, carbonate apatite, and β-tricalcium phosphate, it was found that carbonate apatite was the most stable and had the most bone formation compared to the other two compositions [42]. The features of these biomaterials can be improved by several modifications. The addition of cation strontium and magnesium to the tricalcium phosphate scaffold improved osteogenesis ability [43]. Hydroxyapatite composition with strontium substitution and the addition of alginate showed an improved bone formation ability *in vivo* compared to calcium phosphate material [44].

Further modification to these materials to enhance their suitability can be applied. Nanotopography technology by means of oxidative anodization was applied on the surface of alumina, which produced different pore diameters [45]. This improved the interaction between the biomaterial and recipient tissue in terms of higher cell adhesion and viability, thus, better bone healing and regeneration. The surface of alumina and zirconia can also be treated chemically and coated biomimetically with calcium-phosphate, which makes the surface become bioactive. In a previous study, the mixture of aluminium oxide (Al_2O_3) and zirconium dioxide (ZrO_2) was treated with several chemicals and coated with calcium phosphate. These modifications caused changes in the roughness of the surface, leading to favorable conditions for bone implants [46]. Modifications of bioceramics using nanotechnology, *i.e.*, nanostructured bioceramics and nanocomposites, have been shown to improve its properties, such as biocompatibility, osteoconductivity, biodegradation, and bioactivity. However certain disadvantages were also reported, such as poor mechanical properties and limited osteoinductivity [47].

Polymers

There are varieties of polymers that can be used in bone tissue engineering, which are categorized according to their sources: natural, synthetic, and semi-synthetic [48]. Natural polymers are mainly composed of proteins (collagen, silk fibroin) and polysaccharides (chitosan, alginate, hyaluronic acid, and cellulose). The properties that made them suitable for bone tissue engineering are bioactivity, biomimetic surface, and natural remodelling. However, there are also limitations, such as microbial contamination, reduced tunability, uncontrollable degradation rate, and weak mechanical strength [49]. Natural polymers can be either from plants (such as starch and cellulose) or animals/fungi (such as collagen, glycosaminoglycan, and keratin). Examples of synthetic polymers are poly(lactic acid), poly(glycolic acid), and poly(vinyl alcohol), while semi-synthetic polymers include methylcellulose and ethylcellulose. Collagen was reported as the most cited polymer for the development of bone tissue regeneration scaffolds, followed by gelatin, chitosan, poly (lactic-co-glycolic acid) (PLGA), polycaprolactone, alginates, hyaluronic acid, and polyvinyls [13].

The major protein present in the body is collagen which plays a role as connective tissue in many body parts, including bone. The use of collagen as a biomaterial in tissue engineering is favored due to its excellent biological features and physicochemical properties [50]. Collagen also mimics the natural environment for cells, which mediates cell attachment, and has high biocompatibility and low immunogenicity [51]. Pure collagen scaffolds need to be incorporated with other biomaterials to improve mechanical strength and osteoconductivity, for example, natural polymers such as glycosaminoglycans and silk fibroin. Chondroitin sulfate, which is a glycosaminoglycan acts as a coating material that improves the binding of osteoblasts and osteoclasts and attracts growth factors onto materials and cell surfaces. Another glycosaminoglycan, *i.e.*, hyaluronan, has the effect of recruiting osteoblast precursor cells from the bone marrow as well as regulating bone remodeling and osteogenic differentiation [52]. Collagen can also be incorporated with ceramics to improve strength, osteoconductive ability, and dimensional stability and increase the surface area for cell attachment [53]. Combination of human mesenchymal stem cells isolated from adipose tissue on collagen/Mg doped hydroxyapatite scaffold leads to an increase in the osteogenic process [54].

Several fabrication methods can be applied to develop collagen-based scaffolds which can be used in bone regeneration. Collagen molecules can undergo fibrillogenesis and exist in the form of a hydrogel that can be used as a bone scaffold with the advantage of promoting the adhesion, migration, and proliferation of bone marrow stromal cells [55]. Hydrogel displays superior mechanical strength and can provide nutrient environments suitable for endogenous cell growth [56]. Hydrogels have the ability to absorb huge amounts of water or biological fluids and swell without dissolving. Hydrogels which have absorbed water are soft and rubbery, which resemble living tissues [6]. It is reported that hydrogel mimics the properties of the extracellular cell matrix (ECM) of host tissue [57]. This environment is suitable for cellular proliferation and differentiation, allows the growth of bone cells in the hydrogel and secretion of new ECM, and subsequently restores bone tissue [58]. Other fabrication methods for collagen-based scaffolds include plastic compression, freeze-drying, compression molding and porogen leaching, electrospinning, and electrochemical fabrication. Each with its own advantages and disadvantages [51].

Silk fibroin polymer has high biocompatibility, can be modified for a regulated degradation rate, and can be processed into several forms, such as hydrogels, sponges, fibers, and microspheres [59], which provide suitable attributes as a bone scaffold. Unlike collagen, silk fibroin lacks the peptide which served as a recognition site for the binding of $\alpha 2 \beta 1$ integrin, which mediates osteoblast [60]. However, both polymers displayed similar efficacy in promoting bone regeneration [61]. The silk fibroin scaffold can be pre-seeded with pre-differentiated mesenchymal stem cells which display higher bone regenerative potential [62]. Another modification includes adding hydroxyapatite to the silk fibroin scaffold, which improves the mechanical properties as well as promotes mesenchymal stem cell differentiation and bone regeneration [63].

Synthetic polymers can be synthesized specifically so that it possesses the desired physicochemical and biological characteristics. The most commonly used synthetic polymers are Poly(ε-caprolactone) (PCL), polylactide (PDLA, PLLA), and Poly(lactide-co-glycolide acid) (PLGA) [49]. However, cell recognition sites and osteoconductivity are still lacking with pure synthetic polymers. The performance of these synthetic polymers can be improved further by incorporating them with other materials, such as bioactive molecules or nanoparticles [64]. PCL/alginate composite scaffold which was seeded with pre-osteoblasts, showed increased biological activities compared to pure PCL scaffolds [65]. The addition of hydroxyapatite to PLA scaffold improved mechanical properties and displayed higher cell adhesion, proliferation, and osteo-differentiation [66]. PLGA is a copolymer that consists of lactic (LA) and glycolic (GA) acids, which can be prepared at varied ratios. PLGA is preferred compared to PLA or PGA due to its wide range of degradation rates [67]. Similar to other synthetic polymers, PLGA can be modified with the addition of other materials, such as ceramics, to improve its properties and hence improved bone regeneration [68]. Table **2** lists the types of biomaterials used for bone tissue engineering and a brief description of their advantages and limitations.

NATURAL PRODUCTS AS BONE SCAFFOLD FOR BONE REGENERATION

Studies on plants as alternative materials for tissue engineering are on the rise. Fabrication of scaffolds from plants or plant-based materials is considered green chemistry since the materials used are safe and clean. Using plant-based scaffolds have advantages since the materials are renewable and can be mass-produced easily and inexpensively [78]. Plant tissue has an advantage over synthetic polymer or animal-derived material due to its unique cellulose skeleton that can act as a scaffold for mammalian cells [79].

Table 2. Types of biomaterials

Types of Biomaterials	Advantages	Limitations
Bioceramic: Calcium phosphate	Good bone conductivity [69]	High brittleness and limited mechanical strength [70].
Bioceramic: Bioactive glass	Excellent osteoinductive properties and the ability to promote osteogenesis [71]	Low mechanical strength and fracture toughness [72].
Metallic	High mechanical strength and fracture toughness [73]	Corrosion leads to toxicity and fatigue failure [74].
Biopolymers	Biocompatibility, high toughness, and plasticity [75]	Risks of immunogenic response and microbial contamination, as well as poor mechanical strength [49].
Composite materials (combination of two or more materials)	Improved porosity, stability, osteoinductivity, and osteogenicity [76]	Data on *in vivo* and clinical studies are still lacking; need more studies on different material combinations [77].

Different plant tissues vary in terms of morphological, physical, and mechanical properties; thus, different plants may be developed for tissue-specific scaffolds. Three different plant tissues (*i.e.*, apple, carrot, and celery) were investigated for the regeneration of adipose tissue, bone tissue, and tendons, respectively. Due to the different properties of these plants, the potential of these plants to be used for different tissue regeneration was established [80]. In a recent study, extracts of grape seed, pomegranate peel, and jabuticaba peel were combined with nanohydroxyapatite and anionic collagen for bone tissue repair. The extracts were used as collagen crosslinker agents and were able to increase the enzymatic resistance and thermal stability of collagen [81]. Other medicinal plants, such as *Spinacia oleracea* and *Eucomis autumnalis* extracts, were incorporated with natural biopolymers in the fabrication of a scaffold and were observed to have the potential for bone regeneration. The scaffold with *Spinacia oleracea* showed cellular biocompatibility [82], while *Eucomis autumnalis* scaffold showed osteoinductivity properties [83].

In another study, mangosteen peel was used in the development of a scaffold together with collagen from Tilapia fish skin, which was subjected to a phosphorylation process. The produced scaffold possessed thermal stability, and mineralization was able to occur, which signified its potential in bone tissue regeneration [84]. One of the properties of biomaterial used for the bone scaffold is biodegradation to allow *in vivo* tissue regeneration. The usage of plant tissue for bone scaffolds poses a challenge in terms of cellulose degradation. Plants that are subjected to decellularization and chemical oxidation processes were shown to have enhanced biocompatibility and biodegradation [85].

BONE SCAFFOLDS AS DELIVERY SYSTEM

Bone scaffolds do not just serve as a platform for new bone growth in bone regeneration but also can act as a delivery system for drugs, hormones, or growth factors which can enhance bone healing. Growth factors such as bone morphogenetic protein-2 (BMP-2) have been incorporated with a hydrogel which was fabricated with the addition of other polymers. It was observed that BMP-2 was released successfully from the system and caused an increase in alkaline phosphatase and mineralization [86]. Parathyroid hormone bound to modified hydrogel was able to induce bone formation comparable to autologous bone graft implantation [87]. For instance, hydrogel loaded with an agent that has anti-inflammatory and anti-osteoclastogenic effects was shown to enhance the osteogenic differentiation of rat bone marrow-derived mesenchymal stem cells and inhibit osteoclast formation [88].

Drugs can be loaded onto scaffolds *via* several methods: i) Mixing directly with scaffold material before fabrication [89], ii) Drugs entrapped in a basic drug carrier which is then added to scaffold material [90], iii) Coating the fabricated scaffold in a polymer or composite solution [91] and iv) Drugs impregnated on the fabricated scaffold [92]. When designing scaffolds for drug delivery, the scaffolds must be able to allow drug delivery to the tissues at a controlled rate in order to maintain drug concentration at the target sites. Drug levels must also be maintained at a level so that no excessive drug activity occurs at the target site that may lead to drug toxicity. The type of drug will determine the selection of compounds to be used for scaffold fabrication [93].

Besides drugs, bone scaffolds can also be the delivery system for other compounds, such as antioxidants. In one study, quercetin was incorporated into thermosensitive beta-glycerophosphate (bGP) chitosan/collagen hydrogels. It was observed that this system was effective as a scaffold for bone tissue engineering and able to sustain the release of natural flavonoids, which promote the growth of human periodontal ligament stem cells [94]. In another study, curcumin, which is an antioxidant and anti-inflammatory, was loaded onto β tricalcium phosphate scaffold to determine its effects on bone regeneration *in vivo*. Bone formation was enhanced in the presence of curcumin which indicates the success of curcumin release, which affects tissue regeneration [95]. Polyphenolic mixture extracted from a plant that possesses antioxidant and anti-inflammatory properties has also been incorporated into a ceramic biomaterial. It was observed that the phenolic was able to downregulate inflammation in macrophages, stimulate the expression of genes involved in bone matrix deposition, and decrease the RANKL/OPG ratio [96].

CHALLENGES AND THE FUTURE OF BONE TISSUE ENGINEERING

One of the challenges in bone tissue engineering is the selection of materials. As mentioned earlier, bone tissue engineering requires three key components, *i.e.*, cells, scaffolds, and signaling molecules. The selection of cell type, materials for scaffold, and combination of signaling molecules pose a challenge for optimum bone regeneration [97]. Even though single material such as bone scaffold has been proven beneficial in bone tissue engineering, no single material has all the properties to ensure efficient bone healing. There are many combinations and modifications that can be applied to materials that require further investigation [98]. The application of biomaterials or implants to heal bone defects may be challenging and may result in failure of healing, especially in aged or postmenopausal individuals. Coating the implant with specific small interfering RNA (siRNA) enables the controlled release of siRNA which can target a specific protein. In one study, a siRNA that targets cathepsin K was used, and it was observed that osteoclastic differentiation was inhibited and osteogenesis was promoted [99].

Another major challenge with regard to the bone scaffold is its translation to clinical settings. Bone scaffolds need to have the right design and right size with suitable materials, which have to be customized according to types of bone defects and fracture sites. Three-dimensional printing technologies enable the fabrication of bone scaffolds that can be tailored to the intended usage [100]. Optimization and improvement of 3D printing are made possible by means of artificial intelligence technology such as machine learning. Machine learning provides predictions which optimise printing parameters and maximise structure's properties. In addition, the quality of the printing can also be assessed [101].

The usage of conventional scaffolds had its advantages, such as limited compatibility and the inability to replicate the biological environment, which eventually affected the effectiveness and sustainability of bone regeneration. Earlier in this chapter, allograft and its limitation in use for bone healing were briefly described. The safety in the use of allograft can be enhanced by applying the decellularisation technique. Decellularized tissue can be the alternative to conventional scaffolds with the advantages of preserving its biomimetic property [102] and allowing better interaction between cells as opposed to conventional biomaterials [103]. Acellular bone tissue, which was seeded with bone marrow mesenchymal stem cells and used as bone allograft, showed osteogenic differentiation of cells [104]. Apart from using animal sources for decellularized tissue, plant-derived tissues have also been studied and have been described earlier. However, more exploration needs to be done due to the varieties of plants and their different features.

CONCLUSION

Much has been studied on biomaterials used for bone regeneration however, much is yet to be explored. Bone biomaterials have evolved from just a mere bone template to a bone regeneration system. The flexibility of the structure of scaffolds that can be modified and the ability of the scaffolds to be incorporated with various components open up endless possibilities in tissue engineering. Biocompatibility, osteoconductivity, and osteoinductivity of the scaffolds can be further improved with these modifications, which then facilitate interactions with cells and integration with host tissues and eventually enhance bone repair.

REFERENCES

[1] Affshana MM, Priya J. Healing mechanism in bone fracture. Journal of Pharmaceutical Sciences and Research 2015; 7(7): 441-2.

[2] Sheen JR, Garla VV. Fracture Healing Overview.StatPearls. Treasure Island, FL: StatPearls Publishing 2021. Updated 2021 May 12 Internet

[3] Dimitriou R, Mataliotakis GI, Angoules AG, Kanakaris NK, Giannoudis PV. Complications following autologous bone graft harvesting from the iliac crest and using the RIA: A systematic review. Injury 2011; 42 (Suppl. 2): S3-S15.
[http://dx.doi.org/10.1016/j.injury.2011.06.015] [PMID: 21704997]

[4] Delloye C, van Cauter M, Dufrane D, Francq BG, Docquier PL, Cornu O. Local complications of massive bone allografts: an appraisal of their prevalence in 128 patients. Acta Orthop Belg 2014; 80(2): 196-204.
[PMID: 25090792]

[5] Harsini SM, Tafti AK. Bone Regenerative Medicine and Bone Grafting. J Tissue Sci Eng 2018; 9: 220.

[6] Murphy CM, O'Brien FJ, Little DG, Schindeler A. Cell-scaffold interactions in the bone tissue engineering triad. Eur Cell Mater 2013; 26: 120-32.
[http://dx.doi.org/10.22203/eCM.v026a09] [PMID: 24052425]

[7] Baino F, Novajra G, Vitale-Brovarone C. Bioceramics and Scaffolds: A Winning Combination for Tissue Engineering. Front Bioeng Biotechnol 2015; 3: 202.
[http://dx.doi.org/10.3389/fbioe.2015.00202] [PMID: 26734605]

[8] Iaquinta M, Mazzoni E, Manfrini M, *et al.* Innovative Biomaterials for Bone Regrowth. Int J Mol Sci 2019; 20(3): 618.
[http://dx.doi.org/10.3390/ijms20030618] [PMID: 30709008]

[9] Li L, Li Y, Yang L, *et al.* Polydopamine coating promotes early osteogenesis in 3D printing porous Ti6Al4V scaffolds. Ann Transl Med 2019; 7(11): 240.
[http://dx.doi.org/10.21037/atm.2019.04.79] [PMID: 31317010]

[10] Yu J, Xia H, Ni QQ. A three-dimensional porous hydroxyapatite nanocomposite scaffold with shape memory effect for bone tissue engineering. J Mater Sci 2018; 53(7): 4734-44.
[http://dx.doi.org/10.1007/s10853-017-1807-x]

[11]   Ge Z, Jin Z, Cao T. Manufacture of degradable polymeric scaffolds for bone regeneration. Biomed Mater 2008; 3(2): 022001.
[http://dx.doi.org/10.1088/1748-6041/3/2/022001] [PMID: 18523339]

[12]   Alvarez K, Nakajima H. Metallic Scaffolds for Bone Regeneration. Materials (Basel) 2009; 2(3): 790-832.
[http://dx.doi.org/10.3390/ma2030790]

[13]   Girón J, Kerstner E, Medeiros T, *et al.* Biomaterials for bone regeneration: an orthopedic and dentistry overview. Braz J Med Biol Res 2021; 54(9): e11055.
[http://dx.doi.org/10.1590/1414-431x2021e11055] [PMID: 34133539]

[14]   Glenske K, Donkiewicz P, Köwitsch A, *et al.* Applications of Metals for Bone Regeneration. Int J Mol Sci 2018; 19(3): 826.
[http://dx.doi.org/10.3390/ijms19030826] [PMID: 29534546]

[15]   Vasconcellos LMR, Leite DO, Oliveira FN, Carvalho YR, Cairo CAA. Evaluation of bone ingrowth into porous titanium implant: histomorphometric analysis in rabbits. Braz Oral Res 2010; 24(4): 399-405.
[http://dx.doi.org/10.1590/S1806-83242010000400005] [PMID: 21180959]

[16]   Khorasani AM, Goldberg M, Doeven EH, Littlefair G. Titanium in biomedical applications—properties and fabrication: a review. J Biomater Tissue Eng 2015; 5(8): 593-619.
[http://dx.doi.org/10.1166/jbt.2015.1361]

[17]   Saini M, Singh Y, Arora P, Arora V, Jain K. Implant biomaterials: A comprehensive review. World J Clin Cases 2015; 3(1): 52-7.
[http://dx.doi.org/10.12998/wjcc.v3.i1.52] [PMID: 25610850]

[18]   Budei DV, Vaireanu DI, Prepelita P, Popescu-Pelin G, Mincu M, Ciobotaru I-A. A comparative morphological study of titanium dioxide surface layer dental implants. Open Chem 2021; 19(1): 189-98.
[http://dx.doi.org/10.1515/chem-2021-0197]

[19]   Sáenz de Viteri V, Fuentes E. Titanium and Titanium Alloys as Biomaterials.Tribology Fundamentals and Advancements. IntechOpen 2013.
[http://dx.doi.org/10.5772/55860]

[20]   Anchieta RB, Baldassarri M, Guastaldi F, *et al.* Mechanical property assessment of bone healing around a titanium-zirconium alloy dental implant. Clin Implant Dent Relat Res 2014; 16(6): 913-9.
[http://dx.doi.org/10.1111/cid.12061] [PMID: 23527994]

[21]   Shah FA, Trobos M, Thomsen P, Palmquist A. Commercially pure titanium (cp-Ti) versus titanium alloy (Ti6Al4V) materials as bone anchored implants — Is one truly better than the other? Mater Sci Eng C 2016; 62: 960-6.
[http://dx.doi.org/10.1016/j.msec.2016.01.032] [PMID: 26952502]

[22]   Agapovichev A, Sotov A, Kokareva V, Smelov V. Possibilities and limitations of titanium alloy additive manufacturing. Matec Web Conf.
[http://dx.doi.org/10.1051/matecconf/201822401064]

[23]   Ataee A, Li Y, Brandt M, Wen C. Ultrahigh-strength titanium gyroid scaffolds manufactured by selective laser melting (SLM) for bone implant applications. Acta Mater 2018; 158: 354-68.
[http://dx.doi.org/10.1016/j.actamat.2018.08.005]

[24]   Li Y, Ding Y, Munir K, *et al.* Novel β-Ti35Zr28Nb alloy scaffolds manufactured using selective laser melting for bone implant applications. Acta Biomater 2019; 87: 273-84.
[http://dx.doi.org/10.1016/j.actbio.2019.01.051] [PMID: 30690210]

[25]   Guo Y, Wu J, Xie K, *et al.* Study of Bone Regeneration and Osteointegration Effect of a Novel Selective Laser-Melted Titanium-Tantalum-Niobium-Zirconium Alloy Scaffold. ACS Biomater Sci Eng 2019; 5(12): 6463-73.

[http://dx.doi.org/10.1021/acsbiomaterials.9b00909] [PMID: 33417799]

[26] Wang H, Zhao BJ, Yan RZ, Wang C, Luo CC, Hu M. [Evaluation of biocompatibility of Ti-6Al-4V scaffolds fabricated by electron beam melting]. Chung Hua Kou Chiang Hsueh Tsa Chih 2016; 51(11): 667-72.
[PMID: 27806759]

[28] Jia B, Yang H, Han Y, *et al.* In vitro and *in vivo* studies of Zn-Mn biodegradable metals designed for orthopedic applications. Acta Biomater 2020; 108: 358-72.
[http://dx.doi.org/10.1016/j.actbio.2020.03.009] [PMID: 32165194]

[29] Castellani C, Lindtner RA, Hausbrandt P, *et al.* Bone–implant interface strength and osseointegration: Biodegradable magnesium alloy versus standard titanium control. Acta Biomater 2011; 7(1): 432-40.
[http://dx.doi.org/10.1016/j.actbio.2010.08.020] [PMID: 20804867]

[30] Bahraminasab M, Sahari BB, Edwards KL, Farahmand F, Arumugam M. Aseptic loosening of femoral components – Materials engineering and design considerations. Mater Des 2013; 44: 155-63.
[http://dx.doi.org/10.1016/j.matdes.2012.07.066]

[31] Li J, Li P, Lu H, *et al.* Digital design and individually fabricated titanium implants for the reconstruction of traumatic zygomatico-orbital defects. J Craniofac Surg 2013; 24(2): 363-8.
[http://dx.doi.org/10.1097/SCS.0b013e3182701243] [PMID: 23524694]

[32] Liu CF, Lee TH, Liu JF, *et al.* A unique hybrid-structured surface produced by rapid electrochemical anodization enhances bio-corrosion resistance and bone cell responses of β-type Ti-24Nb-4Zr-8Sn alloy. Sci Rep 2018; 8(1): 6623.
[http://dx.doi.org/10.1038/s41598-018-24590-x] [PMID: 29700340]

[33] Abdel-Haq J, Karabuda CZ, Arısan V, Mutlu Z, Kürkçü M. Osseointegration and stability of a modified sand-blasted acid-etched implant: an experimental pilot study in sheep. Clin Oral Implants Res 2011; 22(3): 265-74.
[http://dx.doi.org/10.1111/j.1600-0501.2010.01990.x] [PMID: 20946211]

[34] Patel S, Butt A, Tao Q, *et al.* Novel functionalization of Ti-V alloy and Ti-II using atomic layer deposition for improved surface wettability. Colloids Surf B Biointerfaces 2014; 115: 280-5.
[http://dx.doi.org/10.1016/j.colsurfb.2013.11.038] [PMID: 24384144]

[35] Bartmański M, Pawłowski Ł, Belcarz A, *et al.* The Chemical and Biological Properties of Nanohydroxyapatite Coatings with Antibacterial Nanometals, Obtained in the Electrophoretic Process on the Ti13Zr13Nb Alloy. Int J Mol Sci 2021; 22(6): 3172.
[http://dx.doi.org/10.3390/ijms22063172] [PMID: 33804677]

[36] Roualdes O, Duclos ME, Gutknecht D, Frappart L, Chevalier J, Hartmann DJ. In vitro and *in vivo* evaluation of an alumina–zirconia composite for arthroplasty applications. Biomaterials 2010; 31(8): 2043-54.
[http://dx.doi.org/10.1016/j.biomaterials.2009.11.107] [PMID: 20053439]

[37] Piconi C, Porporati AA. Bioinert Ceramics: Zirconia and Alumina.Handbook of Bioceramics and Biocomposites. Cham: Springer 2016.
[http://dx.doi.org/10.1007/978-3-319-12460-5_4]

[38] Wang M, Guo L, Sun H. Manufacturing Technologies for Biomaterials.Encyclopedia of Biomedical Engineering. Elsevier 2019; pp. 116-34.
[http://dx.doi.org/10.1016/B978-0-12-801238-3.11027-X]

[39] Jones JR, Gibson IR. Ceramics, Glasses, and Glass-Ceramics. In: Wagner WR, Sakiyama-Elbert SE, Zhang G, Yaszemski MJ, Eds. Biomaterials Science. An Introduction to Materials in Medicine Fourth Edition. Academic Press, 2020; 289–306.

[40] Masala S, Taglieri A, Chiaravalloti A, *et al.* Thoraco-lumbar traumatic vertebral fractures augmentation by osteo-conductive and osteo-inductive bone substitute containing strontium–hydroxyapatite: our experience. Neuroradiology 2014; 56(6): 459-66.

[http://dx.doi.org/10.1007/s00234-014-1351-1] [PMID: 24652532]

[41]   Trimeche M. Biomaterials for bone regeneration: an overview. Biomater Tissue Technol 2017; 1(2): 1-5.

[42]   Ishikawa K, Miyamoto Y, Tsuchiya A, Hayashi K, Tsuru K, Ohe G. Physical and Histological Comparison of Hydroxyapatite, Carbonate Apatite, and β-Tricalcium Phosphate Bone Substitutes. Materials (Basel) 2018; 11(10): 1993.
[http://dx.doi.org/10.3390/ma11101993] [PMID: 30332751]

[43]   Tarafder S, Davies NM, Bandyopadhyay A, Bose S. 3D printed tricalcium phosphate scaffolds: Effect of SrO and MgO doping on *in vivo* osteogenesis in a rat distal femoral defect model. Biomater Sci 2013; 1(12): 1250-9.
[http://dx.doi.org/10.1039/c3bm60132c] [PMID: 24729867]

[44]   Sprio S, Dapporto M, Montesi M, *et al.* Novel Osteointegrative Sr-Substituted Apatitic Cements Enriched with Alginate. Materials (Basel) 2016; 9(9): 763.
[http://dx.doi.org/10.3390/ma9090763] [PMID: 28773884]

[45]   Mussano F, Genova T, Serra F, Carossa M, Munaron L, Carossa S. Nano-Pore Size of Alumina Affects Osteoblastic Response. Int J Mol Sci 2018; 19(2): 528.
[http://dx.doi.org/10.3390/ijms19020528] [PMID: 29425177]

[46]   dos Santos KH, Ferreira JA, Osiro D, *et al.* Influence of different chemical treatments on the surface of Al2O3/ZrO2 nanocomposites during biomimetic coating. Ceram Int 2017; 43(5): 4272-9.
[http://dx.doi.org/10.1016/j.ceramint.2016.12.069]

[47]   Lyons JG, Plantz MA, Hsu WK, Hsu EL, Minardi S. Nanostructured Biomaterials for Bone Regeneration. Front Bioeng Biotechnol 2020; 8: 922.
[http://dx.doi.org/10.3389/fbioe.2020.00922] [PMID: 32974298]

[48]   Filippi M, Born G, Chaaban M, Scherberich A. Natural Polymeric Scaffolds in Bone Regeneration. Front Bioeng Biotechnol 2020; 8: 474.
[http://dx.doi.org/10.3389/fbioe.2020.00474] [PMID: 32509754]

[49]   Chocholata P, Kulda V, Babuska V. Fabrication of Scaffolds for Bone-Tissue Regeneration. Materials (Basel) 2019; 12(4): 568.
[http://dx.doi.org/10.3390/ma12040568] [PMID: 30769821]

[50]   Ferreira AM, Gentile P, Chiono V, Ciardelli G. Collagen for bone tissue regeneration. Acta Biomater 2012; 8(9): 3191-200.
[http://dx.doi.org/10.1016/j.actbio.2012.06.014] [PMID: 22705634]

[51]   Nijsure MP, Kishore V. Collagen-Based Scaffolds for Bone Tissue Engineering Applicat ions.Orthopedic Biomaterials Springer. 2017.
[http://dx.doi.org/10.1007/978-3-319-73664-8_8]

[52]   Zhang D, Wu X, Chen J, Lin K. The development of collagen based composite scaffolds for bone regeneration. Bioact Mater 2018; 3(1): 129-38.
[http://dx.doi.org/10.1016/j.bioactmat.2017.08.004] [PMID: 29744450]

[53]   Yunus Basha R, Sampath Kumar TS, Doble M. Design of biocomposite materials for bone tissue regeneration. Mater Sci Eng C 2015; 57: 452-63.
[http://dx.doi.org/10.1016/j.msec.2015.07.016] [PMID: 26354284]

[54]   Calabrese G, Giuffrida R, Fabbi C, *et al.* Collagen-Hydroxyapatite Scaffolds Induce Human Adipose Derived Stem Cells Osteogenic Differentiation In Vitro. PLoS One 2016; 11(3): e0151181.
[http://dx.doi.org/10.1371/journal.pone.0151181] [PMID: 26982592]

[55]   Hesse E, Hefferan TE, Tarara JE, *et al.* Collagen type I hydrogel allows migration, proliferation, and osteogenic differentiation of rat bone marrow stromal cells. J Biomed Mater Res A 2010; 9999A(2): NA.
[http://dx.doi.org/10.1002/jbm.a.32696] [PMID: 20186733]

[56] Bai X, Gao M, Syed S, Zhuang J, Xu X, Zhang XQ. Bioactive hydrogels for bone regeneration. Bioact Mater 2018; 3(4): 401-17.
[http://dx.doi.org/10.1016/j.bioactmat.2018.05.006] [PMID: 30003179]

[57] Geckil H, Xu F, Zhang X, Moon S, Demirci U. Engineering hydrogels as extracellular matrix mimics. Nanomedicine (Lond) 2010; 5(3): 469-84.
[http://dx.doi.org/10.2217/nnm.10.12] [PMID: 20394538]

[58] Kondiah P, Choonara Y, Kondiah P, *et al.* A Review of Injectable Polymeric Hydrogel Systems for Application in Bone Tissue Engineering. Molecules 2016; 21(11): 1580.
[http://dx.doi.org/10.3390/molecules21111580] [PMID: 27879635]

[59] Melke J, Midha S, Ghosh S, Ito K, Hofmann S. Silk fibroin as biomaterial for bone tissue engineering. Acta Biomater 2016; 31: 1-16.
[http://dx.doi.org/10.1016/j.actbio.2015.09.005] [PMID: 26360593]

[60] Mizuno M, Fujisawa R, Kuboki Y. Type I collagen-induced osteoblastic differentiation of bone-marrow cells mediated by collagen-?2?1 integrin interaction. J Cell Physiol 2000; 184(2): 207-13.
[http://dx.doi.org/10.1002/1097-4652(200008)184:2<207::AID-JCP8>3.0.CO;2-U] [PMID: 10867645]

[61] Kim JY, Yang BE, Ahn JH, Park SO, Shim HW. Comparable efficacy of silk fibroin with the collagen membranes for guided bone regeneration in rat calvarial defects. J Adv Prosthodont 2014; 6(6): 539-46.
[http://dx.doi.org/10.4047/jap.2014.6.6.539] [PMID: 25551015]

[62] Meinel L, Betz O, Fajardo R, *et al.* Silk based biomaterials to heal critical sized femur defects. Bone 2006; 39(4): 922-31.
[http://dx.doi.org/10.1016/j.bone.2006.04.019] [PMID: 16757219]

[63] McNamara SL, Rnjak-Kovacina J, Schmidt DF, Lo TJ, Kaplan DL. Silk as a biocohesive sacrificial binder in the fabrication of hydroxyapatite load bearing scaffolds. Biomaterials 2014; 35(25): 6941-53.
[http://dx.doi.org/10.1016/j.biomaterials.2014.05.013] [PMID: 24881027]

[64] Shi C, Yuan Z, Han F, Zhu C, Li B. Polymeric biomaterials for bone regeneration. Ann Joint 2016; 1(9): 27.
[http://dx.doi.org/10.21037/aoj.2016.11.02]

[65] Kim MS, Kim G. Three-dimensional electrospun polycaprolactone (PCL)/alginate hybrid composite scaffolds. Carbohydr Polym 2014; 114: 213-21.
[http://dx.doi.org/10.1016/j.carbpol.2014.08.008] [PMID: 25263884]

[66] Holmes B, Bulusu K, Plesniak M, Zhang LG. A synergistic approach to the design, fabrication and evaluation of 3D printed micro and nano featured scaffolds for vascularized bone tissue repair. Nanotechnology 2016; 27(6): 064001.
[http://dx.doi.org/10.1088/0957-4484/27/6/064001] [PMID: 26758780]

[67] Gentile P, Chiono V, Carmagnola I, Hatton P. An overview of poly(lactic-co-glycolic) acid (PLGA)-based biomaterials for bone tissue engineering. Int J Mol Sci 2014; 15(3): 3640-59.
[http://dx.doi.org/10.3390/ijms15033640] [PMID: 24590126]

[68] Pan Z, Ding J. Poly(lactide- *co* -glycolide) porous scaffolds for tissue engineering and regenerative medicine. Interface Focus 2012; 2(3): 366-77.
[http://dx.doi.org/10.1098/rsfs.2011.0123] [PMID: 23741612]

[69] Fukuda N, Tsuru K, Mori Y, Ishikawa K. Fabrication of self-setting β-tricalcium phosphate granular cement. J Biomed Mater Res B Appl Biomater 2018; 106(2): 800-7.
[http://dx.doi.org/10.1002/jbm.b.33891] [PMID: 28370963]

[70] Castro AGB, Polini A, Azami Z, *et al.* Incorporation of PLLA micro-fillers for mechanical reinforcement of calcium-phosphate cement. J Mech Behav Biomed Mater 2017; 71: 286-94.
[http://dx.doi.org/10.1016/j.jmbbm.2017.03.027] [PMID: 28376362]

[71]   Jia W, Lau GY, Huang W, Zhang C, Tomsia AP, Fu Q. Bioactive Glass for Large Bone Repair. Adv Healthc Mater 2015; 4(18): 2842-8.
[http://dx.doi.org/10.1002/adhm.201500447] [PMID: 26582584]

[72]   Kaur G, Kumar V, Baino F, *et al.* Mechanical properties of bioactive glasses, ceramics, glass-ceramics and composites: State-of-the-art review and future challenges. Mater Sci Eng C 2019; 104: 109895.
[http://dx.doi.org/10.1016/j.msec.2019.109895] [PMID: 31500047]

[73]   Bazaka O, Bazaka K, Kingshott P, *et al.* Metallic Implants for Biomedical Applications.The Chemistry of Inorganic Biomaterials. RSC Publishing 2021; pp. 1-98.
[http://dx.doi.org/10.1039/9781788019828-00001]

[74]   Chen Q, Thouas GA. Metallic implant biomaterials. Mater Sci Eng Rep 2015; 87: 1-57.
[http://dx.doi.org/10.1016/j.mser.2014.10.001]

[75]   Kashirina A, Yao Y, Liu Y, Leng J. Biopolymers as bone substitutes: a review. Biomater Sci 2019; 7(10): 3961-83.
[http://dx.doi.org/10.1039/C9BM00664H] [PMID: 31364613]

[76]   Tang G, Liu Z, Liu Y, *et al.* Recent Trends in the Development of Bone Regenerative Biomaterials. Front Cell Dev Biol 2021; 9: 665813.
[http://dx.doi.org/10.3389/fcell.2021.665813] [PMID: 34026758]

[77]   Jahan K, Tabrizian M. Composite biopolymers for bone regeneration enhancement in bony defects. Biomater Sci 2016; 4(1): 25-39.
[http://dx.doi.org/10.1039/C5BM00163C] [PMID: 26317131]

[78]   Iravani S, Varma RS. Plants and plant-based polymers as scaffolds for tissue engineering. Green Chem 2019; 21(18): 4839-67.
[http://dx.doi.org/10.1039/C9GC02391G]

[79]   Bilirgen AC, Toker M, Odabas S, Yetisen AK, Garipcan B, Tasoglu S. Plant-Based Scaffolds in Tissue Engineering. ACS Biomater Sci Eng 2021; 7(3): 926-38.
[http://dx.doi.org/10.1021/acsbiomaterials.0c01527] [PMID: 33591719]

[80]   Contessi Negrini N, Toffoletto N, Farè S, Altomare L. Plant Tissues as 3D Natural Scaffolds for Adipose, Bone and Tendon Tissue Regeneration. Front Bioeng Biotechnol 2020; 8: 723.
[http://dx.doi.org/10.3389/fbioe.2020.00723] [PMID: 32714912]

[81]   Garcia CF, Marangon CA, Massimino LC, Klingbeil MFG, Martins VCA, Plepis AMG. Development of collagen/nanohydroxyapatite scaffolds containing plant extract intended for bone regeneration. Mater Sci Eng C 2021; 123: 111955.
[http://dx.doi.org/10.1016/j.msec.2021.111955] [PMID: 33812583]

[82]   Sharmila G, Muthukumaran C, Kirthika S, Keerthana S, Kumar NM, Jeyanthi J. Fabrication and characterization of Spinacia oleracea extract incorporated alginate/carboxymethyl cellulose microporous scaffold for bone tissue engineering. Int J Biol Macromol 2020; 156: 430-7.
[http://dx.doi.org/10.1016/j.ijbiomac.2020.04.059] [PMID: 32294496]

[83]   Alaribe FN, Motaung SCKM. Fabrication of herbal scaffold for bone tissue engineering using *Eucomis autumnalis* plant extract. J Bioeng Biomed Sci 2016; 6(4) (Suppl.): 48.

[84]   Milan EP, Rodrigues MÁV, Martins VCA, Plepis AMG, Fuhrmann-Lieker T, Horn MM. Mineralization of Phosphorylated Fish Skin Collagen/Mangosteen Scaffolds as Potential Materials for Bone Tissue Regeneration. Molecules 2021; 26(10): 2899.
[http://dx.doi.org/10.3390/molecules26102899] [PMID: 34068232]

[85]   S H A, Mohan CC, P S U, Krishnan AG, Nair MB. Decellularization and oxidation process of bamboo stem enhance biodegradation and osteogenic differentiation. Mater Sci Eng C 2021; 119: 111500.
[http://dx.doi.org/10.1016/j.msec.2020.111500] [PMID: 33321600]

[86]   Kim HK, Shim WS, Kim SE, *et al.* Injectable *in situ*-forming pH/thermo-sensitive hydrogel for bone

tissue engineering. Tissue Eng Part A 2009; 15(4): 923-33.
[http://dx.doi.org/10.1089/ten.tea.2007.0407] [PMID: 19061427]

[87]   Jung RE, Cochran DL, Domken O, *et al.* The effect of matrix bound parathyroid hormone on bone regeneration. Clin Oral Implants Res 2007; 18(3): 319-25.
[http://dx.doi.org/10.1111/j.1600-0501.2007.01342.x] [PMID: 17386063]

[88]   Zhou W, Li Q, Ma R, *et al.* Modified Alginate-Based Hydrogel as a Carrier of the CB2 Agonist JWH133 for Bone Engineering. ACS Omega 2021; 6(10): 6861-70.
[http://dx.doi.org/10.1021/acsomega.0c06057] [PMID: 33748600]

[89]   Meng ZX, Zheng W, Li L, Zheng YF. Fabrication, characterization and in vitro drug release behavior of electrospun PLGA/chitosan nanofibrous scaffold. Mater Chem Phys 2011; 125(3): 606-11.
[http://dx.doi.org/10.1016/j.matchemphys.2010.10.010]

[90]   Bennet D, Marimuthu M, Kim S, An J. Dual drug-loaded nanoparticles on self-integrated scaffold for controlled delivery. Int J Nanomedicine 2012; 7: 3399-419.
[PMID: 22888222]

[91]   Kim HW, Knowles JC, Kim HE. Development of hydroxyapatite bone scaffold for controlled drug release via poly(?-caprolactone) and hydroxyapatite hybrid coatings. J Biomed Mater Res 2004; 70B(2): 240-9.
[http://dx.doi.org/10.1002/jbm.b.30038] [PMID: 15264306]

[92]   Kundu B, Soundrapandian C, Nandi SK, *et al.* Development of new localized drug delivery system based on ceftriaxone-sulbactam composite drug impregnated porous hydroxyapatite: a systematic approach for in vitro and *in vivo* animal trial. Pharm Res 2010; 27(8): 1659-76.
[http://dx.doi.org/10.1007/s11095-010-0166-y] [PMID: 20464462]

[93]   Mouriño V, Cattalini JP, Li W, *et al.* Multifunctional scaffolds for bone tissue engineering and in situ drug delivery. In Boccaccini AR, Ma PX. Eds. Tissue Engineering Using Ceramics and Polymers, Elsevier, 2014; pp. 648–675.

[94]   Arpornmaeklong P, Sareethammanuwat M, Apinyauppatham K, Boonyuen S. Characteristics and biologic effects of thermosensitive quercetin☐chitosan/collagen hydrogel on human periodontal ligament stem cells. J Biomed Mater Res B Appl Biomater 2021; 109(10): 1656-70.
[http://dx.doi.org/10.1002/jbm.b.34823] [PMID: 33644957]

[95]   Bose S, Sarkar N, Banerjee D. Effects of PCL, PEG and PLGA polymers on curcumin release from calcium phosphate matrix for *in vitro* and *in vivo* bone regeneration. Mater Today Chem 2018; 8: 110-20.
[http://dx.doi.org/10.1016/j.mtchem.2018.03.005] [PMID: 30480167]

[96]   Iviglia G, Torre E, Cassinelli C, Morra M. Functionalization with a Polyphenol-Rich Pomace Extract Empowers a Ceramic Bone Filler with In Vitro Antioxidant, Anti-Inflammatory, and Pro-Osteogenic Properties. J Funct Biomater 2021; 12(2): 31.
[http://dx.doi.org/10.3390/jfb12020031] [PMID: 34063147]

[97]   Amini AR, Laurencin CT, Nukavarapu SP. Bone tissue engineering: recent advances and challenges. Crit Rev Biomed Eng 2012; 40(5): 363-408.
[http://dx.doi.org/10.1615/CritRevBiomedEng.v40.i5.10] [PMID: 23339648]

[98]   Riester O, Borgolte M, Csuk R, Deigner HP. Challenges in Bone Tissue Regeneration: Stem Cell Therapy, Biofunctionality and Antimicrobial Properties of Novel Materials and Its Evolution. Int J Mol Sci 2020; 22(1): 192.
[http://dx.doi.org/10.3390/ijms22010192] [PMID: 33375478]

[99]   Xing H, Wang X, Xiao G, *et al.* Hierarchical assembly of nanostructured coating for siRNA-based dual therapy of bone regeneration and revascularization. Biomaterials 2020; 235: 119784.
[http://dx.doi.org/10.1016/j.biomaterials.2020.119784] [PMID: 31981763]

[100] Bahraminasab M. Challenges on optimization of 3D-printed bone scaffolds. Biomed Eng Online 2020;

19(1): 69.
[http://dx.doi.org/10.1186/s12938-020-00810-2] [PMID: 32883300]

[101]   Conev A, Litsa EE, Perez MR, Diba M, Mikos AG, Kavraki LE. Machine Learning-Guided Three-Dimensional Printing of Tissue Engineering Scaffolds. Tissue Eng Part A 2020; 26(23-24): 1359-68.
[http://dx.doi.org/10.1089/ten.tea.2020.0191] [PMID: 32940144]

[102]   Urciuolo A, Urbani L, Perin S, *et al.* Decellularised skeletal muscles allow functional muscle regeneration by promoting host cell migration. Sci Rep 2018; 8(1): 8398.
[http://dx.doi.org/10.1038/s41598-018-26371-y] [PMID: 29849047]

[103]   Williams DF. Challenges With the Development of Biomaterials for Sustainable Tissue Engineering. Front Bioeng Biotechnol 2019; 7: 127.
[http://dx.doi.org/10.3389/fbioe.2019.00127] [PMID: 31214584]

[104]   Smith CA, Board TN, Rooney P, Eagle MJ, Richardson SM, Hoyland JA. Correction: Human decellularized bone scaffolds from aged donors show improved osteoinductive capacity compared to young donor bone. PLoS One 2017; 12(11): e0187783.
[http://dx.doi.org/10.1371/journal.pone.0187783] [PMID: 29095911]

CHAPTER 11

Decellularised Natural Cancellous Trabecular Bone Scaffold in Tissue Engineering

Kok-Lun Pang[1], **Sophia Ogechi Ekeuku**[1] and **Kok-Yong Chin**[1,*]

[1] Department of Pharmacology, Faculty of Medicine, Universiti Kebangsaan Malaysia, 56000 Cheras, Kuala Lumpur, Malaysia

Abstract: Delayed fracture healing and non-union fractures are major orthopaedic issues that have become a significant healthcare burden. Among many approaches, bone grafts facilitate the healing of non-union fractures. Native cancellous bones represent a more viable and advantageous source of bone grafts due to structural and biochemical similarity with natural bone. They also provide a large surface-to-volume ratio to host cells and for the formation of the vasculature. Given these advantages, we aimed to review some of the recent innovations in native cancellous bone graft production, such as bone selection, decellularisation, demineralisation, and *in vitro* and *in vivo* testing. Some endogenous and processing factors affecting performance are also highlighted. In addition, innovations such as the coadministration of interleukin-4, and impregnation of the scaffold with platelet-rich plasma are introduced to increase scaffold performance. A brief overview of skeletal properties and metabolism, fracture healing, and essential features of bone grafts is provided to appreciate these innovations.

Keywords: Bone fracture, Bone graft, Fracture healing, Osteoblast, Osteoporosis, Scaffold.

INTRODUCTION

Non-union and delayed fracture healing continue to be a challenge for orthopaedic surgeons. Although many papers cited 10% incidence rate of non-union fractures [1], National prospective data over a 5-year period in a Scottish population found a significantly lower incidence, which is approximately 1.9% [2, 3]. Nevertheless, non-union fractures significantly impair function and may leave emotional trauma [4]. Patients with non-union fractures are prone to refracture within 2 years and are subject to more intensive therapy and prolonged length of opioid therapy [5]. The high costs of non-union fracture and delayed fracture healing come from the

---

*** Corresponding author Kok-Yong Chin**: Department of Pharmacology, Faculty of Medicine, Universiti Kebangsaan Malaysia, 56000 Cheras, Kuala Lumpur, Malaysia; E-mail:chinkokyong@ppukm.ukm.edu.my

Mohd Fauzi Mh Busra, Daniel Law Jia Xian, Yogeswaran Lokanathan and Ruszymah Haji Idrus (Eds.)

direct medical and hospitalisation cost and the loss of productivity and employment [6]. Given the gravity of this condition, innovations in facilitating fracture healing are ongoing.

Bone grafts are used to promote the healing of large bone defects [7]. Both natural and synthetic graft materials have been investigated and used [8]. This chapter will focus on the use of decellularised native bone grafts, because they are readily available biomaterials with natural properties that promote successful engraftment. Native cancellous bone grafts have become a focus of research because their porous nature is suitable for cell attachment, revascularisation, and final dissociation upon the completion of fracture healing, despite their lower mechanical strength compared with cortical bones [7]. This chapter will discuss the bone mechanism and the mechanism underlying fracture healing. A discourse on native cancellous bone scaffold preparation is presented, along with some insights offered by investigations performed in the recent five years.

Structure and Metabolism of Bone

Bone is one of the strongest tissues in the human body. Mineralised structures in bone carry out the functions of locomotion, protection, and support. Bone comprises compact and cancellous bone tissues. Compact bone makes up the dense and rigid outer layer, whereas cancellous bone consists of sponge-like structures with a trabecular network and cavities [9]. The bone extracellular matrix comprises the following: inorganic components, such as calcium and phosphorus; and organic components, including type 1 collagen (around 90%) and some minor non-collagenous proteins, such as proteoglycans, osteocalcin, osteonectin, osteopontin and bone morphogenetic proteins (BMPs) [10-12]. Non-collagenous proteins help in bone mineralisation and bridge the connection between collagen and mineral components [10, 11].

Bone contains four main bone cells, including osteocytes, osteoblasts, osteoclasts, and bone lining cells [11]. Bone lining cells are the quiescent dedifferetiated osteoblasts that cover bone surfaces. Osteoblasts originate from mesenchymal stem cells from bone marrow stroma and eventually differentiate to mature osteocytes. Osteoblasts synthesise the bone extracellular matrix and initiate the calcification process [13]. They can be reactivated rapidly into osteoblasts upon stimulation [13]. Osteoclasts, the main mediators of bone resorption, originate from hematopoietic precursor cells from monocyte/macrophage lineage [14]. Osteoclasts also secrete proangiogenic factors, such as vascular endothelial growth factor (VEGF) [15], which can promote subsequent angiogenesis and osteoclast differentiation [16].

Bone is a dynamic tissue that undergoes continuous formation and resorption, despite its high tensile strength and rigid structure. Bone growth and development during childhood involve the bone modelling process, which involves the removal of bone from one site and the formation of a new bone in a different site [17, 18]. Bone remodelling is relatively important in adult bone homeostasis to maintain bone health and strength with continuous regeneration and localised replacement of old bone tissues [17]. Bone remodelling is greatly dependent on the balance between osteoclast and osteoblast activities. Higher bone resorption than formation ultimately weakens the skeletal structures and increases the risk of osteoporosis and bone fracture. Osteoclastogenesis and osteoclast activation are regulated by several effectors, like receptor activators of nuclear factor kappa-B ligand (RANKL) and osteoprotegerin (decoy receptor for RANKL) [15, 19]. Osteoblastogenesis and osteoblast differentiation are regulated by insulin-like growth factor (IGF), fibroblast growth factor, BMP, Wnt, and Notch signalling pathway [20, 21]. Transcription factors, such as runt-related transcription factor 2 (RUNX2) and osterix, are also essential in osteoblast differentiation [22-24].

Fracture Healing

Understanding the various processes involved in fracture healing is indispensable in selecting or designing treatments for fractures, particularly large bone defects [25]. Fracture healing aims to rebuild mineralised tissue that resembles the intact bone at the fracture site and to restore the mechanical strength and integrity of the injured bone [26]. Bone regeneration ability is critical in restoring original tissue morphology and function. Apart from fracture type and fixation methods, the biomaterial or graft used to repair the damaged region, and the additional pharmacological agents will determine bone healing success [25].

Fracture healing can be classified as primary (direct) or secondary (indirect) in classic histological terminology, depending on the fixing method used [27, 28]. The distinction between these two pathways is that primary healing necessitates total stabilisation and the absence of interfragmentary motion. By contrast, indirect healing necessitates the appearance of interfragmentary motion at the site of the fracture, which causes relative stability. Secondary healing occurs when mechanical stimulation combined with the activity of inflammatory molecules results in a fractured callus, which is accompanied by woven tissue that is gradually remodelled as lamellar bone [29].

Fracture recovery occurs in stages, as follows: hematoma development, inflammation, proliferation, differentiation, ossification, and remodelling (Fig. **1**) [30]. The vascular damage to the periosteum, endosteum, and underlying soft tissue causes hypoperfusion in the immediate region immediately after a fracture occurs. The coagulation cascade is triggered, resulting in the development of platelet and macrophage-rich hematoma. The macrophages synthesise cytokines that induce inflammatory responses, including increased blood flow and vascular permeability at the fracture site. Subsequent results are determined by mechanical and molecular signals [29].

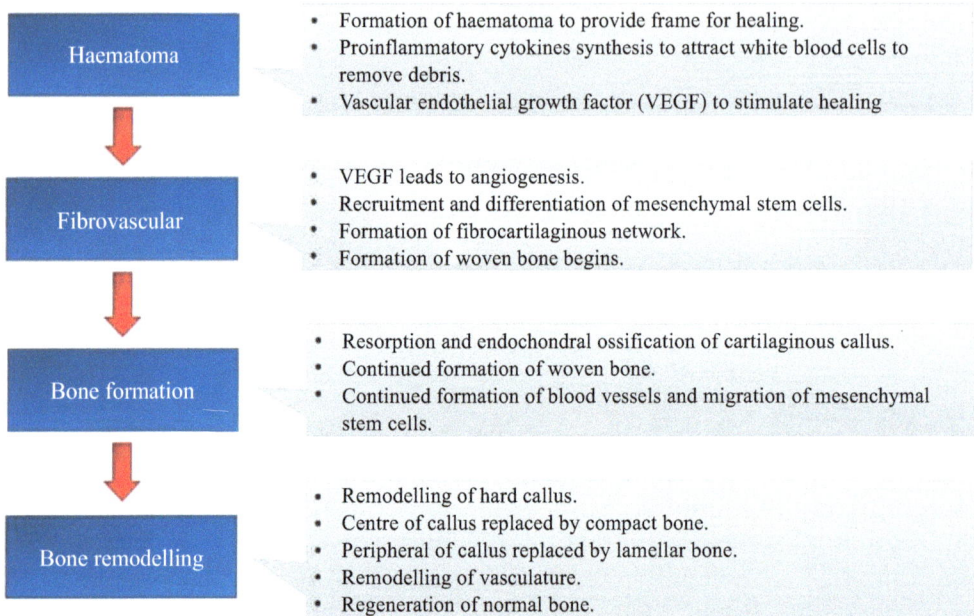

Haematoma
- Formation of haematoma to provide frame for healing.
- Proinflammatory cytokines synthesis to attract white blood cells to remove debris.
- Vascular endothelial growth factor (VEGF) to stimulate healing

Fibrovascular
- VEGF leads to angiogenesis.
- Recruitment and differentiation of mesenchymal stem cells.
- Formation of fibrocartilaginous network.
- Formation of woven bone begins.

Bone formation
- Resorption and endochondral ossification of cartilaginous callus.
- Continued formation of woven bone.
- Continued formation of blood vessels and migration of mesenchymal stem cells.

Bone remodelling
- Remodelling of hard callus.
- Centre of callus replaced by compact bone.
- Peripheral of callus replaced by lamellar bone.
- Remodelling of vasculature.
- Regeneration of normal bone.

Fig. (1). Normal fracture healing process.

These diverse pathways are coordinated on the molecular level by the secretion of various cytokines and proinflammatory factors. The initial inflammatory response is mediated by tumour necrosis factor (TNF), interleukin-1 (IL-1), IL-6, IL-11, and IL-18 [31]. These mediators stimulate the migration of mesenchymal stem cells from the surrounding soft tissue and induce their differentiation into osteogenic cells, which are responsible for the formation of cartilaginous and periosteal bony callus [26]. Revascularisation, an important component of bone healing, occurs through various molecular pathways that require either angiopoietin or VEGF [32]. In the second step of bone regeneration, growth factors induce the development of granulation tissue, resulting in the formation of a soft callus, which is accompanied by the formation of a hard callus [29]. Mechanical loading, such as weight-bearing and aerobic activity, also promotes the differentiation of mesenchymal stem cells into fibroblasts, chondroblasts, and osteoblasts [28]. Thus, effective fracture healing demands a harmonious interaction between biological and biomechanical forces.

Small bone injuries, such as stable fractures, can heal on their own without orthopaedic surgery. However, the normal fracture healing process may be inadequate to repair large bone defects. Fracture healing may also be complicated by local (nature of fracture, infections, and blood supply) and systemic factors (diabetes, menopause, obesity, aging, and smoking) [33]. The conventional therapy for a non-union fracture involves surgical intervention and autologous bone grafting [34]. Low-intensity pulsed ultrasound is another conservative and alternative approach to managing a non-union fracture [35]. Several local and systematic interventional approaches, such as the administration of growth factors, stem cells, biologics and grafting of natural or synthetic scaffold to fill the bone defects, have been designed to improve the healing response [34, 36]. This chapter will focus on designing and testing a native cancellous scaffold.

Characteristics of an Ideal Bone Scaffold

Bone scaffold properties could be evaluated based on several aspects, as follows: (1) Osteoconductivity, *i.e.*, the ability of the bone graft to host cells and allow bone growth on the surface or inside the porous structure; (2) Osteoinductivity, *i.e.*, the ability of the bone graft to recruit mesenchymal stem cells and promote their differentiation to osteoblasts, depending on bone morphogenetic proteins; and (3) Osteogenic, *i.e.*, the ability to promote de novo bone formation by the cells in the grafts or from the host, depending on cellular elements, growth factors, matrix, and angiogenesis. In addition, the bone graft needs to be biocompatible; it should not have immunogenic proteins, DNA, and any other cellular residues that can stimulate an immune response from the host. It should also offer mechanical strength similar to the native bone to support the fracture site. Lastly, it should be cost-effective so that it can be adopted clinically [37, 38].

The main types of natural bone scaffolds currently available are autografts, allografts, and xenografts. Autografts harvested from patients remain the gold standard in bone grafting. They offer good osteogenic, osteoconductivity, and osteoinductive properties and do not lead to potential immunological reactions [39]. A study revealed that patients implanted with autografts achieved complete fracture healing earlier and had a lower risk of infection than those implanted with allografts or a combination of autografts and allograft [40]. However, harvesting autografts would require the performance of an additional surgical operation, which could cause complications and morbidity on the site of harvest. Additionally, only a limited amount of bone could be harvested from the patients [39]. Allograft harvested from other human donors represents an alternative to autograft. Allografts have broader source availability, are time-saving, have higher customisability, and do not lead to donor complications. However, allografts might have lower osteoinductivity, osteogenic properties, and rejection risk compared with autografts. Improper processing might also increase the risk of human disease transmission [39]. Additionally, the production of allografts is costly [39]. An estimation study performed in 2014 in Switzerland showed that the production costs of commercialised human femoral head allografts were €1672 and €2149, whereas the in-house production cost was €1367 [41]. Xenografts harvested from animals offer an unlimited supply of bone grafts and are very cost-effective. However, they might lack osteogenic properties and could lead to rejection [39].

In the following sections, we focused on the preparation of native cancellous bone scaffolds, mostly allogenic and xenogenic. The articles published on this topic within the past 5 years are evaluated.

Preparation of Natural Cancellous Trabecular Bone Scaffold

Source of Bone Scaffold

As mentioned in the previous section, the source of bone graft could be human (autografts or allografts) or animal species (xenografts). The pros and cons of autografts, allografts, and xenografts have been discussed previously. For allografts, bone scaffold materials could be obtained from individuals undergoing total hip replacement therapy [42-44]. Informed consent and ethical issues should be given careful consideration when obtaining samples from living subjects. The regional sample is usually the femoral head/caput femoris [42-44], which is rich in trabeculae. Subchondral bone from the metacarpal region of a human cadaver had also been used [45]. For xenografts, bone scaffold materials are from porcine or bovine sources. The common bone segments used are a metaphyseal or epiphyseal region of the femur [46-49], the subchondral bone of the knees [50], or the costa/rib [51-53]. The animal bone samples are usually obtained from slaughterhouses [47,49, 51]; thus, ethical issues are minimised. The physical differences between human and animal native bone scaffolds have been elucidated previously. Sladkova *et al.* compared decellularised human and bovine subchondral bone from the metacarpal region and showed that both had similar microstructural, topographical and elemental (calcium to phosphate ratio) characteristics, except that human bone seemed to have larger pores. Although some studies established bone scaffold with a defined geometrical shape, several studies used homogenised or granulalised bone samples [49, 54].

Decellularisation

In decellularisation, dead cells and other cellular materials that can cause immunological reactions are removed (Fig. **2**). In particular, bone tissues from non-primates contain alpha(α)-Gal epitopes, which are not expressed in humans.

However, humans produce anti-α-Gal antibodies which can lead to the rejection of tissues from α-Gal-expressing donors [55]. Apart from α-Gal, the major histocompatibility complex (MHC), other cellular contents, and infectious pathogens of the residual cells could cause rejection, fibrosis, and failure of bone scaffold implantation [56]. Decellularisation of bone tissue is complicated because osteocytes, which are the most abundant cells in bone, are embedded deep inside the bone matrix [57]. They might not be moved adequately through chemical agents. Maintaining the structural and mechanical integrity of the bone scaffold after decellularisation is essential to ensure that it can well support the fracture site [45].

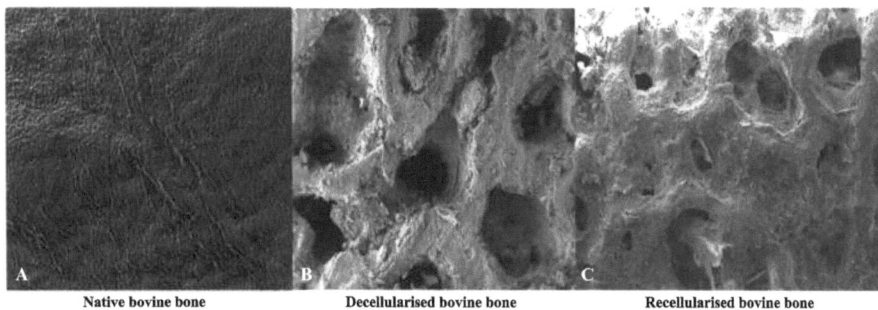

Native bovine bone   Decellularised bovine bone   Recellularised bovine bone

Fig. (2). Surface features of native (A), decellularised (B), and recellularised bovine bone (C) obtained from scanning electron microscope. The native bovine bone is fully covered with an extracellular matrix. The decellularised bovine bone appears porous, while the recellularised bovine bone is partially covered in cellular matrix. Images courtesy of Nur Farhana Mohd Fozi.

Various approaches have been attempted to decellularise bone tissues. Chemical decellularisation using detergent is one of the most common methods. Bracey *et al.* treated the bone scaffold with trypsin to detach cells from the native bone scaffold, after which 1.5% peracetic acid (oxidising agent) and 2% Triton X-100 (non-ionic detergent) were used to disrupt the cells/pathogens, and washing was repeated [46-48]. The decellularised bone scaffold had similar surface topographical features to native bone, except that the pores were larger [47]. The decellularised bone scaffold's mineral density was lower than that of native bone, but the structural characteristics were retained [47]. The decellularisation process removed all the bone marrow content and osteocytes, but retained the major matrix protein in the matrix, such as chondroadherin, collagens 1 and 2, pigment epithelium-derived factor, albumin, α-2HS-glycoprotein, lumican and biglycan [47]. However, the mechanical strength of decellularised bone scaffold was slightly altered, as indicated by reduced Young's Modulus and stiffness and high strain [47]. The process removed viruses, bacteria, and 98.5% of the α-Gal protein from the scaffold [48]. As a result, the scaffold did not induce an immune cell reaction [48].

Combining sonication and chemical decellularisation for complete cell lysis and cellular content removal is common. Leng *et al.* combined sonication for debris and fat removal, immersion with dispase, Triton-X, and Tris-hydrochloride acid (HCl) to lyse cells and denature the protein in scaffold processing [58]. The porcine bone-cancellous scaffold showed low α-Gal and collagen content but similar mechanical strength compared with native bone [58].

Extreme temperature changes could break the cells and denature proteins. Thus, thermal shock and repeated freeze/dry cycles have been incorporated into the decellularisation process. Rashmi *et al.* put a bovine bone cancellous scaffold through a freeze/thaw cycle, followed by 3% hydrogen peroxide and enzymatic solution to remove the antigen [59]. The resultant decellularised bone scaffold was more porous than native bone and was devoid of cells [59]. Smith *et al.* subjected human cancellous bone from the femoral head to a freeze/thaw cycle, sonication, and treatment with 3% hydrogen peroxide and 0.02% peroxyacetic acid [43, 44]. The resultant bone scaffolds showed detached fine meshwork in the marrow space, the absence of cells on the bone surface, and few remaining osteocytes [44]. Immunohistology showed decreased MHC class 1-staining in the processed scaffold compared with native bone [44]. Mechanical testing showed slightly decreased deflected yield and increased Young's Modulus in the processed bone compared with native bone [44].

Decellularisation through high hydrostatic pressure (HHP) was previously attempted [50, 52, 53]. Nakamura *et al.* subjected porcine cancellous bone to HHP, rinsing, and sterilisation in 80% ethanol [52, 53]. The HHP procedures retained the reticular and adipose tissues in the marrow space and some osteocytes in the bone scaffold [52, 53]. They also compared the scaffolds processed using HHP and conventional chemical decellularisation process using EDTA (a series of concentrations), 0.1% sodium dodecyl sulphate (SDS, a strong ionic detergent), and Tris-HCl [52]. The chemical methods removed all cellular, protein, and DNA content in the bone [52]. Despite the higher efficacy, the authors argued that removing protein content effectively eliminates the scaffolds' osteogenic potential [52]. This aspect is discussed in the following section.

In addition to HHP, You *et al.* used supercritical carbon dioxide and irradiation to remove cellular materials and pathogens in the scaffold [50]. Supercritical carbon dioxide has the advantage of being non-toxic and non-flammable, and it does not leave any residue on the scaffold [60]. As evidence, the implantation of the scaffold produced by You *et al.* in the abdominal cavity of mice did not elicit an immunological response, as marked by unaltered pro- or anti-inflammatory cytokine, immunoglobulin levels, and white population in the blood (T- and B-cells) and in the peritoneal fluid (macrophages). The spleen and kidney weight of the rats bearing the implants also remained unchanged [50].

A combination of decellularisation methods, including temperature (freeze/thaw or thermal shock), HHP, sonication, and chemical and supercritical carbon dioxide, could effectively remove potential immunogens and pathogens from the cancellous bone scaffold.

Demineralisation

Demineralisation using acid is an optional process in creating scaffold materials (Fig. **3**). This process reduces the mechanical strength of the decellularised bone scaffold. Thus, it is not commonly performed. Otherwise, the structure of demineralised and decellularised human cancellous bone scaffolds could be similar [42]. Lee *et al.* compared the demineralised (using HCl) and non-demineralised bone scaffolds [54]. Demineralised bone scaffolds apparently had a more fibrous structure and larger pores for potential cell attachment [54]. Through X-ray spectroscopy analysis, the demineralisation process showed that the protein amide group was previously hidden under the inorganic matrix [54]. These properties might promote the osteogenic properties of the scaffold. Additionally, the demineralised scaffold showed higher bone morphogenetic protein-2 and -7 levels but lower DNA and α-Gal epitope levels compared with the non-demineralised scaffolds [54].

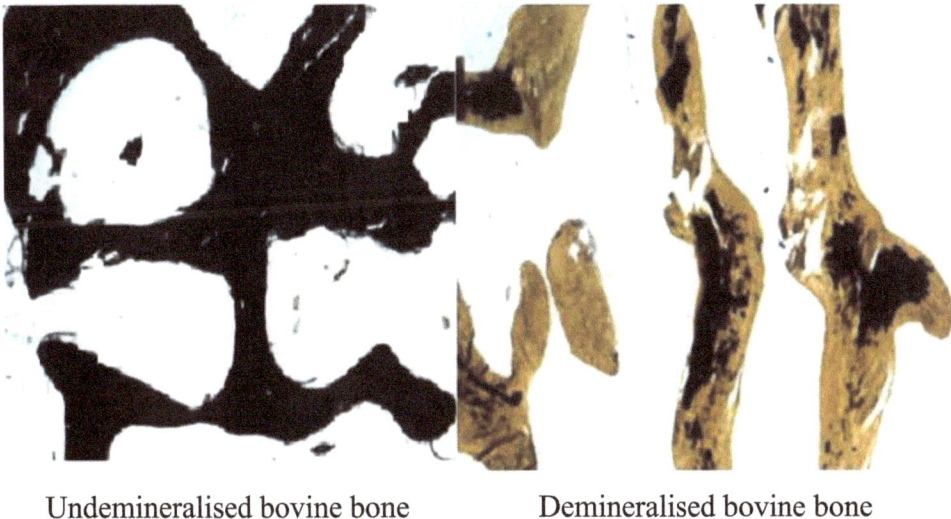

Undemineralised bovine bone   Demineralised bovine bone

Fig. (3). Undermineralised and demineralised bovine bone stained with silver nitrate, which binds with the phosphate in the bone tissue. A darker staining reflects a higher mineral content. Images courtesy of Nur Farhana Mohd Fozi.

Assessment of Osteogenic Properties of Bone Scaffold in Vitro

After processing, the decellularised/demineralised bone scaffold must retain the osteoinductivity, osteoconductivity, and osteogenic properties of the native bone. These properties of the processed scaffold could be tested by culturing bone cells onto the scaffold. Bracey *et al.* compared the effects of decellularised porcine bone scaffold and commercialised bone scaffold and Gelform on the growth and differentiation of C2C12 mouse myoblasts, which could differentiate into osteoblasts and MC3T3-E1 mouse preosteoblasts [46]. Despite showing the lowest pro-proliferation effects among the scaffolds tested, the decellularised porcine bone scaffold stimulated higher early and late osteogenic differentiation, as marked by increased RANKL expression in MC3T3-E1 cells and alkaline phosphatase (ALP) activity in C2C12 cells [46].

Several endogenous and processing factors affect the osteogenic properties of the cancellous bone scaffolds. Smith *et al.* compared the age of allograft donors on osteogenic properties of the bone scaffold from the human femoral head [43]. They seeded the scaffolds with primary human mesenchymal cells (hMSCs) and demonstrated that these cells exhibited a higher rate of differentiation on scaffolds from old donors, as indicated by higher gene expressions of RUNX2, osteopontin and osteocalcin and higher ALP activity [43]. Although bone samples from old and young donors showed similar IGF-1 and -2 levels, the authors found a lower IGF-1 binding protein (IGFBP-1) level in the scaffold from older donors. IGF is essential for the terminal differentiation of mesenchymal stem cells into osteoblasts [61] and a determinant of bone mass [62]. Thus, the antagonistic effects of IGFBPs on IGFs could limit the pro-osteogenic actions of IGFs [63] and lower the osteogenic properties of allografts from young donors. Allografts from old donors had lower mineral density and bone volume and were more porous compared with those from young donors [43].

The interspecies difference in the osteogenic properties of cancellous bone scaffold (allograft vs. xenograft) was also noteworthy. Sladkova *et al.* cultured mesenchymal progenitor cells from human induced pluripotent stem cells (line 1013A) on bovine and human scaffold derived from subchondral bone [45]. They reported that seeding efficacy was higher in the human bone scaffold compared with the bovine scaffold, but cell viability was similar between the two scaffolds [45]. However, expressions of osteogenic genes, such as *RUNX-2, COL1A1, ALPL, BSP, OPN,* and *PDGFRB*, were higher in cells seeded on the bovine scaffold [45]. ALP activities and staining for osteogenic proteins in histology sections (bone sialoprotein, osteopontin, and osteocalcin) and the release of osteocalcin into the media were higher in the human scaffold [45]. The disparity between gene and protein expressions could be due to the different assessment methods; however, the absence of time series data precluded any conclusion from this study [45]. The authors suggested that the bovine bone scaffold had smaller pores than the human scaffold, thereby promoting cell aggregation and differentiation. The larger pores of the human scaffold facilitated cell proliferation into the scaffold. Thus, the higher protein expressions and osteocalcin release are due to satisfactory cell number and attachment efficacy [45]. The structural parameters dictate the osteogenic properties of the scaffold from the donor of a different species.

Scaffold processing methods also determine the efficacy of recellularisation. For example, if the bone scaffold is not cleansed from cellular debris, proliferation, viability, and osteogenic differentiation of hMSC seeded would be affected, as indicated by Smith *et al.* [44]. The HHP-processed bone scaffold produced by Nakamura *et al.* retained reticular and adipose tissue. Rat mesenchymal stem cells (rMSC) and hMSCs that were seeded could not penetrate the scaffold efficiently compared with commercialised collagen scaffold [53]. The authors also showed that a brief culture period at a lower temperature (1.5 h at 4 °C) would help cells penetrate the scaffold [53]. However, the differentiation of hMSC into osteogenic cells, which was marked by osteopontin expression, was better in the HHP-washed scaffold compared with the SDS-washed scaffold [52]. However, penetration was not an issue for completely decellularised bone scaffolds [64]. Otherwise, the use of a bioreactor with a dynamic medium flow can facilitate cell survival. In a study by Liu *et al.*, who examined spontaneous lumen formation of epithelial cells in the cancellous bone scaffold, lumen distribution was more evident throughout the scaffold with the bioreactor [51].

Ethanol immersion is usually performed to de-fat and dehydrate the scaffold. Gardin compared air-dried and ethanol-processed homogenised bone scaffolds and found that ethanol processing leads to less cell toxicity and enables osteogenic differentiation of adipose stem cells. This observation could be due to the fact that ethanol removes residual lipids and detergents, which could potentially impede cell survival in the bone scaffold [49].

Nie *et al.* compared the attachment and osteogenic properties of non-demineralised and decellularised scaffold sampled from porcine rib subjected to processing, *i.e.*, heating, sonication, and detergent-washing and β-tricalcium phosphate (β-TCP) [65]. The attachment and proliferation of hMSCs seeded on the bone scaffold were better than on β-TCP [65]. However, the bone scaffold did not significantly promote osteogenic differentiation, which was marked by *RUNX-2, ALP,* and *OCN*, compared with β-TCP [65]. In fact, BSP expression increased early for cells seeded on β-TCP, which might be related to the fact that osteogenic protein in the bone scaffold is possibly hidden by the inorganic matrix, thus impairing its osteogenic properties.

Implantation

Implantation of bone scaffold seeded with cells subcutaneously or at the site of bone defect in laboratory animals is the standard approach for assessing the performance of a scaffold. Using a subcutaneously implanted and detergent-washed porcine scaffold to examine the effects of prior cell seeding on bone formation in mice, Bracey *et al*. showed increased osteoblast differentiation marked by the gene expressions of ALP, BMP-2, and BMP-7 in scaffold seeded with MC3T3-E1 murine preosteoblasts [46]. However, bone volume and trabecular thickness of the scaffold increased regardless of prior cell seeding. In addition, signs of pre-osteoclasts and angiogenesis were apparent [46].

Subcutaneous implantation of HHP-processed porcine rib scaffold with or without hMSCs could induce the formation of red bone marrow and sustain haematopoietic stem cells [52]. The scaffold also caused the migration of granulocytes and macrophages after 1 week, but the inflammatory response decreased afterward [52]. The inflammatory response was less for SDS-washed and hydroxyapatite scaffolds [52]. Neovascularisation was enhanced in the HHP-processed scaffold because reticular tissue inside the scaffold prevented the invasion of fibroblasts, thereby blocking the migration of other cells into the scaffold [52]. Serial transplantation of the scaffolds from normal mice to irradiated mice showed that they carried haematopoietic stem cells that can differentiate from other cells [52].

Lee *et al*. showed that implantation of homogenised, demineralised, and decellularised scaffold was cleared using hydrogen peroxide-induced bone formation at the mouse calvarial bone defect, as marked by increased bone volume and mineral density. It did not induce inflammation at the site of implantation [54]. Wong *et al*. implanted demineralised and decellularised porcine bone scaffold seeded or unseeded with allogenic bone marrow mesenchymal stem cells at the critical size defect on the radius of rabbit [64]. Implantation of seeded scaffold led to increased bone density and volume at the defect site compared with the unseeded scaffold [64]. It also facilitated the bony union. However, oestrogen deficiency induced by ovariectomy compromised the effects of scaffold implantation, which was attributed to increased osteoclastogenesis [64]. Therefore, this factor should be taken into account in case of postmenopausal women receiving bone grafts.

The combination of growth stimulants with bone scaffold might prevent the occurrence of the abovementioned problem. Leng *et al*. combined porcine bone scaffold with platelet-rich plasma (PRP), containing platelet-derived growth factor, basic fibroblast growth factor, insulin-like growth factor 1, and vascular endothelial growth factor under negative pressure. PRP impregnation promoted osteointegration and bone regeneration at the defect site at the radius of rabbits [58]. It also facilitated angiogenesis and hindered fibrosis [58]. Overall, rabbits implanted with PRP-impregnated scaffold showed higher radiological, collagen, and histological scores compared with a normal decellularised bone scaffold [58]. The authors suggested that during scaffold processing (sonication, dispase digestion, and washing with detergent), most osteogenic proteins are denatured, and PRP can overcome such limitations [58].

Excessive inflammation is an important factor leading to the failure of osteointegration and scaffold rejection. Zheng *et al.* implanted a porcine bone scaffold cleaned by 70% ethanol and phosphate buffer saline at the cranial defect created in Wistar rats and administered interleukin-4 (IL-4) indirectly to the implantation site to stop inflammation [66]. Increased bone formation was found in the IL-4-treated group, and the defect was completely filled after 12 weeks [66]. Histological examination at the defect site revealed both bone growth engulfing the scaffold and inside it, which led to better osteointegration [66]. These observations could be attributed to IL-4-induced macrophage polarisation to the M2 phenotype and reduction in the M1 phenotype [66]. M2 macrophages are associated with healing, whereas M2 macrophages are associated with killing pathogens, often with collateral damage in the surrounding tissue [67]. Cytokines secreted by M2 macrophages (VEGF, BMP-2, and transforming growth factor-β) are associated with osteoblastogenesis and bone formation [68,69]. At the implantation site, IL-4 treatment also reduced inflammation, *i.e.*, it increased the IL-10 and reduced the tumour necrosis-alpha, and cellular apoptosis, *i.e.*, it reduced the DNA fragmentation and caspase-3 activation [66]. Moreover, IL-4 treatment attracted migration to the scaffold and osteogenic differentiation of mesenchymal cells [66]. However, a critical range for the therapeutic effects of IL-4 exists (10–50 ng in this study) [66], as excessive M2 polarisation is associated with the fusion of macrophages [70], which may lead to osteoclast formation.

Vascularisation of bone graft is critical in ensuring the supply of progenitor cells and nutrients and the removal of waste for fracture healing [71]. Huang *et al.* adopted an *in vivo* bioreactor approach to allow the formation of blood vessels before implantation at the defect site [42]. They inserted decalcified irradiated human scaffold into the rabbit pedicled periosteal flab or muscle pouch. After some time, the scaffolds were wrapped with the periosteum and muscle tissue [42]. Both scaffolds showed higher bone volume and mineral density compared with their respective baselines [42]. Osteoid and new blood vessel formation were evident for both scaffolds [42]. These changes were more prominent in the periosteal-wrapped scaffold, which demonstrated higher mechanical strength [42].

Pre-seeded or unseeded native cancellous bone scaffolds promote bone regeneration and do not induce inflammation *in vivo*. The incorporation of bone scaffolds with PRP or IL-4 could further enhance fracture healing by supporting the bone formation and suppressing inflammation. Pre-vascularisation of the scaffold with *in vivo* bioreactor approach can also improve engraftment efficiency (Table **1**).

Table 1. Examples of studies demonstrating successful engraftment of cancellous bone grafts.

Studies	Scaffold design	Findings
Wang *et al.* 2015 (64)	Porcine caput femoris, degreased, dialysed, demineralised, and then seeded with allogenic foetal rabbit bone marrow mesenchymal stem cells from femurs and tibiae.	A critical size defect was created in the radius of the rabbit. X-ray: Dense structure in the DDS+MSC group compared with the DDS group. Bone union was seen in an intact group compared with the OVX group. DDS+MSC in the intact group led to higher bone density and volume compared with DDS-implanted OVX rabbits. Histology: DDS+MSC led to bony union and bone lacunae formation. Adipocyte formation was noted in the OVX group that received DDS+MSC. In the DCM alone group with OVX, undegraded scaffold particles were present.
Huang *et al.* 2017 (42)	Human femoral head bones from replacement surgery. Subjected to degreasing, decalcification, removal of non-collagen protein, and sterilisation by gamma-radiation.	*In vivo* bioreactor: bone scaffold was inserted into rabbit pedicled periosteal flap or muscle pouch. µCT: ↑ BV, BMC, and BMD vs. pre-baseline for both implantation approaches. The values of periosteal > muscle pouch except for BMD. ↑ Tb.N and Tb.Th, and ↓ Tb.Sp in the periosteal group vs. muscle pouch group. Histology: Apparent new osteoid deposition, mineralisation, and angiogenesis. The effects of periosteal group > muscle pouch group. Young's modulus: periosteal group > muscle pouch group
You *et al.* 2018 (50)	Subchondral bone of bovine knee joint. HHP, Triton X-100 immersion, supercritical CO_2 treatment (30 Mpa for 30 min, at 50 °C), and finally, irradiation.	DS was implanted into the abdominal cavity of the mice. NC in spleen index, kidney weight, macrophages, and neutrophils in peripheral blood. NC in T-cells and B-cells in peritoneal fluid and peripheral blood, splenocyte activation, pro/anti-inflammatory cytokines level in the peritoneal fluid and peripheral blood, and immunoglobulin levels.

(Table 1) cont.....

Studies	Scaffold design	Findings
Zheng *et al.* 2018 (66)	Porcine caput femoris was processed with 70% ethanol and rinsed with PBS.	Cranial defects were created in Wistar rats. ↑ New bone tissue formation (6th week) and vascular networks (12th week) with IL-4 (10–50 ng) administration. *In situ* growth was not observed in DS without IL-4. ↑ bone formation and osteointegration with IL-4 over DS alone. ↑ polarisation of macrophages to M2 types and ↓ M1 types with IL-4. ↑ IL-10 and ↓ TNF-α with IL-4. ↓ tissue apoptosis with IL-4. ↑ MSC migration to DS and osteogenic differentiation with IL-4.
Nakamura *et al.* 2019 (52)	Cancellous bone of porcine costae. Processed with HHP, immersion with DNAase, antibiotics, and 80% ethanol. Another group was processed with graded series of EDTA, 01% sodium dodecyl sulphate (SDS), and Tris-HCl.	Subcutaneous implantation of HHP-DS with or without hMSC-induced red bone marrow formation and sustained haematopoietic stem cells. Migration of inflammatory cells (granulocytes and macrophages) was observed in the HHP-DS group (1st week) and was reduced after 4 weeks. Degree of neovascularisation: HHP>SDS=HA. Transplantation of HHP-DS and HA from normal mice to irradiated mice showed a carryover of haematopoietic stem cells. Marrow transplantation of 2nd generation mice showed the presence of multipotent cells, which were marked with a tracer from the 1st generation mice. Effects of HHP>HA.
Lee *et al.* 2020 (54)	Bone femur (region of interest unknown). The bone was homogenised, defatted with H_2O_2, demineralised with HCl, decellularised with citric acid, freeze-dried and lyophilised.	DDS ↑ bone formation, BV, and BMD at the mouse calvarial bone defects. Histology: DDS did not induce inflammation and fibrosis as a natural bone scaffold.
Leng *et al.* 2020 (58)	Porcine femoral cancellous bone combined with rabbit PRP under negative pressure. The bone was sonicated and soaked in dispase, Triton-X, and Tris-HCL.	↑ Osteointegration and bone regeneration by DS+PRP at rabbit radius defect. DS+PRP promoted new bone formation *in situ* and angiogenesis and limited fibrosis at the defect site. Healing was not completed.

Abbreviation: BV, bone volume; BMC, bone mineral content; BMD, bone mineral density; DS, decellularised scaffold; DDS, demineralised decellularised scaffold; HA, hydroxyapatite; HHP, high hydrostatic pressure; human MSC, mesenchymal stem cells; IL-interleukin; MSC, mesenchymal stem cells; OVX, ovariectomy; PRP, platelet-rich plasma; Tb.N, trabecular number; Tb.Th, trabecular thickness; Tb.Sp, trabecular separation; TNF-α, tumour necrosis factor-alpha.

Methods			
• Chemical • Sonication • HPP • Freeze/Thaw • Supercritical CO_2	• Strong/weak acid	• Seeding with mesenchymal/ adipose stem cells	• Subcutaneous • Defect site

| | Decellularisation | Demineralisation | Recellularisation | Implantation |

Purpose			
To remove potential immunogens, cellular debris and pathogens	To expose mineral embedded osteogenic proteins	To assess the viability, proliferation and osteogenic differentiation of cells	To assess immunological reaction and osteointegration

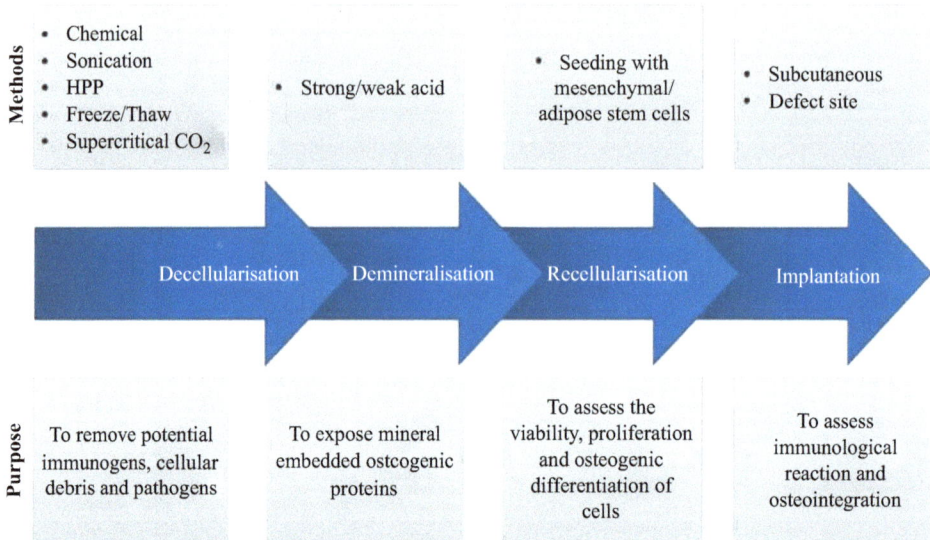

Fig. (4). Summary of processing native cancellous bone grafts

CONCLUSION

Continuous innovation in the production of native cancellous bone grafts will help in the healing of non-union fractures. The advantages of native cancellous bone grafts are apparent compared with other types of scaffolds in terms of structural similarity with living bone, natural ability to promote osteointegration and bone formation, and the ready availability of xenografts. Nevertheless, standardisation and optimisation of the production process are crucial to ensure the performance and safety of native bone grafts. This chapter highlighted some of the recent innovations in scaffold production from decellularisation, demineralisation, recellularisation assay, and *in vivo* testing (Fig. **4**), which we hope will help the readers select and design their approach for native cancellous scaffold production.

ACKNOWLEDGEMENTS

The authors thank Universiti Kebangsaan Malaysia for the funding *via* Research University Grant (GUP-2020-021).

REFERENCES

[1]   Zimmermann G, Moghaddam A. Trauma: Non-Union: New Trends. In: Bentley G, editor. European Instructional Lectures: Volume 10, 2010; 11th EFORT Congress, Madrid, Spain. Berlin, Heidelberg: Springer Berlin Heidelberg; 2010. p. 15-9

[2]   Mills LA, Aitken SA, Simpson AHRW. The risk of non-union per fracture: current myths and revised figures from a population of over 4 million adults. Acta Orthop 2017; 88(4): 434-9.
[http://dx.doi.org/10.1080/17453674.2017.1321351] [PMID: 28508682]

[3]   Mills LA, Simpson AHRW. The relative incidence of fracture non-union in the Scottish population (5.17 million): a 5-year epidemiological study. BMJ Open 2013; 3(2): e002276.
[http://dx.doi.org/10.1136/bmjopen-2012-002276] [PMID: 23396560]

[4]   Johnson L, Igoe E, Kleftouris G, Papachristos IV, Papakostidis C, Giannoudis PV. Physical Health and Psychological Outcomes in Adult Patients with Long-bone Fracture Non-unions: Evidence Today. J Clin Med 2019; 8(11): 1998.
[http://dx.doi.org/10.3390/jcm8111998] [PMID: 31731803]

[5]   Antonova E, Le TK, Burge R, Mershon J. Tibia shaft fractures: costly burden of nonunions. BMC Musculoskelet Disord 2013; 14(1): 42.
[http://dx.doi.org/10.1186/1471-2474-14-42] [PMID: 23351958]

[6]   Ekegren C, Edwards E, de Steiger R, Gabbe B. Incidence, Costs and Predictors of Non-Union, Delayed Union and Mal-Union Following Long Bone Fracture. Int J Environ Res Public Health 2018; 15(12): 2845.
[http://dx.doi.org/10.3390/ijerph15122845] [PMID: 30551632]

[7]   Roberts TT, Rosenbaum AJ. Bone grafts, bone substitutes and orthobiologics. Organogenesis 2012; 8(4): 114-24.
[http://dx.doi.org/10.4161/org.23306] [PMID: 23247591]

[8]   Pereira HF, Cengiz IF, Silva FS, Reis RL, Oliveira JM. Scaffolds and coatings for bone regeneration. J Mater Sci Mater Med 2020; 31(3): 27.
[http://dx.doi.org/10.1007/s10856-020-06364-y] [PMID: 32124052]

[9]   Currey JD. The structure and mechanics of bone. J Mater Sci 2012; 47(1): 41-54.
[http://dx.doi.org/10.1007/s10853-011-5914-9]

[10]   Florencio-Silva R, Sasso GRS, Sasso-Cerri E, Simões MJ, Cerri PS. Biology of Bone Tissue: Structure, Function, and Factors That Influence Bone Cells. BioMed Res Int 2015; 2015: 1-17.
[http://dx.doi.org/10.1155/2015/421746] [PMID: 26247020]

[11]   Mohamed AM. An overview of bone cells and their regulating factors of differentiation. Malays J Med Sci 2008; 15(1): 4-12.
[PMID: 22589609]

[12]   Wang RN, Green J, Wang Z, et al. Bone Morphogenetic Protein (BMP) signaling in development and human diseases. Genes Dis 2014; 1(1): 87-105.
[http://dx.doi.org/10.1016/j.gendis.2014.07.005] [PMID: 25401122]

[13]   Dirckx N, Moorer MC, Clemens TL, Riddle RC. The role of osteoblasts in energy homeostasis. Nat Rev Endocrinol 2019; 15(11): 651-65.
[http://dx.doi.org/10.1038/s41574-019-0246-y] [PMID: 31462768]

[14]   Boyce B, Yao Z, Xing L. Osteoclasts have multiple roles in bone in addition to bone resorption. Crit Rev Eukaryot Gene Expr 2009; 19(3): 171-80.
[http://dx.doi.org/10.1615/CritRevEukarGeneExpr.v19.i3.10] [PMID: 19883363]

[15]   Cackowski FC, Anderson JL, Patrene KD, et al. Osteoclasts are important for bone angiogenesis. Blood 2010; 115(1): 140-9.
[http://dx.doi.org/10.1182/blood-2009-08-237628] [PMID: 19887675]

[16]   Aldridge SE. Lennard Tw Fau - Williams JR, Williams Jr Fau - Birch MA, Birch MA. Vascular endothelial growth factor receptors in osteoclast differentiation and function. (0006-291X (Print)).

[17]   Siddiqui JA, Partridge NC. Physiological Bone Remodeling: Systemic Regulation and Growth Factor Involvement. Physiology (Bethesda) 2016; 31(3): 233-45.
[http://dx.doi.org/10.1152/physiol.00061.2014] [PMID: 27053737]

[18]   Manolagas SC. Cell number versus cell vigor--what really matters to a regenerating skeleton? Endocrinology 1999; 140(10): 4377-81.

[http://dx.doi.org/10.1210/endo.140.10.7129] [PMID: 10499488]

[19]   Tobeiha M, Moghadasian MH, Amin N, Jafarnejad S. RANKL/RANK/OPG Pathway: A Mechanism Involved in Exercise-Induced Bone Remodeling. BioMed Res Int 2020; 2020: 1-11.
[http://dx.doi.org/10.1155/2020/6910312] [PMID: 32149122]

[20]   Shahi M, Peymani A, Sahmani M. Regulation of Bone Metabolism. Rep Biochem Mol Biol 2017; 5(2): 73-82.
[PMID: 28367467]

[21]   Zuo C, Huang Y, Bajis R, Sahih M, Li YP, Dai K, *et al.* Osteoblastogenesis regulation signals in bone remodeling Osteoporosis international : a journal established as result of cooperation between the European Foundation for Osteoporosis and the National Osteoporosis Foundation of the USA 2012; 23(6): 1653-63.
[http://dx.doi.org/10.1007/s00198-012-1909-x]

[22]   Komori T. Regulation of Proliferation, Differentiation and Functions of Osteoblasts by Runx2. Int J Mol Sci 2019; 20(7): 1694.
[http://dx.doi.org/10.3390/ijms20071694] [PMID: 30987410]

[23]   Tang W, Li Y, Osimiri L, Zhang C. Osteoblast-specific transcription factor Osterix (Osx) is an upstream regulator of Satb2 during bone formation. J Biol Chem 2011; 286(38): 32995-3002.
[http://dx.doi.org/10.1074/jbc.M111.244236] [PMID: 21828043]

[24]   Komori T. Regulation of osteoblast differentiation by Runx2. Adv Exp Med Biol 2009; 658: 43-9.
[http://dx.doi.org/10.1007/978-1-4419-1050-9_5] [PMID: 19950014]

[25]   Oryan A, Alidadi S, Moshiri A. Current concerns regarding healing of bone defects. Hard Tissue 2013; 2(2): 13.
[http://dx.doi.org/10.13172/2050-2303-2-2-374]

[26]   Marsell R, Einhorn TA. The biology of fracture healing. Injury 2011; 42(6): 551-5.
[http://dx.doi.org/10.1016/j.injury.2011.03.031] [PMID: 21489527]

[27]   Cottrell JA, Turner JC, Arinzeh TL, O'Connor JP. The Biology of Bone and Ligament Healing. Foot Ankle Clin 2016; 21(4): 739-61.
[http://dx.doi.org/10.1016/j.fcl.2016.07.017] [PMID: 27871408]

[28]   LaStayo PC, Winters KM, Hardy M. Fracture healing: Bone healing, fracture management, and current concepts related to the hand. J Hand Ther 2003; 16(2): 81-93.
[http://dx.doi.org/10.1016/S0894-1130(03)80003-0] [PMID: 12755160]

[29]   Morshed S. Current Options for Determining Fracture Union. Adv Med 2014; 2014: 1-12.
[http://dx.doi.org/10.1155/2014/708574] [PMID: 26556422]

[30]   Harwood PJ, Newman JB, Michael ALR II. (ii) An update on fracture healing and non-union. Orthop Trauma 2010; 24(1): 9-23.
[http://dx.doi.org/10.1016/j.mporth.2009.12.004]

[31]   Gerstenfeld LC, Cullinane DM, Barnes GL, Graves DT, Einhorn TA. Fracture healing as a post-natal developmental process: Molecular, spatial, and temporal aspects of its regulation. J Cell Biochem 2003; 88(5): 873-84.
[http://dx.doi.org/10.1002/jcb.10435] [PMID: 12616527]

[32]   Tsiridis E, Upadhyay N, Giannoudis P. Molecular aspects of fracture healing: which are the important molecules?

[33]   Sheen JR, Garla VV. Fracture Healing Overview 2020. https://www.ncbi.nlm.nih.gov/books/NBK551678/

[34]   Schlickewei CW, Kleinertz H, Thiesen DM, *et al.* Current and Future Concepts for the Treatment of Impaired Fracture Healing. Int J Mol Sci 2019; 20(22): 5805.
[http://dx.doi.org/10.3390/ijms20225805] [PMID: 31752267]

[35]   Leighton R, Watson JT, Giannoudis P, Papakostidis C, Harrison A, Steen RG. Healing of fracture nonunions treated with low-intensity pulsed ultrasound (LIPUS): A systematic review and meta-analysis. Injury 2017; 48(7): 1339-47.
[http://dx.doi.org/10.1016/j.injury.2017.05.016] [PMID: 28532896]

[36]   Einhorn TA, Gerstenfeld LC. Fracture healing: mechanisms and interventions. Nat Rev Rheumatol 2015; 11(1): 45-54.
[http://dx.doi.org/10.1038/nrrheum.2014.164] [PMID: 25266456]

[37]   Schmidt AH. Autologous bone graft: Is it still the gold standard? Injury 2021; 52 (Suppl. 2): S18-22.
[http://dx.doi.org/10.1016/j.injury.2021.01.043] [PMID: 33563416]

[38]   Wang W, Yeung KWK. Bone grafts and biomaterials substitutes for bone defect repair: A review. Bioact Mater 2017; 2(4): 224-47.
[http://dx.doi.org/10.1016/j.bioactmat.2017.05.007] [PMID: 29744432]

[39]   Sohn HS, Oh JK. Review of bone graft and bone substitutes with an emphasis on fracture surgeries. Biomater Res 2019; 23(1): 9.
[http://dx.doi.org/10.1186/s40824-019-0157-y] [PMID: 30915231]

[40]   Flierl MA, Smith WR, Mauffrey C, *et al.* Outcomes and complication rates of different bone grafting modalities in long bone fracture nonunions: a retrospective cohort study in 182 patients. J Orthop Surg Res 2013; 8(1): 33.
[http://dx.doi.org/10.1186/1749-799X-8-33] [PMID: 24016227]

[41]   Benninger E, Zingg PO, Kamath AF, Dora C. Cost analysis of fresh-frozen femoral head allografts: is it worthwhile to run a bone bank? Bone Joint J 2014; 96-b(10): 1307-1.
[http://dx.doi.org/10.1302/0301-620X.96B10.33486]

[42]   Huang RL, Tremp M, Ho CK, Sun Y, Liu K, Li Q. Prefabrication of a functional bone graft with a pedicled periosteal flap as an *in vivo* bioreactor. Sci Rep 2017; 7(1): 18038.
[http://dx.doi.org/10.1038/s41598-017-17452-5] [PMID: 29269864]

[43]   Smith CA, Board TN, Rooney P, Eagle MJ, Richardson SM, Hoyland JA. Correction: Human decellularized bone scaffolds from aged donors show improved osteoinductive capacity compared to young donor bone. PLoS One 2017; 12(11): e0187783.
[http://dx.doi.org/10.1371/journal.pone.0187783] [PMID: 29095911]

[44]   Smith CA, Richardson SM, Eagle MJ, Rooney P, Board T, Hoyland JA. The use of a novel bone allograft wash process to generate a biocompatible, mechanically stable and osteoinductive biological scaffold for use in bone tissue engineering. J Tissue Eng Regen Med 2015; 9(5): 595-604.
[http://dx.doi.org/10.1002/term.1934] [PMID: 24945627]

[45]   Sladkova M, Cheng J, Palmer M, *et al.* Comparison of Decellularized Cow and Human Bone for Engineering Bone Grafts with Human Induced Pluripotent Stem Cells. Tissue Eng Part A 2019; 25(3-4): 288-301.
[http://dx.doi.org/10.1089/ten.tea.2018.0149] [PMID: 30129897]

[46]   Bracey DN, Jinnah AH, Willey JS, *et al.* Investigating the Osteoinductive Potential of a Decellularized Xenograft Bone Substitute. Cells Tissues Organs 2019; 207(2): 97-113.
[http://dx.doi.org/10.1159/000503280] [PMID: 31655811]

[47]   Bracey D, Seyler T, Jinnah A, *et al.* A Decellularized Porcine Xenograft-Derived Bone Scaffold for Clinical Use as a Bone Graft Substitute: A Critical Evaluation of Processing and Structure. J Funct Biomater 2018; 9(3): 45.
[http://dx.doi.org/10.3390/jfb9030045] [PMID: 30002336]

[48]   Bracey DN, Seyler TM, Jinnah AH, *et al.* A porcine xenograft☐derived bone scaffold is a biocompatible bone graft substitute: An assessment of cytocompatibility and the alpha☐Gal epitope. Xenotransplantation 2019; 26(5): e12534.
[http://dx.doi.org/10.1111/xen.12534] [PMID: 31342586]

[49] Gardin C, Ricci S, Ferroni L, *et al.* Decellularization and Delipidation Protocols of Bovine Bone and Pericardium for Bone Grafting and Guided Bone Regeneration Procedures. PLoS One 2015; 10(7): e0132344.
[http://dx.doi.org/10.1371/journal.pone.0132344] [PMID: 26191793]

[50] You L, Weikang X, Lifeng Y, Changyan L, Yongliang L, Xiaohui W, *et al.* et al. in vivo immunogenicity of bovine bone removed by a novel decellularization protocol based on supercritical carbon dioxide. Artificial Cells, Nanomedicine, and Biotechnology. 2018; 46((sup2): 334-44.

[51] Liu X, Jakus AE, Kural M, *et al.* Vascularization of Natural and Synthetic Bone Scaffolds. Cell Transplant 2018; 27(8): 1269-80.
[http://dx.doi.org/10.1177/0963689718782452] [PMID: 30008231]

[52] Nakamura N, Kimura T, Nam K, *et al.* Induction of *in Vivo* Ectopic Hematopoiesis by a Three-Dimensional Structured Extracellular Matrix Derived from Decellularized Cancellous Bone. ACS Biomater Sci Eng 2019; 5(11): 5669-80.
[http://dx.doi.org/10.1021/acsbiomaterials.8b01491] [PMID: 33405698]

[53] Nakamura N, Saito K, Kimura T, Kishida A. Recellularization of decellularized cancellous bone scaffolds using low-temperature cell seeding. Tissue Cell 2020; 66: 101385.
[http://dx.doi.org/10.1016/j.tice.2020.101385] [PMID: 32933708]

[54] Lee MS, Lee DH, Jeon J, Tae G, Shin YM, Yang HS. Biofabrication and application of decellularized bone extracellular matrix for effective bone regeneration. J Ind Eng Chem 2020; 83: 323-32.
[http://dx.doi.org/10.1016/j.jiec.2019.12.005]

[55] Huai G, Qi P, Yang H, Wang Y. Characteristics of α-Gal epitope, anti-Gal antibody, α1,3 galactosyltransferase and its clinical exploitation (Review). Int J Mol Med 2016; 37(1): 11-20.
[http://dx.doi.org/10.3892/ijmm.2015.2397] [PMID: 26531137]

[56] Sun X, Liu C, Shi Y, *et al.* The assessment of xenogeneic bone immunotoxicity and risk management study. Biomed Eng Online 2019; 18(1): 108.
[http://dx.doi.org/10.1186/s12938-019-0729-z] [PMID: 31727050]

[57] Goldring SR. The osteocyte: key player in regulating bone turnover RMD Open 2015; 1(Suppl 1)): e000049-e..
[http://dx.doi.org/10.1136/rmdopen-2015-000049]

[58] Leng Y, Ren G, Cui Y, *et al.* Platelet-rich plasma-enhanced osseointegration of decellularized bone matrix in critical-size radial defects in rabbits. Ann Transl Med 2020; 8(5): 198.
[http://dx.doi.org/10.21037/atm.2020.01.53] [PMID: 32309345]

[59] Rashmi PR, Pathak R, Amarpal , *et al.* Evaluation of tissue-engineered bone constructs using rabbit fetal osteoblasts on acellular bovine cancellous bone matrix. Vet World 2017; 10(2): 163-9.
[http://dx.doi.org/10.14202/vetworld.2017.163-169] [PMID: 28344398]

[60] García-González CA, Concheiro A, Alvarez-Lorenzo C. Processing of Materials for Regenerative Medicine Using Supercritical Fluid Technology. Bioconjug Chem 2015; 26(7): 1159-71.
[http://dx.doi.org/10.1021/bc5005922] [PMID: 25587916]

[61] Crane JL, Zhao L, Frye JS, Xian L, Qiu T, Cao X. IGF-1 Signaling is Essential for Differentiation of Mesenchymal Stem Cells for Peak Bone Mass. Bone Res 2013; 1(2): 186-94.
[http://dx.doi.org/10.4248/BR201302007] [PMID: 26273502]

[62] Chin KY, Ima-Nirwana S, Mohamed IN, *et al.* Insulin-like growth factor-1 is a mediator of age-related decline of bone health status in men. Aging Male 2014; 17(2): 102-6.
[http://dx.doi.org/10.3109/13685538.2014.896895] [PMID: 24593848]

[63] Kawai M, Rosen CJ. The insulin-like growth factor system in bone: basic and clinical implications. Endocrinol Metab Clin North Am 2012; 41(2): 323-333, vi.
[http://dx.doi.org/10.1016/j.ecl.2012.04.013] [PMID: 22682633]

[64]   Wang ZX, Chen C, Zhou Q, *et al.* The Treatment Efficacy of Bone Tissue Engineering Strategy for Repairing Segmental Bone Defects Under Osteoporotic Conditions. Tissue Eng Part A 2015; 21(17-18): 2346-55.
[http://dx.doi.org/10.1089/ten.tea.2015.0071] [PMID: 26066049]

[65]   Nie Z, Wang X, Ren L, Kang Y. Development of a decellularized porcine bone matrix for potential applications in bone tissue regeneration. Regen Med 2020; 15(4): 1519-34.
[http://dx.doi.org/10.2217/rme-2019-0125] [PMID: 32441554]

[66]   Zheng Z, Chen Y, Wu D, *et al.* Development of an Accurate and Proactive Immunomodulatory Strategy to Improve Bone Substitute Material-Mediated Osteogenesis and Angiogenesis. Theranostics 2018; 8(19): 5482-500.
[http://dx.doi.org/10.7150/thno.28315] [PMID: 30555559]

[67]   Ley K. M1 Means Kill; M2 Means Heal. J Immunol 2017; 199(7): 2191-3.
[http://dx.doi.org/10.4049/jimmunol.1701135] [PMID: 28923980]

[68]   Gong L, Zhao Y, Zhang Y, Ruan Z. The Macrophage Polarization Regulates MSC Osteoblast Differentiation *in vitro.* Ann Clin Lab Sci 2016; 46(1): 65-71.
[PMID: 26927345]

[69]   Muñoz J, Akhavan NS, Mullins AP, Arjmandi BH. Macrophage Polarization and Osteoporosis: A Review. Nutrients 2020; 12(10): 2999.
[http://dx.doi.org/10.3390/nu12102999] [PMID: 33007863]

[70]   Kao WJ, McNally AK, Hiltner A, Anderson JM. Role for interleukin-4 in foreign-body giant cell formation on a poly(etherurethane urea)*in vivo.* J Biomed Mater Res 1995; 29(10): 1267-75.
[http://dx.doi.org/10.1002/jbm.820291014] [PMID: 8557729]

[71]   Roux BM, Cheng MH, Brey EM. Engineering clinically relevant volumes of vascularized bone. J Cell Mol Med 2015; 19(5): 903-14.
[http://dx.doi.org/10.1111/jcmm.12569] [PMID: 25877690]

CHAPTER 12

3D-Scaffold Design of Biodegradable Nanofibers for Tissue Regeneration and Drug Delivery

Wan Kartini binti Wan Abdul Khodir[1,2] and **Mohd Reusmaazran bin Yusof**[3,*]

[1] *Department of Chemistry, Kulliyyah of Science, International Islamic University Malaysia Kuantan Campus, Bandar Indera Mahkota, Kuantan 25200, Pahang, Malaysia*

[2] *SYNTOF, Kulliyyah of Science, International Islamic University Malaysia Kuantan Campus, Bandar Indera Mahkota, Kuantan 25200, Pahang, Malaysia*

[3] *Material Technology Group, Agensi Nuclear Malaysia, Bangi, 43000, Selangor, Malaysia*

Abstract: Materials with specific properties and structures are required for 3D nanofibers scaffold to perform well during tissue regeneration and drug delivery applications. When designing and fabricating 3D scaffolds, it is crucial to consider how the biomaterials interact with the native tissue structures and how they function in the surrounding environment. This chapter provided a brief discussion on the fabrication methods used to construct 3D biodegradable polymeric nanofibers scaffolds through electrospinning from 2D structures. Further, it extended to the characterisation required for the scaffold to be used in either tissue engineering or drug delivery. Additionally, this chapter presented recent progress in the practical application of 3D scaffolds that incorporate different therapeutic agents.

Keywords: 3D scaffold, Electrospinning, Nanofibers, Tissue regenerations, Drug delivery.

INTRODUCTION

According to Wilson *et al.* [1] and Barhoum *et al.* [2], nanofibers can have an outer diameter below 1000 nm and an aspect ratio of less than 50 nm. Nanofibers consist of two external dimensions at the nanoscale, with the third dimension being larger. The development of nanofibers has progressively led to scaffold materials, specifically in tissue engineering and drug delivery system applications. The limited cellular infiltration in 2D scaffolds is a major issue due to the closed-pack arrangement of the scaffold, which inhabits some of the functions similar to native tissue. Unstable cellular infiltration leads to distorted cell migration into the scaffold, resulting in non-uniform cellular distribution, limitations in vascularisa-

* **Corresponding author Mohd Reusmaazran bin Yusof:** Material Technology Group, Agensi Nuclear Malaysia, Bangi, 43000, Selangor, Malaysia; E-mail: reusmaazran@nuclearmalaysia.com

tion and compromised cell regeneration. Thus, the 3D nanofibers scaffold provides biomimetic structures for cell activities in the microenvironment [3 - 5]. Given the limitations that arise from a 2D nanofibers scaffold, many research groups are interested in developing 3D scaffolds for tissue engineering to overcome these limitations.

Electrospinning

Electrospinning has emerged as a suitable technique for creating a 3D structure from a nanofibers scaffold as shown in Fig. (**1**). The transformation of this technology into a 3D structure has been a great challenge and interest to many research groups. Combining this technique with other methods or post-processing techniques has also shown promise in producing 3D nanofiber structures. Recently, Vyas *et al.* [6] used a combination of 3D printing and electrospinning to create a complex hierarchical structure of polycaprolactone (PCL) micro/nanofibers. Chen *et al.* [7] utilised a hybridisation of electrospinning and freeze-drying technique to produce 3D scaffold structures. During the fabrication process, they used an electrospun mat with the foaming agent sodium borohydride to construct the 3D structure, which was then freeze-dried to obtain a 3D structure with better integrity.

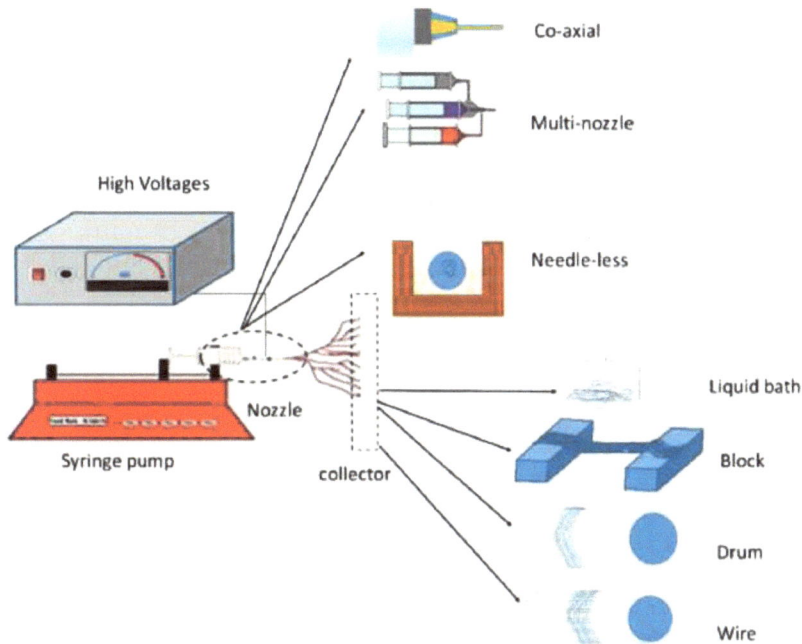

Fig. (1). The versatile configuration of electrospinning with different features.

The electrospinning technique is versatile, low-cost, easy to set up, making it an attractive method to produce a porous scaffold that mimics natural tissue. The basic electrospinning set-up consists of a high-voltage unit, nozzle and collector, which can be configured vertically or horizontally with stationery or rotary collectors. Other modifications to electrospinning include core-axial electrospinning, needless electrospinning and multi-nozzle feature, which can be used to create various scaffold structures. Co-axial electrospinning has been used to create core-sheath structure nanofibers, which are suitable for drug delivery applications [8]. This method involves the use of a dual nozzle system with a smaller diameter nozzle positioned inside a larger diameter nozzle. The larger nozzle is used to produce= the sheath structure, while the core structure is constructed by the smaller diameter nozzle.

In tissue regeneration, both single and multi-nozzles were used to produce different structures of fibres. Yusof *et al.* [9] used nozzle electrospinning with a dual polymer system to produce biodegradable polymeric nanofibers. The electrospinning mechanism involves several stages before the nanofibers are deposited onto the collector. The first stage of electrospinning involves applying high voltage to create a potential difference between the needle tips and the collector, which generates an electrostatic field between them. Subsequently, the polymer solution is pushed towards the end of the needle tips. In the second stage of electrospinning, the polymer solution at the tips becomes electrically charged. In the next stage of electrospinning, the polymer solution forms a polymer jet that is attracted toward the collector by the electric force. At a critical voltage, the charges on the polymer solution break the surface tension, causing the jet to drive toward the collector [10]. During this process, the polymer jet may experience winding instability, resulting from existing repulsive forces in the jet [11, 12]. This instability causes the jet to break into smaller jets until it reaches the nanoscale, resulting in the formation of nanofibers. The final stage of electrospinning is the deposition of dry fibres on the collector. As the polymer jet travels towards the collector, the solvent in the polymer solution evaporates, causing the fibre to dry being deposited onto the collector.

Optimization of Electrospinning Parameter

The formation of nanofiber scaffolds is influenced by numerous factors, including system and process parameters. System parameters include the properties of the polymer solution such as electrical conductivity, solvent properties and surface tension. On the other hand, process parameters consist of voltages, flow rate, distance and collector types. In addition to system and process parameters, other environmental factors such as humidity and temperature may also influence nanofiber formation. All of these parameters collectively affect the morphology of the resulting nanofibers. For instance, the characteristics of the polymer solution used can directly impact the formation of the nanofiber scaffold during fabrication.

Meanwhile, the type and molecular weight of the polymer used can impact the degree of entanglement in the resulting nanofibers. Therefore, it is crucial to optimise various parameters to design nanofibers with the desired structure and properties. Table **1** describes the parameters that can influence the properties of the nanofibers.

Table 1. The electrospinning parameters that influence the nanofibers properties

Parameters	Scaffold Properties	References
Concentration	An increase in polymer solution concentration results in an increase in nanofiber diameter, along with a greater likelihood of bead formation. Conversely, if the concentration is too low, electrospraying may occur.	[13-15]
Electrical Conductivity	The electrical conductivity of the polymer solution determines the density of charges that accumulate within it. A higher electrical conductivity results in a smaller nanofiber diameter as it increases the tensile force in the polymer jet during electrospinning.	[7,16]
Surface Tension	An increase in surface tension generally leads to a larger nanofiber diameter. Additionally, the Rayleigh instability phenomenon, which occurs as the polymer jet travels from the nozzle to the collector, can result in the formation of beads on the fibers.	[17, 18]
Voltages	The voltage induces charges and forms an electrical field. Increasing the voltage will reduce the diameter of fibres produced.	[19-22]
Flowrates	The critical flow rate of the polymer solution can be determined to produce nanofibers free from beads. Increasing the flow rate results in larger fiber diameter and may lead to the formation of beads. However, a higher flow rate can also negatively affect the stability of the polymer jet, resulting in non-uniform nanofibers.	[12, 23, 24]
Distances	Increasing the distance between the nozzle and collector will result in smaller diameter fibers. This factor can interact with other parameters since greater distance means a longer travel time for the polymer jet. The evaporation of polymer solution plays a role during the jet travel.	[6, 25]
Collector Type (a) Rotary (b) Stationary	Collectors determine the type of nanofibers produced. A stationary collector produces non-woven fibers, while a rotary collector generates aligned nanofibers.	[26]

Biodegradable Polymeric as 3D Scaffold Materials

A vast range of materials are used to design and fabricate scaffold materials for tissue regeneration applications. Material selection must consider the scaffold's functionality, including the single-phase polymeric material, polymer blend and polymer composite related to the spin ability to form the 3D electrospun mat. Biodegradability, surface hydrophilic, swelling behaviour, crystallinity and mechanical properties of the material have become a significant concern in designing the scaffold. The selected material for a scaffold must be biocompatible and should not cause any local or systemic adverse biological responses [27]. In addition, the material should be non-toxic, non-carcinogenic and non-mutagenic. The ability of the materials to interact chemically with other materials in the composition phase can influence the scaffold's biodegradation properties and surface chemistry, which can promote cell adhesion.

Synthetic Polymer

A wide range of synthetic polymeric materials have been used to construct 3D scaffolds due to their mechanical integrity, spinnability, tunability of diameters and cost-effectiveness. Examples of these materials include aliphatic polyester, PCL, poly (l-lactide acid) (PLLA), poly (vinyl alcohol) (PVA), Poly (glycolide) (PGA), poly (ethylene oxide) (PEO), which have been used to produce the electrospun nanofibers for tissue engineering. For instance, PLLA has been widely used in biomaterials and tissue engineering materials for its biocompatibility and excellent tensile properties, which typically range from 40-70 MPa. Additionally, PLLA exhibits semi-crystalline properties of about 40-50%, and a glass transition temperature of 60-80°C [28]. PLLA is also known to be biodegradable. Chen *et al.* [29] created a 3D structure using PLLA incorporated with gelatine, resulting in a high-porosity scaffold with a randomly distributed pore structure. The treated sample achieved a compressive strength of about 1000 kPa, and the scaffold demonstrated excellent absorbent capability while maintaining its original 3D structure during immersion. Additionally, the scaffold showed excellent biocompatibility, with cells adhering to the 3D surface and integrating with one another to form a sheet of cells. In other studies, PLA was combined with silk fibroin to produce 3D scaffolds for nerve regeneration [30]. The layered structure of the scaffold was successfully created with an interlayer space ranging from 20 to 150 mm. The fibers, with a diameter ranging from 50 to 500 nm, are randomly arranged in a 3D structure. The wall thickness is between 10 and 20 mm, and the unique orientation and random nanofibers structure make it suitable for peripheral nerve regeneration. The scaffold was reported to promote cell adhesion and the proliferation of Schwann cells.

Natural Polymer

Natural polymers are in great demand and subject to extensive research around the globe due to their excellent biocompatibility, desirable biodegradable properties and sufficient mechanical integrity. Polysaccharides and protein source materials are commonly used to fabricate 3D electrospun nanofibers. Polysaccharides such as starch, cellulose, chitin, chitosan and alginate have been used to fabricate nanofibers, whereas protein sources include collagen, elastin, elastin, silk fibroin and fibrinogen. 3D scaffolds are often incorporated with various natural polymers in blending or composite form. For example, 28 types of collagen have been discovered, but only types 1 to IV and XI involve fibrous structures. Collagen is the major protein of the ECM and plays a vital role in regulating cell function and providing structural support to the tissue. Collagen has been successfully fabricated into nanofibers scaffolds that mimic the structure and biological properties of natural collagen ECM, with fibers diameters ranging from 50 to 500 nm as found in the native tissue [31]. Shih *et al.* [32] produced 3D scaffolds from type I collagen with diameters ranging from 50 to 1000 nm. The scaffold supported *in vitro* adhesion, growth and differentiation of mesenchymal stem cells (MSCs). Incorporating biomolecules such as growth factors, cytokines, DNA, RNA and drugs in electrospun nanofibers enhances their functionality by improving the interaction between cells and materials [33].

DESIGN OF 3D ELECTROSPUN NANOFIBERS BASED-SCAFFOLDS FOR TISSUE ENGINEERING

Tissue regeneration requires a specialised material structure that mimics the native tissue as a temporary scaffold in a specific microenvironment. Besides the structure, materials, either single or hybrid, are crucial for the scaffold to serve its purpose. Ideally, tissue engineering scaffolds must meet both the form and function of the native extracellular matrix (ECM). However, the native ECM is complex, dynamic and tissue-specific [4]. A successful tissue engineering scaffold must possess certain criteria such as sufficient porosity to allow for cellular migration and penetration. The surface area of the scaffold must have an appropriate surface area and proper surface chemistry to enhance adhesion, growth, migration and differentiation. The surface properties of the scaffold dictate cell anchorage and cellular response as well as other cellular corresponding functions.

The material used for the scaffold must have biodegradability with a comparable rate to that of the native ECM to promote better tissue ingrowth. The ECM structures have a diameter ranging from 50 to 500 nm and are composed of 3-dimensional arrays of polysaccharides, collagen, elastin, fibronectin and other natural polymers. The scaffold design for tissue engineering applications should consider the properties of the existing material in the native tissue. For example, the collagen matrix provides the cell-matrix and matrix-matrix interaction, making it a critical component of tissue architecture, whereas fibrinogen promotes cell proliferation, migration and hemostasis.

A construct of a 3D architecture is crucial in creating contact with cells to grow on the 3D structures and provide enough mechanical support. There are several techniques to construct the 3D scaffold based on electrospinning technology. Miszuk *et al.* [34] used innovative electrospun-based thermally induced self-agglomeration (TISA) for tissue regeneration. PCL nanofibers were immersed in a solution of water, gelatin and ethanol at 55°C. During this process, the nanofibers spontaneously agglomerated into 3D structures. Direct electrospinning was successfully used to fabricate 3D nanofibers without undergoing post-processing from 2D electrospun membranes. Fig. (**2**) shows an illustration of the fabrication of 3D nanofibers using freeze-dried and electrospinning techniques.

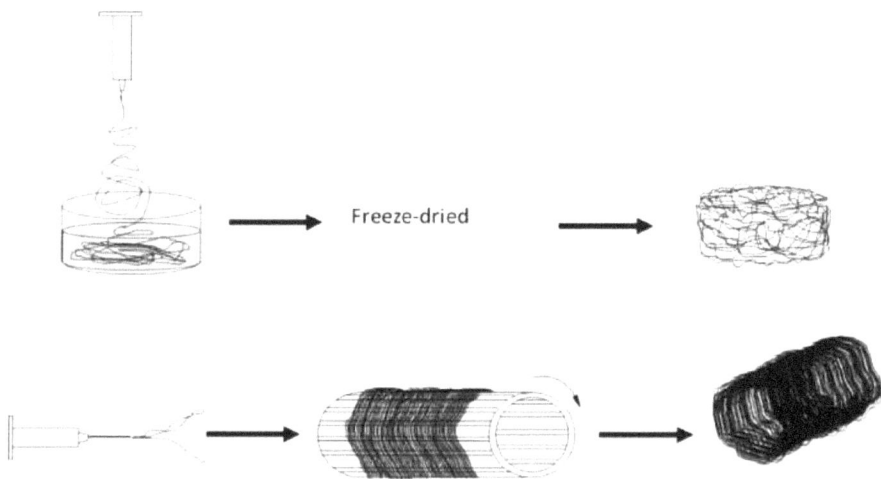

Fig. (2). Illustration of electrospun 3D scaffolds using freeze-dried and electrospinning technique.

Chen *et al.* [35] developed 3D nanofibers for cartilage tissue regeneration by dispersing nanofibers made of poly (lactide acid) (PLA)/gelatin in a tert-butanol solution. The mixture was then frozen at -20°C to allow for the growth of 3D structures in the solution. The freeze-dried nanofiber scaffolds were heated at 190°C. The resulting 3D nanofibers were collected in the middle of the jet flow using a roller collector. They were then freeze-dried to remove the rotary pin. Gas foaming coupled with electrospinning was successful in producing the 3D scaffold from 2D membranes. For example, the use of a $NaBH_4$ aqueous solution successfully transformed 2D nanofibers into 3D electrospun nanofibers. The pore structures and thickness of the 3D architectures depend on the nanofibers fabrication time with a gas bubble-forming solution. Similar techniques were used by Kim *et al.* [36] to fabricate the 3D structure of PCL by using azodicarbonamide as a chemical blowing agent to produce a highly porous structure through decomposition at 100°C. Different collectors can be used to manipulate the electrospinning process and create 3D structures. The insulating gap technique can be used as a supplementary collector to allow fibers to deposit longitudinally and form 3D structures [37]. Table **2** demonstrates materials and applications of 3D scaffolds produced by various techniques using synthetic and natural polymers for tissue regeneration purposes.

The 3D structure provides a larger contact area for cell adhesion and a more efficient transport mechanism through the porous structure. Nanofibers-based scaffolds can be fabricated using various techniques such as phase separation, drawing, gas formation, 3D printing, self-assembly, template synthesis and electrospinning. These techniques have continued to evolve and improve over time, thus achieving remarkable performance in specific sites of application for tissue regeneration.

CHARACTERIZATION OF 3D NANOFIBERS SCAFFOLDS FOR TISSUE ENGINEERING APPLICATION

The performance of a scaffold relies on the design structure during the fabrication process, making it crucial to characterise its geometry. The morphology and structure of the scaffold are categorised as physical or geometrical features. Geometrical features are primarily influenced by processing and fabrication parameters, while physical characteristics significantly predict performance as reflected by the mechanical integrity of the scaffold'. Geometrical features include nanofibers' diameter, porosity, structure, diameter distribution and surface architecture. Standard tools for characterising these features include scanning electron microscopy (SEM) or field emission scanning electron microscopy (FESEM) to determine surface morphology, pore structure, dimension of the diameter, and investigation of 3D scaffold nanofibers. Atomic force microscopy (AFM) is necessary for investigating surface architecture.

The analysis of mechanical properties is considered essential in the design and fabrication of 3D scaffolds. The ability of the scaffold to withstand loads during tissue growth or to support cell regulation is crucial for the regeneration mechanism. The scaffold needs to maintain its shape and structural integrity to avoid a collapsed structure in the *in vivo* environment. The porous structure needs to remain rigid during processes such as blood flow. The fibre struts need to have sufficient strength to support the porous structure. Excellent mechanical properties are necessary for the dynamic loading of tissues such as cartilage and tendon. Wu *et al.* [55] found that the aligned fibre exhibited higher tensile strength compared to the random 3D structure. Several tests have been conducted to obtain the mechanical properties of the scaffold such as tensile, compression, micro tensile and three-point bending tests.

The chemical interaction between components in scaffold materials can be determined by Fourier transform infrared (FTIR) and nuclear magnetic resonance (NMR) techniques. These techniques can reveal the bonding between specific locations of functional groups, which may change during processing, heat treatment and surface treatment of the scaffold. The transformation of chemical bonding can lead to modification in the biodegradability of the scaffold. For example, the study conducted by Huang *et al.* [56] indicated the formation of a new structure by mixing PEO and collagen, which was as shown in NMR analysis based on the formation of a new hydrogen bond in PEO. The crystallization nucleated from the processing method of dissolving techniques can be traced by x-ray diffraction (XRD) and wide-angle x-ray diffraction (WAXD). Both analyses can measure changes in the crystal size of the scaffold regarding various processing parameters. A combination of XRD and differential scanning calorimetry (DSC) analysis techniques could refine the investigation of the crystallinity of polymer nanofibers, which can affect the mechanical properties of the scaffolds. The current trend of using composite or hybrid materials in constructing 3D scaffold structures demands chemical analysis of the molecular structure and requires more complex analysis.

The scaffold in tissue regeneration acts as a temporary site for cell regulation and regeneration. Therefore, the scaffold must have the ability to degrade in the *in vivo* environment. The biodegradation process aids the regeneration mechanism. Polymeric materials degrade through the ester hydrolysis process, enzymatic hydrolysis and photolytic cleavage of the polymer chains [3]. Different materials exhibit different biodegradation rates. For example, the natural polymer collagen has a higher degradation rate than the synthetic PLLA polymer. Thus, it is crucial to design the scaffold with specific degradation behaviour. Treatment with ionizing radiation has also exhibited changes in the *in vitro* environment subject to the ionizing radiation fluency. Therefore, it is possible to use ionizing radiation to control the biodegradation rate of the scaffold [57]. The biodegradability of the scaffold can be evaluated by measuring the weight loss during biodegradation in a phosphate buffer (PBS) solution for a specified duration. Samadian *et al.* [58] reported an increase in weight loss of PLA/PCL/gelatin nanofibers with different compositions of Tau after 30 and 60 days. The weight loss is related to the biodegradation process, which occurs based on the hydrophilicity of the scaffold.

3D ELECTROSPUN POLYMERIC NANOFIBERS FOR DRUG DELIVERY

Controlled-release drug delivery technology was used instead of conventional dosage form and offered a predetermined rate and specific duration in a controlled manner, maintaining optimum drug plasma levels and optimising therapeutic efficacy [59, 60]. Recently, 3D electrospun scaffold polymeric nanofibers have emerged as an exciting strategy in drug delivery applications, specifically for antibacterial treatment, wound dressing and local cancer treatments. The 3D electrospun nanofibers used as drug carriers have an excellent reputation due to their unique properties such as a high surface area with interconnected pores, high loading capacity, high encapsulation efficiency, and the ability to support the controlled release of embedded drug molecules. Moreover, the ease of operation and tunability of polymeric fibers as macroscopic bulk materials give them the potential to be used in the local delivery of therapeutic agents [61-63]. 3D nanofibers scaffold can act as a reservoir matrix and protect the drug from the degradation medium, and the microstructure of nanofibers allows for robust control over the drug release profiles [62]. In order to meet specific therapeutic needs, different drug release profiles such as rapid, biphasic, zero-order, sequential and spatiotemporal release have been introduced. Electrospun nanofibers have been incorporated with antibiotics, anticancer, protein, DNA and RNA to achieve a controlled release profile [63]. In this article, the design strategies and the characterization of 3D scaffold nanofibers would be described, specifically in drug delivery applications.

Design and Strategies of 3D Electrospun Polymeric Nanofibers

Researchers have recently made significant efforts to develop 3D electrospun nanofibers scaffolds for drug delivery applications using various nozzle and add-on techniques as described in Table **3**. Simultaneous and sequential electrospraying, 3D printing, gas foaming, freeze-drying and centrifugal electrospinning have been employed. Simultaneous and sequential deposition techniques that integrate electrospinning and electrospraying offer multifunctional properties compared to single electrospinning. Guarino and his co-worker [62, 64] designed PCL nanofibers decorated with chitosan nanoparticles with amoxicillin and tetracycline hydrochloride using a simultaneous and sequential deposition. They demonstrated an improvement in drug entrapment and sustained the release of antibiotics [62, 64]. An electrospinning-electrospraying configuration produces multilayer membranes and provides spatiotemporal drug delivery [65, 67]. Recently, Liu *et al.* [68] designed core-sheath nanofibers with a 3D hierarchical structure made from hyaluronic acid/theophylline with PLA by using water/oil (w/o) emulsion electrospinning. The drug was released sustainably for nearly 30 days *via* the diffusion path and polymer matrix degradation mechanism.

Recent studies reported that 3D electrospinning technology-assisted 3D printing has been developed to enrich the fiber scaffold by controlling the scaffold composition, hierarchical architecture structure and shape. Liu *et al.* [69] created a PCL mesh using 3D printing and encapsulated PLGA core-shell nanofibers encapsulated with antibiotics (estradiol, lidocaine, metronidazole) and connective tissue growth factor. Using 3D printing as additive manufacturing provides sufficient mechanical strength, and the drugs can sustain release for up to 30 days. However, this technology has specific limitations such as materials, shapes and fibers orientation (random fibers) [74, 75].

Table 3. Recent literature on the design of 3D electrospun nanofibers for controlled release application.

Technique	Materials design	Prospective application	References
Simultaneous/ sequential electrospinning and electrospraying technique	PCL nanofibers decorated with Amoxicillin trihydrate and tetracycline hydrochloride loaded chitosan nano reservoirs.	Antibacterial treatment	[62,64]
	Rhodamine-loaded PLA nanofibers with PEG microparticles.	Drug delivery	[65]
	PLA nanofibers embedded iron-based particles with naproxen (drug).	Drug delivery	[66]
	PLGA fiber loaded with Rhodamine B (RhB) layered sandwich between PCL fibers.	Postoperative therapy	[67]
3D core-sheath emulsion electrospinning	w/o emulsion of hyaluronic acid/theophylline with PLA in 3D core-sheath nanofibers.	Drug delivery	[68]
Electrospinning with 3D printing	PCL mesh and multiple drugs, and growth factor loaded PLGA core-shell nanofibers.	Pelvic organ prolapse repair	[69]
Electrospinning with gas foaming technique	3D Chitosan/PVA layered nanofibers sponges.	Wound healing	[70]
	Silver nanoparticles decorated with 3D cellulose nanofibers.	Antibacterial treatment	[71]
Electrospinning and freeze-drying	3D SiO_2 nanofibers into elastic hydrogels scaffold.	Drug delivery	[72]
Centrifugal electrospinning and co-axial electrospinning	Emulsion centrifugal electrospinning of Pluronic F-68 loaded protein/PCL.	Deliver growth factor	[73]
	Ibuprofen and human epidermal growth factors (EGF) were loaded into CCS/PEO shell layer and core layer.	Wound healing	[74]

The gas foaming method was used to prepare a 3D porous sponge, which was combined with electrospinning using a H_2 bubble generator and $NaBH_4$ solution to produce 3D nanofibers sponges scaffolds. Zhang *et al.* [70] successfully prepared 3D layered chitosan/PVA nanofibers sponges for haemostasis and wound healing using the electrospinning integrated gas foaming method. The 3D sponges produced can absorb up to 60 times their weight in solution. Similarly, Kim *et al.* [71] produced silver nanoparticles decorated with 3D cellulose nanofibers using simultaneous gas foaming. It showed that the decorated 3D cellulose nanofibers had an excellent antibacterial effect on *Staphylococcus aureus* and *Escherichia Coli* with the help of silver nanoparticles. Ding *et al.* [72] reported the reconstruction of 3D SiO_2 nanofibers into elastic hydrogels scaffold using the freeze-drying method. A combination of electrospinning and freeze-drying method is used to build 3D porous structures, absorb more water content, organize cellular architecture, and have good mechanical properties.

Another recent strategy for creating a 3D nanofibers scaffold involves using nozzle-free centrifugal spinning technology that uses a rotating platform with centrifugal force [75]. The polymer solution is jetted toward the collector and produces fluffy mesh-like cocoon structures that allow for good cellular infiltration into the electrospun nanofiber. Buzgo *et al.* [73] and Kong *et al.* [74] used core-shell centrifugal spinning to protect therapeutic agents such as proteins and anti-inflammatory agents and release them properly at the site of action. The feasibility of delivering growth factors for wound healing applications using the centrifugal electrospinning technique has shown remarkable results in drug delivery.

Characterization of 3D Nanofibers Scaffold for Drug Delivery Application

Generally, the characterization of 3D electrospun polymeric nanofibers can provide insight into drug-polymer solvent interactions that may inform the properties of the final solid dispersion and drug release kinetics. Therefore, several techniques have been identified to investigate the final product. Table 4 summarises the characterization techniques for 3D nanofibers reported in several studies. Scanning electron microscopy (SEM) and transmission electron microscopy (TEM) are standard techniques used to measure fiber size, shape, surface features and fiber alignment. To confirm the core-sheath structure, TEM analysis can be used to analyse nanofibers [69]. The diameters of the nanofibers can be measured using ImageJ software (NIH, USA) from the morphological images [62, 76]. When the drug is loaded into nanofibers, the size diameters also increase [76]. Statistical data of the 3D nanofibers should be considered to obtain a reasonable estimation of the average fiber diameters of the scaffold.

A multi-functional materials scaffold can have a variety of structures. It requires a deep understanding of the material structure and properties to modulate the kinetics of drug release. Thus, it is necessary to investigate the physicochemical properties of 3D nanofibers using various techniques. Fourier transform infrared spectroscopy (FTIR) is used to analyse functional groups present in the polymer/drug and the absorption spectrum is recorded in the wavenumber range of 400 to 4000cm^{-1}. In the X-ray diffraction (XRD) technique, an X-ray, which acts as a source beam, is aimed at the samples and the diffraction pattern is observed. The crystallinity of the polymeric materials can be obtained from the XRD diffractogram.

Table 4. Summary of characterization techniques 3D nanofibers scaffold in the recent literature

Materials	SEM	TEM	FTIR	XRD	DSC	WCA	Tensile test	drug release	Other methods	References
PCL nanofibers decorated with chitosan/drugs.	x	x	-	-	-	-	-	x	Antibacterial test	[62,64]
Rhodamine-loaded PLA nanofibers with PEG microparticles	x	-	-	-	x	x	-	x	-	[65]
PLA nanofibers embedded iron-based particles with naproxen	x	-	x	x	-	x	x	x	ICP-AES, TGA	[66]
PVP/loratadine nanofibers 3D printed	x	-	x	x	x	-	-	x	-	[81]
HA/ theophylline with PLA in 3D core-sheath nanofibers	x	x	x	x	x	-	-	x	TGA	[68]
3D PCL mesh with drugs-loaded PLGA core-shell nanofibers.	x	x	x	-	-	x	x	x	Fatigue test, confocal microscopy	[69]
3D cellulose nanofibers decorated with silver nanoparticles	x	-	x	x	x	-	x	-	swelling ratio test, antibacterial test	[82]
Ibuprofen and hEGF loaded CCS/PEO shell layer and core layer	x	x	x	-	x	x	-	x	Viscosity, TGA, antibacterial test	[74]

Abbreviations: scanning electron microscopy (SEM), transmission electron microscopy (TEM), Fourier transform infrared spectroscopy (FTIR), X-ray diffraction (XRD), differential scanning calorimetry (DSC), water contact angle (WCA), inductive coupled plasma- atomic emission plasma (ICP-AES), thermogravimetric analysis (TGA), polycaprolactone (PCL), polylactic acid(PLA), polyethylene glycol (PEG), polyvinylpyrrolidone (PVP), hyaluronic acid (HA), polyethylene glycol (PLGA), human epidermal growth factor (hEGF), carboxylated chitosan (CCS), polyethylene oxide (PEO).

Bikiaris *et al.* [77] reported that polymers with a low degree of crystallinity exhibit higher drug release rates. The thermal properties and crystallinity of nanofibers can be measured using differential scanning calorimetry (DSC). A sample weighing around 5 mg was heated from 30 °C with a heating rate of 10 °C/ min. It was observed that 3D core-sheath nanofibers that were prepared using co-axial centrifugal spinning exhibited two endothermic peaks, indicating the occurrence of two-stage crystallization [78]. The hydrophilicity of the surface of electrospun nanofibers with drugs can be determined to characterize the water wettability and spreading capability of the material's surface and verify their release properties. If the contact angle is greater than 90°, the material is hydrophobic, and if the contact angle is less than 90°, the material is hydrophilic [79].

The mechanical properties of electrospun polymeric nanofibers are limited by their relatively low stiffness and strength due to their porous structure. Several factors affect the mechanical properties, including the diameter of the fiber size, defects on the bead and fiber alignment. Therefore, it is imperative to design 3D polymeric nanofibers as their mechanical properties are independent of their drug-release behaviours. Instead, mechanical properties can influence drug loading, drug-polymer interaction, release behaviour, drug partitioning and polymer degradation. Chen *et al.* [69] demonstrated that 3D printed PCL nanofibers exhibited comparable strength to non-degradable materials used for pelvic organ prolapse. In another study, the enhancement of the mechanical properties of 3D core-shell nanofibers showed an improvement in molecular alignment in polymer chains [80]. However, the mechanical properties of 3D cellulose acetate nanofibers loaded with silver nanoparticles, which were prepared using electrospinning integrated with gas foaming, showed significantly lower Young's modulus and ultimate tensile strength (UTS) values compared to 2D cellulose acetate nanofibers. The physical impact of the H_2 gas on the 3D fibers during the gas foaming process caused the 3D fibers to be separated from each other, thereby reducing their mechanical properties [71]. This shows that the various techniques used in the design of the 3D scaffold methods can affect the mechanical properties.

In vitro drug release performance must be studied to determine whether the drug concentration can be controlled to maintain the therapeutic effect of the drug. It has been accepted that drug-release properties from electrospun nanofibers would be significantly affected by the diameter of fiber. The electrospinning processing parameter influences the morphology of the final 3D nanofibers structure. By optimising the design parameters, sustained release for hydrophilic and hydrophobic drugs at high loadings can be achieved [81, 82]. Loratadine is known as a poorly water-soluble drug with low availability. Thus, Rita el al [81]. used polyvinylpyrrolidone (PVP) as a drug carrier and fabricated it using electrospinning and 3D printing (electrospun nanofibers have a higher surface area to volume ratio). During the first 10 minutes, around 66% of the drug was released from the nanofibers, and the controlled release pattern showed a higher release than the conventional sample, which only released 4% of the drug. This indicates faster drug release and higher dissolution for the poorly water-soluble loratadine, making it potentially useful for topical dosage forms. Rafiei *et al.* [83] prepared PCL-loaded bovine serum albumin (BSA) into 3D core-shell structures and 2D structures using co-axial wet electrospinning and blend electrospinning. The 3D electrospun scaffold showed superior performance by sustaining the protein release for 12 days compared to the conventional 2D forms of nanofibers due to their porosity and hydrophilicity properties. By using 3D nanofibers, researchers could tune the size of the fibers and porosity to suit the desired application.

CONCLUSION AND FUTURE PERSPECTIVE

The evolution of scaffolds from 2D to 3D nanofiber structures promises a prominent contribution to tissue generation and drug delivery applications. The limitations of 2D structure such as packing density can be overcome with scaffolds that can perform in a complex 3D microenvironment. Optimising various fabrication parameters and techniques ensures the production of scaffolds with a homogenous, porous structure that mimics the native tissue architecture. The improved structure and dimensions of these scaffolds encourage cell infiltration and homogenous tissue regeneration. Recently, 3D nanofiber structures have been successfully used in tissue regeneration for bone, tendon cartilage, muscle and ligament. In drug delivery applications, co-axial electrospinning techniques have been practically used to produce homogenous encapsulation of numerous drugs in core-sheath structures along the nanofibers to ensure sustained drug release. Previous studies also indicated that the core-sheath structure preserves the activity of drugs loaded into the fibre and release mechanism. In addition, the hybrid material used in the 3D construct has demonstrated its effectiveness in cell and material interaction in various studies, whether in tissue regeneration or drug delivery systems.

Characterising both the materials and structure design continues to be essential for specific scaffold applications. Some of the characterisations focus on understanding the fundamental properties and performance of materials, while others focus on structure design, which also plays an important role. For example, the physical structure, including pore size, pore and diameter distribution, and surface architecture, is known to have a great influence on the transport mechanism for both tissue engineering and drug release applications.

Although significant progress has been made in developing 3D structures from 2D constructs, many challenges remain to be resolved in future development to suit the dynamic microenvironment. One issue is combining bioactive molecules with current fabrication techniques while maintaining the efficacy of the biomolecules beneath the scaffold struts. Future study can also focus on developing hierarchical structures of different scales biomimetically to reflect the function of cell migration and proliferation.

REFERENCES

[1]   Wilson A. 1 - The formation of dry, wet, spunlaid and other types of non-wovens. In: Chapman RA, Ed. Applications of Non-wovens in Technical Textiles. Woodhead Publishing 2010; pp. 3-17.
[http://dx.doi.org/10.1533/9781845699741.1.3]

[2]   Barhoum A, Rasouli R, Yousefzadeh M, Rahier H, Bechelany M. Nanofiber Technology: History and Developments. In: Barhoum A, Bechelany M, Makhlouf A, Eds. Handbook of Nanofibers. Cham: Springer International Publishing 2018; pp. 1-42.

[3]   Han S, Nie K, Li J, *et al.* 3D Electrospun Nanofiber-Based Scaffolds: From Preparations and Properties to Tissue Regeneration Applications. Stem Cells Int 2021; 2021: 1-22.
[http://dx.doi.org/10.1155/2021/8790143] [PMID: 34221024]

[4]   Khorshidi S, Solouk A, Mirzadeh H, *et al.* A review of key challenges of electrospun scaffolds for tissue-engineering applications. J Tissue Eng Regen Med 2016; 10(9): 715-38.
[http://dx.doi.org/10.1002/term.1978] [PMID: 25619820]

[5]   Zhong S, Zhang Y, Lim CT. Fabrication of large pores in electrospun nanofibrous scaffolds for cellular infiltration: a review. Tissue Eng Part B Rev 2012; 18(2): 77-87.
[http://dx.doi.org/10.1089/ten.teb.2011.0390] [PMID: 21902623]

[6]   Vyas C, Ates G, Aslan E, Hart J, Huang B, Bartolo P. Three-Dimensional Printing and Electrospinning Dual-Scale Polycaprolactone Scaffolds with Low-Density and Oriented Fibers to Promote Cell Alignment. 3D Printing and Additive Manufacturing. 2020; 7: 105-3.

[7]   Chen Y, Shafiq M, Liu M, Morsi Y, Mo X. Advanced fabrication for electrospun three-dimensional nanofiber aerogels and scaffolds. Bioact Mater 2020; 5(4): 963-79.
[http://dx.doi.org/10.1016/j.bioactmat.2020.06.023] [PMID: 32671291]

[8]   Pant B, Park M, Park SJ. Drug Delivery Applications of Core-Sheath Nanofibers Prepared by Coaxial Electrospinning: A Review. Pharmaceutics 2019; 11(7): 305.
[http://dx.doi.org/10.3390/pharmaceutics11070305] [PMID: 31266186]

[9]   Yusof MR, Shamsudin R, Abdullah Y, Yalcinkaya F, Yaacob N. Electrospinning of carboxymethyl starch/poly(L-lactide acid) composite nanofiber. Polym Adv Technol 2018; 29(6): 1843-51.
[http://dx.doi.org/10.1002/pat.4292]

[10]   Bhardwaj N, Kundu SC. Electrospinning: A fascinating fiber fabrication technique. Biotechnol Adv 2010; 28(3): 325-47.
[http://dx.doi.org/10.1016/j.biotechadv.2010.01.004] [PMID: 20100560]

[11]   Yener F, Yalcinkaya B, Jirsak O. On the measured current in needle- and needleless electrospinning. J Nanosci Nanotechnol 2013; 13(7): 4672-9.
[http://dx.doi.org/10.1166/jnn.2013.7189] [PMID: 23901489]

[12]   Yarin AL, Koombhongse S, Reneker DH. Bending instability in electrospinning of nanofibers. J Appl Phys 2001; 89(5): 3018-26.
[http://dx.doi.org/10.1063/1.1333035]

[13]   Yalcinkaya F, Jirsak O, Gemci R. Effect of Polymer Concentration on Electrospinning System 2010.

[14]   Yener F, Yalcinkaya B. Electrospinning of polyvinyl butyral in different solvents. e-Polymers2013. p. 229.

[15]   Seeram Ramakrishna KF. Wee-Eong Teo. Teik-Cheng Lim & Zuwei Ma. An Introduction to Electrospinning and Nanofibers 2005.

[16]   Haider A, Haider S, Kang IK. A comprehensive review summarizing the effect of electrospinning parameters and potential applications of nanofibers in biomedical and biotechnology. Arab J Chem 2018; 11(8): 1165-88.
[http://dx.doi.org/10.1016/j.arabjc.2015.11.015]

[17]   Casasola R, Thomas NL, Trybala A, Georgiadou S. Electrospun poly lactic acid (PLA) fibres: Effect of different solvent systems on fibre morphology and diameter. Polymer (Guildf) 2014; 55(18): 4728-37.
[http://dx.doi.org/10.1016/j.polymer.2014.06.032]

[18]   Shahreen L, Chase GG. Effects of Electrospinning Solution Properties on Formation of Beads in Tio2 Fibers with PdO Particles. J Eng Fibers Fabrics 2015; 10(3)
[http://dx.doi.org/10.1177/155892501501000308]

[19]   Motamedi AS, Mirzadeh H, Hajiesmaeilbaigi F, Bagheri-Khoulenjani S, Shokrgozar M. Effect of electrospinning parameters on morphological properties of PVDF nanofibrous scaffolds. Prog Biomater 2017; 6(3): 113-23.
[http://dx.doi.org/10.1007/s40204-017-0071-0] [PMID: 28895062]

[20]   Aljehani AK, Hussaini MA, Hussain MA, Alothmany NS, Aldhaheri RW. Effect of electrospinning parameters on nanofiber diameter made of poly (vinyl alcohol) as determined by Atomic Force Microscopy. 2nd Middle East Conference on Biomedical Engineering. 379-81.
[http://dx.doi.org/10.1109/MECBME.2014.6783283]

[21]   Matabola K, Moutloali R. The influence of electrospinning parameters on the morphology and diameter of poly(vinyledene fluoride) nanofibers—Effect of sodium chloride 2013.

[22]   Yalcinkaya F, Komárek M, Lubasova D, sanetrníi f, Maryska J. Preparation of Antibacterial Nanofibre/Nanoparticle Covered Composite Yarns 2016.

[23]   Shamim Z, Bazgir S, Tavakoli A, Rashidi AS, Damerchely R. The Effect of Flow Rate on Morphology and Deposition Area of Electrospun Nylon 6 Nanofiber. J Eng Fibers Fabrics 2012; 7: 8.

[24]   Reneker DH, Yarin AL. Electrospinning jets and polymer nanofibers. Polymer (Guildf) 2008; 49(10): 2387-425.
[http://dx.doi.org/10.1016/j.polymer.2008.02.002]

[25]   Jiang J, Zheng G, Wang X, *et al.* Arced Multi-Nozzle Electrospinning Spinneret for High-Throughput Production of Nanofibers. Micromachines (Basel) 2019; 11(1): 27.
[http://dx.doi.org/10.3390/mi11010027] [PMID: 31878348]

[26]   Ulubayram K, Calamak S, Shahbazi R, Eroglu I. Nanofibers based antibacterial drug design, delivery and applications. Curr Pharm Des 2015; 21(15): 1930-43.
[http://dx.doi.org/10.2174/1381612821666150302151804] [PMID: 25732666]

[27]   Xavier MV, Macedo MF, Benatti ACB, *et al.* PLLA Synthesis and Nanofibers Production: Viability by Human Mesenchymal Stem Cell from Adipose Tissue. Procedia CIRP 2016; 49: 213-21.
[http://dx.doi.org/10.1016/j.procir.2015.11.019]

[28]   Tashiro K, Kouno N, Wang H, Tsuji H. Crystal Structure of Poly(lactic acid) Stereocomplex: Random Packing Model of PDLA and PLLA Chains As Studied by X-ray Diffraction Analysis. Macromolecules 2017; 50(20): 8048-65.
[http://dx.doi.org/10.1021/acs.macromol.7b01468]

[29]   Chen W, Chen S, Morsi Y, *et al.* Superabsorbent 3D Scaffold Based on Electrospun Nanofibers for Cartilage Tissue Engineering. ACS Appl Mater Interfaces 2016; 8(37): 24415-25.

[http://dx.doi.org/10.1021/acsami.6b06825] [PMID: 27559926]

[30]   Rao F, Yuan Z, Li M, *et al.* Expanded 3D nanofibre sponge scaffolds by gas-foaming technique enhance peripheral nerve regeneration. Artif Cells Nanomed Biotechnol 2019; 47(1): 491-500.
       [http://dx.doi.org/10.1080/21691401.2018.1557669] [PMID: 30942090]

[31]   Sell SA, Wolfe PS, Garg K, McCool JM, Rodriguez IA, Bowlin GL. The Use of Natural Polymers in Tissue Engineering: A Focus on Electrospun Extracellular Matrix Analogues. Polymers (Basel) 2010; 2(4): 522-53.
       [http://dx.doi.org/10.3390/polym2040522]

[32]   Shih YRV, Chen CN, Tsai SW, Wang YJ, Lee OK. Growth of mesenchymal stem cells on electrospun type I collagen nanofibers. Stem Cells 2006; 24(11): 2391-7.
       [http://dx.doi.org/10.1634/stemcells.2006-0253] [PMID: 17071856]

[33]   Law JX, Liau LL, Saim A, Yang Y, Idrus R. Electrospun Collagen Nanofibers and Their Applications in Skin Tissue Engineering. Tissue Eng Regen Med 2017; 14(6): 699-718.
       [http://dx.doi.org/10.1007/s13770-017-0075-9] [PMID: 30603521]

[34]   Miszuk J, Liang Z, Hu J, *et al.* Elastic Mineralized 3D Electrospun PCL Nanofibrous Scaffold for Drug Release and Bone Tissue Engineering. ACS Appl Bio Mater 2021; 4(4): 3639-48.
       [http://dx.doi.org/10.1021/acsabm.1c00134] [PMID: 33969280]

[35]   Teo WE, Gopal R, Ramaseshan R, Fujihara K, Ramakrishna S. A dynamic liquid support system for continuous electrospun yarn fabrication. Polymer (Guildf) 2007; 48(12): 3400-5.
       [http://dx.doi.org/10.1016/j.polymer.2007.04.044]

[36]   Kim G, Kim W. Highly porous 3D nanofiber scaffold using an electrospinning technique. J Biomed Mater Res B Appl Biomater 2007; 81B(1): 104-10.
       [http://dx.doi.org/10.1002/jbm.b.30642] [PMID: 16924612]

[37]   Subramanian A, Krishnan UM, Sethuraman S. Fabrication of uniaxially aligned 3D electrospun scaffolds for neural regeneration. Biomed Mater 2011; 6(2): 025004.
       [http://dx.doi.org/10.1088/1748-6041/6/2/025004] [PMID: 21301055]

[38]   Carfi Pavia F, Di Bella MA, Brucato V, *et al.* A 3D☐scaffold of PLLA induces the morphological differentiation and migration of primary astrocytes and promotes the production of extracellular vesicles. Mol Med Rep 2019; 20(2): 1288-96.
       [http://dx.doi.org/10.3892/mmr.2019.10351] [PMID: 31173248]

[39]   Zhang C, Wang X, Zhang E, *et al.* An epigenetic bioactive composite scaffold with well-aligned nanofibers for functional tendon tissue engineering. Acta Biomater 2018; 66: 141-56.
       [http://dx.doi.org/10.1016/j.actbio.2017.09.036] [PMID: 28963019]

[40]   Meng J, Boschetto F, Yagi S, *et al.* Design and manufacturing of 3D high-precision micro-fibrous poly (l-lactic acid) scaffold using melt electrowriting technique for bone tissue engineering. Mater Des 2021; 210: 110063.
       [http://dx.doi.org/10.1016/j.matdes.2021.110063]

[41]   Gregor A, Filová E, Novák M, *et al.* Designing of PLA scaffolds for bone tissue replacement fabricated by ordinary commercial 3D printer. J Biol Eng 2017; 11(1): 31.
       [http://dx.doi.org/10.1186/s13036-017-0074-3] [PMID: 29046717]

[42]   Perez-Puyana V, Wieringa P, Yuste Y, *et al.* Fabrication of hybrid scaffolds obtained from combinations of PCL with gelatin or collagen *via* electrospinning for skeletal muscle tissue engineering. J Biomed Mater Res A 2021; 109(9): 1600-12.
       [http://dx.doi.org/10.1002/jbm.a.37156] [PMID: 33665968]

[43]   Lee SJ, Heo DN, Park JS, *et al.* Characterization and preparation of bio-tubular scaffolds for fabricating artificial vascular grafts by combining electrospinning and a 3D printing system. Phys Chem Chem Phys 2015; 17(5): 2996-9.
       [http://dx.doi.org/10.1039/C4CP04801F] [PMID: 25557615]

[44]   Li Y, Wang J, Qian D, *et al.* Electrospun fibrous sponge *via* short fiber for mimicking 3D ECM. J Nanobiotechnology 2021; 19(1): 131.
[http://dx.doi.org/10.1186/s12951-021-00878-5] [PMID: 33964948]

[45]   Khil MS, Cha DI, Kim HY, Kim IS, Bhattarai N. Electrospun nanofibrous polyurethane membrane as wound dressing. J Biomed Mater Res 2003; 67B(2): 675-9.
[http://dx.doi.org/10.1002/jbm.b.10058] [PMID: 14598393]

[46]   Gugutkov D, Gustavsson J, Cantini M, Salmeron-Sánchez M, Altankov G. Electrospun fibrinogen-PLA nanofibres for vascular tissue engineering. J Tissue Eng Regen Med 2017; 11(10): 2774-84.
[http://dx.doi.org/10.1002/term.2172] [PMID: 27238477]

[47]   Elnaggar MA, El-Fawal HAN, Allam NK. Biocompatible PCL-nanofibers scaffold with immobilized fibronectin and laminin for neuronal tissue regeneration. Mater Sci Eng C 2021; 119: 111550.
[http://dx.doi.org/10.1016/j.msec.2020.111550] [PMID: 33321614]

[48]   Wei L, Wu S, Kuss M, *et al.* 3D printing of silk fibroin-based hybrid scaffold treated with platelet rich plasma for bone tissue engineering. Bioact Mater 2019; 4: 256-60.
[http://dx.doi.org/10.1016/j.bioactmat.2019.09.001] [PMID: 31667442]

[49]   Wu Z, Meng Z, Wu Q, *et al.* Biomimetic and osteogenic 3D silk fibroin composite scaffolds with nano MgO and mineralized hydroxyapatite for bone regeneration. J Tissue Eng 2020; 11
[http://dx.doi.org/10.1177/2041731420967791] [PMID: 33294153]

[50]   Chawla D, Kaur T, Joshi A, Singh N. 3D bioprinted alginate-gelatin based scaffolds for soft tissue engineering. Int J Biol Macromol 2020; 144: 560-7.
[http://dx.doi.org/10.1016/j.ijbiomac.2019.12.127] [PMID: 31857163]

[51]   Giretova M, Medvecky L, Petrovova E, *et al.* Polyhydroxybutyrate/Chitosan 3D Scaffolds Promote *In Vitro* and *In Vivo* Chondrogenesis. Appl Biochem Biotechnol 2019; 189(2): 556-75.
[http://dx.doi.org/10.1007/s12010-019-03021-1] [PMID: 31073980]

[52]   Koffler J, Kaufman-Francis K, Shandalov Y, *et al.* Improved vascular organization enhances functional integration of engineered skeletal muscle grafts. Proc Natl Acad Sci USA 2011; 108(36): 14789-94.
[http://dx.doi.org/10.1073/pnas.1017825108] [PMID: 21878567]

[53]   Zhang F, Qian Y, Chen H, *et al.* The preosteoblast response of electrospinning PLGA/PCL nanofibers: effects of biomimetic architecture and collagen I. Int J Nanomedicine 2016; 11: 4157-71.
[http://dx.doi.org/10.2147/IJN.S110577] [PMID: 27601900]

[54]   Ji Y, Ghosh K, Shu X, *et al.* Electrospun three-dimensional hyaluronic acid nanofibrous scaffolds. Biomaterials 2006; 27(20): 3782-92.
[http://dx.doi.org/10.1016/j.biomaterials.2006.02.037] [PMID: 16556462]

[55]   Wu T, Li D, Wang Y, *et al.* Laminin-coated nerve guidance conduits based on poly(1 -lactide--o-glycolide) fibers and yarns for promoting Schwann cells' proliferation and migration. J Mater Chem B Mater Biol Med 2017; 5(17): 3186-94.
[http://dx.doi.org/10.1039/C6TB03330J] [PMID: 32263716]

[56]   Huang L, Nagapudi K, Apkarian RP, Chaikof EL. Engineered collagen-PEO nanofibers and fabrics. J Biomater Sci Polym Ed 2001; 12(9): 979-93.
[http://dx.doi.org/10.1163/156856201753252516] [PMID: 11787524]

[57]   Yusof MR, Shamsudin R, Zakaria S, *et al.* Electron-Beam Irradiation of the PLLA/CMS/β-TCP Composite Nanofibers Obtained by Electrospinning. Polymers (Basel) 2020; 12(7): 1593.
[http://dx.doi.org/10.3390/polym12071593] [PMID: 32709111]

[58]   Samadian H, Farzamfar S, Vaez A, *et al.* A tailored polylactic acid/polycaprolactone biodegradable and bioactive 3D porous scaffold containing gelatin nanofibers and Taurine for bone regeneration. Sci Rep 2020; 10(1): 13366.
[http://dx.doi.org/10.1038/s41598-020-70155-2] [PMID: 32770114]

[59]   Wang B, Hu L, Siahaan TJ. Drug Delivery: Principles and Applications. New Jersey, 2016.

[60]   Jr Allen LV, Ansel HC. Ansel's pharmaceutical dosage forms and drug delivery systems. 10th ed., Philadelphia 2014.

[61]   Hu X, Liu S, Zhou G, Huang Y, Xie Z, Jing X. Electrospinning of polymeric nanofibers for drug delivery applications 1852014; : 12-21. Journal of Controlled Release. Elsevier
        [http://dx.doi.org/10.1016/j.jconrel.2014.04.018]

[62]   Guarino V, Cruz-Maya I, Altobelli R, *et al.* Electrospun polycaprolactone nanofibres decorated by drug loaded chitosan nano-reservoirs for antibacterial treatments. Nanotechnology 2017; 28(50): 505103.
        [http://dx.doi.org/10.1088/1361-6528/aa9542] [PMID: 29058684]

[63]   Bhattarai SR, Saudi S, Khanal S, Aravamudhan S, Rorie CJ, Bhattarai N. Electrodynamic assisted self-assembled fibrous hydrogel microcapsules: a novel 3D *in vitro* platform for assessment of nanoparticle toxicity. RSC Advances 2021; 11(9): 4921-34.
        [http://dx.doi.org/10.1039/D0RA09189H] [PMID: 35424445]

[64]   Khodir WKWA, Guarino V, Alvarez-Perez MA, Cafiero C, Ambrosio L. Trapping tetracycline-loaded nanoparticles into polycaprolactone fiber networks for periodontal regeneration therapy. J Bioact Compat Polym 2013; 28(3): 258-73.
        [http://dx.doi.org/10.1177/0883911513481133]

[65]   Lavielle N, Hébraud A, Thöny-Meyer L, Rossi RM, Schlatter G. 3D Composite Assemblies of Microparticles and Nanofibers for Tailored Wettability and Controlled Drug Delivery. Macromol Mater Eng 2017; 302(8): 1600458.
        [http://dx.doi.org/10.1002/mame.201600458]

[66]   Figueiredo MP, Layrac G, Hébraud A, *et al.* Design of 3D multi-layered electrospun membranes embedding iron-based layered double hydroxide for drug storage and control of sustained release. Eur Polym J 2020; 131: 109675.
        [http://dx.doi.org/10.1016/j.eurpolymj.2020.109675]

[67]   Milosevic M, Stojanovic DB, Simic V, *et al.* Preparation and modeling of three☐layered PCL/PLGA/PCL fibrous scaffolds for prolonged drug release. Sci Rep 2020; 10(1): 11126.
        [http://dx.doi.org/10.1038/s41598-020-68117-9] [PMID: 32636450]

[68]   Liu M, Hao X, Wang Y, Jiang Z, Zhang H. A biodegradable core-sheath nanofibrous 3D hierarchy prepared by emulsion electrospinning for sustained drug release. J Mater Sci 2020; 55(35): 16730-43.
        [http://dx.doi.org/10.1007/s10853-020-05205-1]

[69]   Chen YP, Lo TS, Lin YT, Chien YH, Lu CJ, Liu SJ. Fabrication of drug-eluting polycaprolactone/ poly(Lactic-co-glycolic acid) prolapse mats using solution-extrusion 3d printing and co-axial electrospinning techniques. Polymers (Basel) 2021; 13(14): 2295.
        [http://dx.doi.org/10.3390/polym13142295]

[70]   Zhang K, Bai X, Yuan Z, *et al.* Layered nanofiber sponge with an improved capacity for promoting blood coagulation and wound healing. Biomaterials 2019; 204: 70-9.
        [http://dx.doi.org/10.1016/j.biomaterials.2019.03.008] [PMID: 30901728]

[71]   Moon JY, Lee J, Hwang TI, Park CH, Kim CS. A multi-functional, one-step gas foaming strategy for antimicrobial silver nanoparticle-decorated 3D cellulose nanofiber scaffolds. Carbohydr Polym 2021; 273.

[72]   Si Y, Wang L, Wang X, Tang N, Yu J, Ding B. Ultrahigh-Water-Content, Superelastic, and Shape-Memory Nanofiber-Assembled Hydrogels Exhibiting Pressure-Responsive Conductivity. Adv Mater 2017; 29(24): 1700339.
        [http://dx.doi.org/10.1002/adma.201700339] [PMID: 28417597]

[73]   Buzgo M, Rampichova M, Vocetkova K, *et al.* Emulsion centrifugal spinning for production of 3D drug releasing nanofibres with core/shell structure. RSC Advances 2017; 7(3): 1215-28.

[http://dx.doi.org/10.1039/C6RA26606A]

[74] Liu M, Duan XP, Li YM, Yang DP, Long YZ. Electrospun nanofibers for wound healing. 2017.
[http://dx.doi.org/10.1016/j.msec.2017.03.034]

[75] Chen S, John JV, McCarthy A, Carlson MA, Li X, Xie J. Fast transformation of 2D nanofiber membranes into pre-molded 3D scaffolds with biomimetic and oriented porous structure for biomedical applications. Appl Phys Rev 2020; 7(2): 021406.
[http://dx.doi.org/10.1063/1.5144808] [PMID: 32494338]

[76] Hamdan N, Darnis DS, Khartini W, Khodir WA. In vitro Evaluation of Crosslinked Polyvinyl Alcohol/Chitosan-Gentamicin Sulfate Electrospun Nanofibers. Vol. 23, Malaysian Journal of Chemistry 2021.

[77] Bikiaris D, Karavelidis , Karavas , Giliopoulos , Papadimitriou . Evaluating the effects of crystallinity in new biocompatible polyester nanocarriers on drug release behavior. Int J Nanomedicine 2011; (Nov): 3021.
[http://dx.doi.org/10.2147/IJN.S26016]

[78] Li Z, Mei S, Dong Y, *et al.* Multi-functional core-shell nanofibers for wound healing. Nanomaterials (Basel) 2021; 11(6): 1546.
[http://dx.doi.org/10.3390/nano11061546] [PMID: 34208135]

[79] Alarifi I, Alharbi A, Khan W, Swindle A, Asmatulu R. Thermal, electrical and surface hydrophobic properties of electrospun polyacrylonitrile nanofibers for structural health monitoring. Materials (Basel) 2015; 8(10): 7017-31.
[http://dx.doi.org/10.3390/ma8105356] [PMID: 28793615]

[80] Merkle V, Zeng L, Teng W, Slepian M, Wu X. Gelatin shells strengthen polyvinyl alcohol core–shell nanofibers. Polymer (Guildf) 2013; 54(21): 6003-7.
[http://dx.doi.org/10.1016/j.polymer.2013.08.056]

[81] Ambrus R, Alshweiat A, Csóka I, Ovari G, Esmail A, Radacsi N. 3D-printed electrospinning setup for the preparation of loratadine nanofibers with enhanced physicochemical properties. Int J Pharm 2019; 567: 118455.
[http://dx.doi.org/10.1016/j.ijpharm.2019.118455] [PMID: 31233846]

[82] Stack M, Parikh D, Wang H, Wang L, Xu M, Zou J, *et al.* Electrospun nanofibers for drug delivery. Electrospinning: Nanofabrication and Applications. Elsevier 2018; pp. 735-64.

[83] Rafiei M, Jooybar E, Abdekhodaie MJ, Alvi M. Construction of 3D fibrous PCL scaffolds by co-axial electrospinning for protein delivery. Mater Sci Eng C 2020; 113.

CHAPTER 13

Bio-based Hydrogels and Their Application for Intervertebral Disc Regeneration

Francesca Agostinacchio[1] and **Antonella Motta**[2,*]

[1] *University of Trento, Department of Industrial Engineering, via Sommarive 9, Trento (TN), 38123 Italy and BIOtech Research Center – Center for Biomedical Technologies, via delle Regole 101, Mattarello (TN), 38123, Italy*

[2] *Biotech Research Center, Department of Industrial Engineering, University of Trento, Mattarello (TN), Italy*

Abstract: The intervertebral disc is a complex hierarchical structure, function-dependent, with the main function to provide support during movements, thus functioning as the shock absorber of the vertebral column. Its properties change from the outer toward the inner part, following the diverse composition. It is avascular with poor self-healing capability. During the degeneration process, the cascade of events causes the rupture of the structure and of the extracellular matrix, not able anymore to sustain load stress, leading to cervical or low back chronic pain. Current clinical treatments aim at pain relief but according to the severity of the disease, it might require spinal fusion or a total disc replacement made of metal or plastic disc substitutes, thus reducing the patient's mobility. Tissue engineering and naturally derived hydrogels are gaining interest as important tools for mimicking and delivering cells or molecules either to regenerate a damaged part of the disc, but also its whole structure. Although in the last due decades several improvements have been achieved , the fabrication of IVD constructs, reproducing its structure and functions, is still challenging. For example the standardization of cell cultures conditions,cell sources, mechanical tests paramters, are fundamental achievements to translate the bio-fabricated products to the clinic.

Keywords: Biomaterials, Degeneration, Hydrogels, Intervertebral disc, Regeneration.

HUMAN INTERVERTEBRAL DISC: STRUCTURE AND FUNCTIONS

The intervertebral disc (IVD) is the biggest human avascular tissue. It provides support and flexibility to the vertebral column during tension, torsion, and extension, thus functioning as the shock absorber of the body. In the human vertebral column, there are 23 discs, helping the load transfer along the body. The

* **Corresponding author Antonella Motta:** Biotech Research Center, Department of Industrial Engineering, University of Trento, Mattarello (TN), Italy; E-mail:antonella.motta@unitn.it

Mohd Fauzi Mh Busra, Daniel Law Jia Xian, Yogeswaran Lokanathan and Ruszymah Haji Idrus (Eds.)

dimension of the disc varies according to the area (cervical, lumbar, etc.), but on average, it exhibits a thickness between 7-10 mm and a diameter equal to 40 mm. It is composed of a central part, the nucleus pulposus (NP) enclosed by the annulus fibrosus (AF) and both are sandwiched between the cartridge endplates (CEP). The NP is a jelly-like, deformable, structure composed of 80% water, 20% of collagen type II and proteoglycans [1]. NPs' main function is to resist compressive load [2] generated by the increasing hydrostatic pressure, which generates tension in the surrounding AF. Fundamental is the role of proteoglycans; they are hydrophilic molecules, negatively charged, able to bind and release water following the load applied to the structure, thus they are responsible for the high-water content and the NP reversible deformation according to the different body positions (Fig. **1**). Collagen type II fibrils serve as reinforcement of the NP, keeping the structure together during the continuous loading. The AF is responsible for the tensile strength, it is an elastic material composed of 2% elastin, 50-70% collagen (type I and type II) and water. It forms 15-25 concentric layers made of collagen I called lamellae with an increasing thickness going from the outer to the inner part (0.05-0.5um), providing support to structure during the load (Fig. **1**). The collagen distribution is different going from the outer to the inner layers (collagen type I in the outer part and collagen II in the inner one until the NP). Regarding the cell types present in the IVD, in the AF, there are cells with long elongation processes, fibroblast-like cells, while in the NP, the cells are more rounded, with a notochordal origin. The different morphology leads to different cell metabolic activities in the NP and AF [3]. Finally, the CEPs provide the anchorage for the collagen fibrils, are vascularized and thanks to a semi-permeable interface that they provide all the nutrients and oxygen supply required to the disc. However, since they are the only vascularized part of the intervertebral disc, the NP and AF cellular environment experiences low oxygen levels from 19.5% to 0.65%, where cell survival seems to be affected more by the glucose level than by low oxygen percentages [4]. Indeed, cellular metabolism is based on anaerobic glycolysis, where glucose consumption is essential for cell survival and metabolism [4, 5]. This kind of metabolism leads to the production of lactate, thus to pH levels with an average between 5.7-7-5 [6].

The IVD is a highly complex function-dependent structure, which provides the right stimuli and support to absorb the shock of the vertebral column during loading. Although the IVD is composed of the NP and the AF, there is not a defined border between the two structures, but a gradient changing in the architecture organization, cellular microenvironment, and the extracellular matrix (ECM) composition, moving from the outer towards the inner part of the disc. There is a strong connection between this complex structure, the biological environment, and the metabolism of the cells, all key factors in the response to the continuous loading applied during movements. Specifically, during daily activities, the NP sustains compression by squeezing, thus increasing its dimensions in the radial direction, and being sustained by the anulus fibrosus; after load, a healthy disc is able to elastically recover its original shape, thanks to the fluid flow along the vertebral body and the capability of proteoglycans to continuously bind and release water under the hydrostatic compression. The elastic deformation and recovery depend on the flow of fluid from the IVD to the vertebral body and vice versa. Giving the fact that the disc allows torsion, twisting, compression, and elongation to the vertebral column, the main stresses applied are compression, tension applied to the structure is compression, tension, hydrostatic pressure, and the osmotic one. A deep understanding of the mechanical stimuli applied to the intervertebral disc is a fundamental requirement to understand the relationship between its composition, functions, and mechanobiology. These stresses stimulating the IVD are responsible for the oxygen and nutrients diffusion, thus the glucose and ATP consumption, the cellular matrix deposition and the synthesis of new collagen type I and II fibrils and proteoglycans. Variations in the stimuli, affect the cellular response, the synthesis of IVD components, thus breaking the delicately balanced microenvironment and as a consequence affecting the whole disc function.

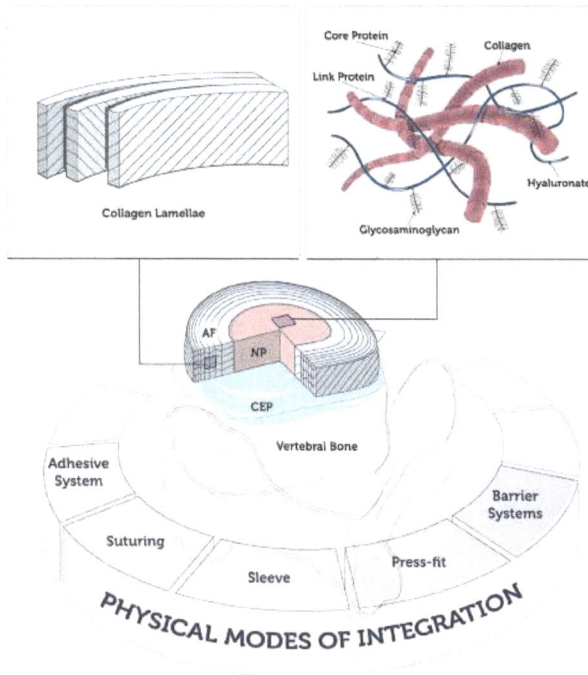

Fig. (1). Intervertebral disc made of nucleus pulposus (NP), annulus fibrosus (AF) and cartilage enplates (CEP), with some of possible strategies to regenerate it. Reproduced from Buckley *et al.*, (4), under the terms of the *Creative Commons CC BY* license.

By the biological point of view, the magnitude and the frequency of the stimuli applied to the disc are critical in dictating cellular responses in terms of gene expression, collagen, and proteoglycan synthesis. Additionally, the different stimuli experienced by the cells according to the disc area, dictate different cytoskeleton rearrangements, cell morphology, and cellular stiffness. Specifically, cells experience the variety of stimuli applied on the disc and this affect mainly the cytoskeleton organization involving, among other, the F-actin proteins. The different cell morphology among the NP and AF is due to a different organization in response to loads, leading to a peripheric distribution of the F-actin around NP cells, while it is elongated exhibiting cellular processes in the AF [6].

Worth noting is the immune privilege of the IVD. Indeed, due to the avascularity of the system, and the AF and CEP surrounding and isolating the NP, the latter results in complete protection from the immune system of the body. Even if, the full mechanisms behind this immune privilege are still unclear, the Blood Nucleus Barrier (BNB) concept has been introduced as a protection system similar to the blood brain barrier (BBB) [7]. However, during damage and degeneration, this complex system can be broken, and the autoimmune response of the body can be activated, leading to a chronic inflammation and pathological consequences. This privilege of the disc is a key factor to be kept into consideration while considering new regenerative approaches [7].

DISC DEGENERATION

The degeneration of the disc is a worldwide diffused problem, affecting almost the 90% of the population over 50 years old [8]. It is associated with lower back pain, reduction in mobility when it implicates the lumbar region of the vertebral column [9, 10], while in the cervical area, it is responsible of neck pain, loss of senses, and a reduction in mobility [11]. The degeneration can be related to age, excessive loading [12], trauma, or risk factors such as obesity, smoking, genetic susceptibility [13]. The result is the structural failure [14]. With age, the composition of the disc changes, where the NP becomes less hydrated, the production of proteoglycans is reduced leading to stiffening of the annulus fibrous, thus to a weaker structure under load [14]. Additionally, the CEPs start to calcify, thus reducing the oxygen, water, nutrient diffusion, and the waste removal, slowly inducing cell death [15, 16]. Inflammation is activated, and cytokines and metalloproteinase (MMPs) result in matrix degradation. The remodeling and changing in the architecture and biochemical composition of the IVD, leads to neo-angiogenesis and neo-innervation phenomena into the annulus fibrosus, apparently contributing to discogenic pain (Fig. **2**) [17, 18].

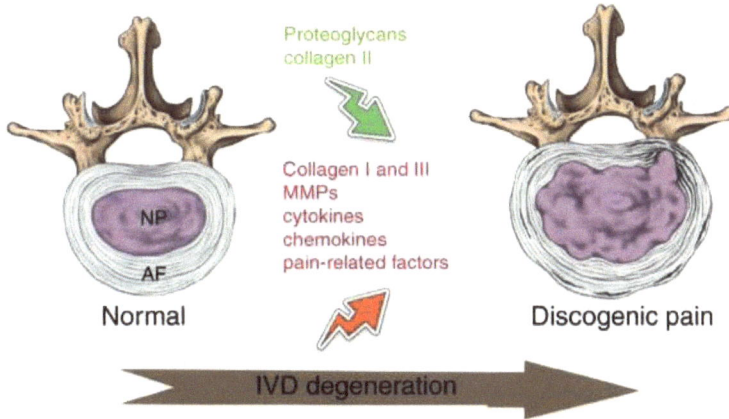

Fig. (2). Degenerative processes during IVD degeneration: decrease in the preotoglycans and collagen II, increasing collagen I and III together with inflammatory molecules like cytokines. Reproduced from Feng-Jan Lyu *et al.* (18), under a Creative Commons Attribution 4.0 International License

Disc degeneration, unbalanced biochemical processes, matrix remodeling and degradation and increased catabolic activity are all related to anatomical changes in the disc. At the starting level, the disc forms a bulge, when the structure becomes larger than its original boundaries but without affecting the nerves [19]. This degenerates into the formation of herniation which creates ruptures and tears into the AF (peripheral, circumferential, radial), not able anymore to support he NP deformations [20]. This can involve nerves, generating pain into the patient. The final effect is the loosening of the integrity of the structure, becoming more thinning, generating chronic pain.

The main therapies aim to the pain relief of the symptomatology related to the degeneration of the disc. However, based on the severity of the degeneration, the clinical approaches are focused on physical activity and physiotherapy, pharmaceuticals, injections, and in severe cases, surgical interventions with minimally invasive procedures to remove small part of the disc, or highly invasive in case of total disc replacement or spinal fusion [21, 22]. The last one is based on the insertion of a metal artificial disc, able to support the spine load. However, even if it might require periodical reoperation or consequences related to the implant, it provides better outcomes compared to the spinal fusion, allowing a better mobility and better clinical outcomes [23, 24].

Although most of the clinical treatments are focused on pain relief, another approach is the one aiming to reduce the severity of the degeneration. Indeed, cellular therapy, gene therapy, and proteins are useful and emerging tools used to alleviate and restore in some ways the microenvironment of the disc. Therapies based on cells transplantation, autologous or not, represent a promising approach. Studies are focusing mainly on mesenchymal cells (MSC) which in the right environment and in the presence of specific growth factors according to disc area, are able to differentiate in the proper cell phenotype [25]. Nonetheless, there are controversial studies about the proper cell types to be used. Indeed, if some works report mesenchymal stem cells as the ideal forefront for the disc regeneration, on the other side other researchers support the use of fully differentiated cells (the NP and AF ones) as more responsive in the repair of the disc homeostasis and microenvironment [17, 25].

TISSUE ENGINEERING

Beside the variety of the current therapeutic approaches, none of them, is able to restore or induce a full repair and regeneration of the IVD. For this reason, tissue engineering (TE) is emerging and gaining attention as a valid approach. TE aims at mimicking the structure and function of native tissue and organs, by combining cells, materials and proper stimuli.

Specifically, intervertebral disc TE represents a great challenge due to the complexity of the microstructure and hierarchical architecture to be reproduced, coupled with varying compositions, functions and cell morphology along the diameter of the disc. An additional challenge is the absence of vascularization and thus of self-healing capabilities. Firstly, the choice of the biomaterial, the form of the scaffold and its fabrications are essential requirements. Additionally, the immune privilege of the disc is a key factor to be kept into consideration since, not only staminal cells might be helpful in the regeneration process, but the biomaterials selected must be formulated in order to avoid any auto-immune reactions [7]. For this reason, natural biomaterials represent a valid alternative and are good candidates for disc applications. Moreover, considering the disc morphology and composition, and the important role of water content on the mechanical response of the disc, hydrogels represent the best option to create architecture for the regenerative purpose [26]. Hydrogels are 3D structures able to retain a high-water content, which can be easily processed with a variety of fabrication processes, and can be modified according to the target application by varying either their concentration and molecular weight [27].

The design and selection of biomaterials are affected by many factors, and among them two alternatives become particularly relevant: reproducing a single scaffold for total disc replacement, or separately producing a scaffold for the NP and one for the AF. An alternative is to engineer injectable hydrogels to restore damaged parts of the disc with minimally invasive procedures. Important criteria for the fabrication of compatible scaffolds for the intervertebral disc are appropriate mechanical properties combined with a slow degradation rate to balance the regenerative capacity of the avascular native disc, cell friendly environment, and a good diffusion of nutrients and oxygen [27]. Natural-derived biomaterials exhibit biocompatibility, low toxicity *in vivo*, tunable properties, and gelation rates, biodegradation and better mimic and resemble the natural composition of the native IVD compared to synthetic biomaterials [19]. Among them, worth noting are silk fibroin, hyaluronic acid, collagen/gelatin, Gellan gum, alginate, and chitosan.

Silk Fibroin

Silk fibroin is a fibrillar protein naturally derived from silkworm, providing structural strength to silk cocoons [28]. It is a fascinating biomaterial which can be fabricated in a variety of forms (hydrogels, films, sponges, fibers, foam). SF is biodegradable, biocompatible, but most importantly it exhibits highly tunable mechanical properties, tunable degradation rates and physical, chemical, and enzymatic gelation processes [29, 30]. In 2019, Costa *et al.*, reported the fabrication of a 3D printed AF made of 3D bio-printed silk fibroin and elastin biomaterials with a patient specific design [31]. Specifically, starting from patient's magnetic resonance images (MRI), applying a reverse engineering approach, a 3D segmentation and reconstruction of the structure have been performed, and the blend of the two biomaterials was printed. Gelation was performed before printing, *via* enzymatic crosslinking mediated by horse radish peroxidase (HRP), and later frozen, freeze-dried and stabilized in ethanol. The structure was fabricated with controlled shape and porosity; mechanical properties were tested through uniaxial compression test and DMA, closely meeting the mechanical requirements of the AF (0.56 ± 0.21 MPa). Biological evaluation was performed solely *in vitro*, up to 21 days using human adipose-derived mesenchymal stem cells (hASC), resulting in good biological outcomes[31].

Silk fibroin has been reported by Park *et al.* [32] in the fabrication of a biphasic composite scaffold for the whole intervertebral disc regeneration. Precisely, it consisted in the AF made of silk fibroin lamellar scaffold, fabricated *via* freeze-drying technique, ringing the NP which was mimicked with a gel of fibrin and hyaluronic acid (HA). A biological study was performed on the scaffold, seeding porcine chondrocytes in the NP hydrogels, and AF porcine cells in the external silk scaffold, cultivating them up to 6 weeks. The results showed that the structure was adequate to resemble the IVD properties by the biological point of view, with cell differentiation and increasing content of GAG and collagen production over the culture time. However, the authors underlined the necessity to perform mechanical properties tests in further studies before the *in vivo* analysis of the fabricated disc [32].

For NP regeneration, an interpenetrating hydrogel made of silk fibroin strain A (rich of tyrosine) and hyaluronic acid was crosslinked with HRP [33].

The authors demonstrated that human-bone-marrow derived mesenchymal stem cells (hBM-MSC)differentiated into a chondrogenic phenotype with an increase of GAG and collagen II production up to 14 days, *in vitro* in the presence of hydrogel, combination of silk fibroin strain A with hyaluronic acid, and the transforming growth factor TGF-β. Additionally, the hydrogels exhibited viscoelasticity similar to the native NP [33].

Hyaluronic Acid

Hyaluronic acid is a glycosaminoglycan, physiologically present in the nucleus pulposus, contributing to shock absorption and lubrifaction, being a negatively charged molecule able to absorb water from $10-10^4$ of its weight mass [34]. In a recent study, Choi *et al.* [35], investigated the effect of Wharton's jelly-derived mesenchymal stromal cells (WJ-MSCs) delivered in rat degenerated NP loaded into an hydrogel of hyaluronan and methyl cellulose. In their work, they demonstrated that the presence of the gel improved cell viability, with respect to the injection of the stand-alone cells, thus reducing the degradation of the extracellular NP matrix. The authors proposed this injectable hydrogel as a possible therapeutic approach for NP repair [35].

Another work aimed at the restoration of NP extracellular matrix, was recently reported [36]. By combining the HA with platelet-rich plasma (PRP) which is rich in growth factors, the authors investigated the delivery of MSCs into *ex vivo* bovine IVD. In details, after the nucleotomy of the NP, the gel, once crosslinked with the batroxobin (BRT) and seeded with cells, was injected and cultured for 7 days (Fig. **3**).

The study demonstrated the availability of the cells with both 1 million and 2 million seeding cells concentration. However, as claimed by the authors, even if after one week, the gels provided a good environment for cell survival and differentiation, the experiment was not performed under dynamic stimuli. The lack of physiological biochemical stimulation should be addressed in further studies, particularly in terms of the integration of the gel and cell metabolism.

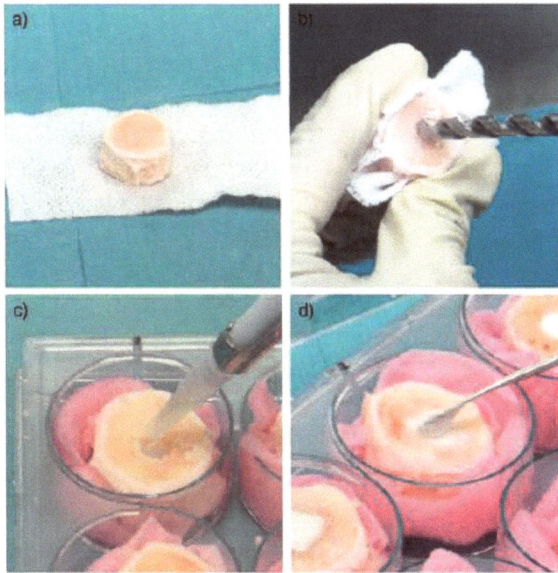

Fig. (3). (a) functional IVD; (b) nucleotomy of the NP; (c) injection of the HAMA gel containing hMSCs; (d) sealing of the injected gel with bone cement and endplate stopper. Reproduced from Choi *et al.* (34), under Creative Commons Attribution License (https://creativecommons.org/licenses/by/4.0/)

Alginate

Alginate is a polysaccharide derived from brown algae. It can be crosslinked in the presence of cations like calcium or, alternatively, it can be chemically crosslinked by a photo-crosslinking process. It is an inert material, but as HA, it is able to retain water [37]. Recently, Ura *et al.* [38], investigated the effect of an ultra-purified alginate gel (UPAL) *in vivo*, on discectomy models of rats and rabbits lumbar IVDs. During chronic inflammation, the main players of IVD degeneration are the tumor necrosis factor α (TNF- α) and the interleukin 6 (IL-6), which stimulate the nerve growth factor (NGF) production, leading to pain development. To reduce this chronic inflammation process and pain, the effect of UPAL gel was investigated, demonstrating a reduction of IL-6 and TGF- α, thus of inflammation, both in herniated disc and after discectomy, making this gel a good option for a therapeutical approach for treating the IVD. In a previous study, the same group, demonstrated the biocompatibility and stimulation of the production of IVD ECM after discectomy due to the herniation in large animals such as sheep models. The UPAL gel presents a much less percentage of endotoxins if compared to commercially available alginate. Additionally, it is bioresorbable and it can stimulate the NP repair also in rabbit models [39]. The UPAL gel is actually in phase I clinical trials, aimed to investigate its safety in patients after discectomy [38].

Collagen and Gelatin

Gelatin is derived from collagen, from which it is extracted and separated through a thermal treatment. Both gelatin and collagen are good candidates in biomedical applications since they can be easily modified and processed. Furthermore, collagen is naturally present in many tissues, including the IVD. However, due to their low viscoelasticity properties and a potentially fast/ease degradation (due to their thermal stability below 37°C) if not chemically modified [27, 37], a second material reinforcement might be also needed.

Gelatin can be chemically modified by adding methacrylic groups (gelatin methacrylate – GelMa), which under a light source and in the presence of a photo-initiator can crosslink in a minutes or seconds timeframe. The level of methacrylation and the photo-crosslinking exposure time might affect its stiffness and the hydrogel final properties. In a recent work [40], GelMa at different concentrations was evaluated to guarantee rats-derived nucleus pulposus chondrocytes' availability, and the proper structure porosity and stiffness to restore NP properties and allow nutrient diffusion. The hydrogels were prepared at three different concentrations, 5%, 10% and 15%, photo-crosslinked under UV light for 12s and characterized. The work (Fig. **3**). demonstrates that pore size decreased by increasing GelMa concentration, like the degradation kinetic, while the compression modulus was the highest in the condition at 15% concentration. However, the 5% GelMa resulted as the most hydrophilic, with the highest wettability, probably not only due to the low concentration but also due to a weaker crosslinking density. Cells injected into the different hydrogels, expressed aggrecan and col II markers in the 5% condition, suggesting that the high hydrophilicity and wettability, which are fundamental requirements in the physiological NP environment, are sensed by cells leading to the tissue-specific ECM components [40].

Concerning collagen, high density gels which were photo-crosslinked *in vitro* were used to evaluate the reparative capability of impaired annulus fibrosus preventing NP herniation [41]. These tests were conducted in *vivo* by using rats tail models, comparing scaffolds with and without annulus fibrosus cells. The results of the study demonstrated that up to 5 weeks, the gels with the cells were able to reduce disc degeneration (moderate severity, grade II compared to the acellular gel resulting in grade IV, that is severe), and preserve disc height, closing the gap of the annular failure site. Nevertheless, as noted by the authors, a longer follow up is needed as well as cell tracking for a deeper understanding of the mechanism behind reparative processes of cellular gels and cell migration and proliferation.

In another work of Friedmann *et al.* [42], collagen was injected *in vivo* into sheep models' damaged disc to study the therapeutic potential. The gel was produced *via* electrospinning, fabricating collagen type I and II fibers, later cut and mixed to a solution of PBS and inactivated serum with an autologous origin. Collagen gels with adipose-derived, autologous, mesenchymal stem cells were injected and followed up for 12 months to test their effect on the disc degeneration 6 weeks after the surgery. The study confirmed that the injection of collagen gels with cells both at 6 and 12 months was able to preserve the disc height and reduce the frequency of the specific histological markers related to the degeneration processes. Sheep models were chosen due to a similar biochemical stress state with respect to the human model [42].

Chitosan

It is a polysaccharide derived from the acetylation of chitin, present mainly in the cytoskeleton of insects and crustaceans. Even if it exhibits low mechanical properties, it is FDA approved, thermally responsive and it exhibits antibacterial properties [37]. Despite the weak mechanical properties, thermo-responsivity of the polysaccharide makes this material a good candidate for injectable hydrogels applications, due to *in situ* gelation. For instance, Alinejad *et al.* [43], overcame the limited mechanical properties, studying the effect of different crosslinker as sodium hydrogen carbonate (SCH), phosphate buffer and/or beta-glycerophosphate (BGP) on chitosan hydrogels suitable for NP scaffolds. They demonstrated an increase in the rheological properties of the formulation composed of chitosan 2% with 0.1M of BGP and 7.5mM of SCH, with proteoglycan synthesis during the culture of human NP cells. The gels were thermo-responsive, physically crosslinked, and stable in water at RT. However, as mentioned by the author, only unconfined compression tests were carried out. Experimental data on the confined compression behavior should be also addressed to reach a complete knowledge on the mechanical properties of the gel with respect to the native NP. The lack of understanding the IVD mechanical properties is still an open issue and the main limitation also due to the nature of the NP, which cannot be ascribed neither to a fully confined or unconfined compression behavior.

CLINICAL TRIALS

After the brief description of the most recent applications of natural biomaterials applied to the disc regeneration, it is evident that most of them aim at the modulation of the degeneration processes, mainly through the development of efficient injectable, cell-seeded hydrogels. Despite the progress in research, the unknown long term clinical outcomes might represent a limitation for the translation into the clinic [19]. On the other side, even if some attempts have been done for the fabrication of total disc replacement [44], the necessity to fabricate composite material emerged, to follow the different composition of the disc and mimic its complex, gradient structure.

Actually, there are many ongoing clinical trials, most of them are based on cell-based therapies [17], or at least on hyaluronic acid as vector as shown in (Table. 1).

Table 1. Some examples of ongoing clinical trials related to IVD regeneration and pain relief.

Gov ID	Responsible	Status	Approach	Country	Cell Type	Estimated Completion Date
NCT03955315	DiscGenics, Inc.	Recruiting	Injections of two doses of IDCT (Discogenic Cells + Sodium Hyaluronate vehicle) or injectable Disc Cell Therapy	Japan	Discogenic cells	August 2021
NCT01640457	Tetec AG	Active, not recruiting	Drug: NOVOCART® Disc plus Autologous Disc Chondrocyte Transplantation System (ADCT)	Austria/Germany	Autologous cells	August 2021
NCT03692221	Salim M Hayek, University Hospitals Cleveland Medical Center	Not yet recruiting	Percutaneous image guided delivery of autologous bone marrow derived mesenchymal stem cells	USA	Autologous bone marrow derived mesenchymal stem cells	September 30, 2022
NCT03367039	Zhu Zhenqi, Peking University People's Hospital	Not yet recruiting	Cervical disc replacement with the ProDisc-C vivo Cervical Disc	China		March 1, 2025
NCT04012996	Centinel Spine	Recruiting	Prodisc C SK and/or Vivo	USA		February 2028
NCT03709901	Vivex Biomedical, Inc.	Active, not recruiting	Active allograft, Injection of viable allograft into the nucleus pulposus of the degenerated disc	USA		January 31, 2022

(Table 1) cont.....

Gov ID	Responsible	Status	Approach	Country	Cell Type	Estimated Completion Date
NCT04414592	Qiang Fu, Shanghai General Hospital, Shanghai Jiao Tong University School of Medicine	Recruiting	Human umbilical cord mesenchymal stem cells for the treatment of lumbar disc degeneration disease	China	Human umbilical cord mesenchymal stem cells	March 2023
NCT03607838	Seikagaku Corporation	Recruiting	Single-dose intervertebral disc injection of SI-6603 drug	Japan		November 2022
NCT02138110	InVivo Therapeutics	Active, not recruiting	Neuro-Spinal Scaffold (poly(lactic-co-glycolic acid)-b-poly(L-lysine) Scaffold)	USA		August 2024

FUTURE PERSPECTIVES

In order to translate the TE approach for IVD regeneration into the clinic, also 3D bio-printing is gaining much attention. Indeed, the fabrication of composite material, for instance by combining electrospun, oriented fiber for the AF, with bio-printed hydrogels for the NP, can be a good alternative to provide the right bio-mechanical environment together with the advantages of 3D bio-printing techniques in fabricating highly complex structures, with high structure resolutions (Fig. **4**). The bioinks, containing cells, could be reinforced with synthetic polymers to provide adequate mechanical strength required for a healthy disc and patients' autologous cells could be used. Although with the complexity of the disc structure, absence of vascularization, poor self-healing process, the 3D bio-printing can open a new frontier to fabricated custom-made constructs, eventually through a reverse TE approach [45].

Sun *et al*. [46], fabricated a 3D bio-printed disc combining biomaterial, MSCs and growth factors, specifically connective tissue growth factor (CTGF) and transforming growth factor β3 (TGF- β3), slowly released from the scaffold to improve the regeneration outcomes. The system *in vitro* and *in vivo* resulted in the differentiation of the cells with the specific phenotype according to the disc area, synthesis of GAG and collagen type II and I, in the central part and outer part of the disc, respectively.

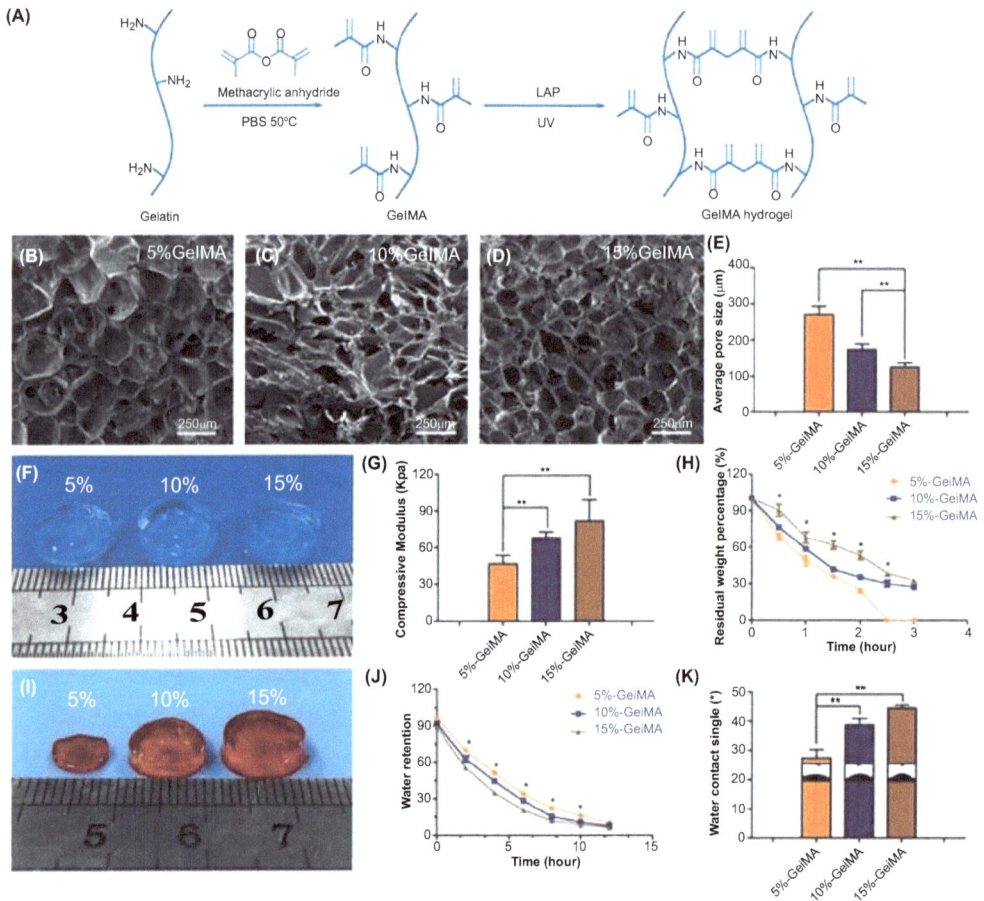

Fig. (4). (A) reaction to obtain GelMa; electron microscopy images of GelMa at 5% (B), 10% (C), and 15% (D). Pore diameter average (E); hydrogels at all the concentrations (F); Compressive modulus of the conditions tested (G); *in vitro* GelMa degradation at different hours (H); Gel-Ma hydrogels at all the concentration after two hours of degradation (I); swelling (J); wettability (K). Reproduced from Xu *et al.*,(40) under the Creative Commons CC BY license.

CONCLUSION

Tissue engineering is a promising field which through the combination of growth factors, cytokines, cells and biomaterials is gaining interest for the regeneration of the IVD. Naturally derived hydrogels are good candidates in mimicking and providing a proper microenvironment with tunable degradation rates, mechanical properties, and ease of modification.

However, this represents a great scientific challenge and many improvements have still to be achieved. Among them, the definition of the best cell sources to activate the correct downstream cellular pathways is fundamental. Indeed, if in some studies MSCs seem an ideal source (both adipose and bone marrow-derived) that is able to differentiate under specific stimuli in IVD phenotype specific cells, other works reports porcine differentiated chondrocytes as better candidates. Additionally, a variety of animal models have been tested, from rats, to goat, primates and sheep, which can present differences in disc dimension, and in the force applied during load [25].

A deep research is required to better define the precise stimuli and mechanisms working in the regulation of the regeneration process in the different area, and also understand the function of the growth factors involved.

The regeneration of anulus fibrous might require the reinforcement of the material by the creation of a composite, with electrospun fibers or just fibers as silk or collagen ones, among others [45].

Moreover, *in vitro* evaluation has also to be improved, considering the anabolic environment, the dynamic stimuli, pH, and low oxygen levels present in healthy physiological conditions at which cells are subjected. The use of bioreactors, hypoxia cultures, reproducing the native microenvironment and stimuli, might help in improving the mimicry of the intervertebral disc structures.

Finally, in the selection of precision biomaterials, among the requirements to be satisfied, a key factor is the evaluation of materials adhesive properties to allow the attachment of the AF and NP to the CEPs, enabling the creation of a unique, continuous structure.

LIST OF ABBREVIATIONS

AF   Annulus fibrosus

BNB   Blood nucleus barrier

BBB   Blood brain barrier

BRT   Batroxobin

CEP   Cartridge endplates

Ctgf   Connective tissue growth factor

ECM   Extracellular matrix

GAG   Glycosaminoglycan

GelMa Gelatin methacrylate

HRP   Horseradish peroxidase

HA   Hyaluronic acid

IVD   Intervertebral disc

IL   Interleukin

MMPs Metalloproteinases

MSCs Mesenchymal cells

MRI Magnetic resonance images

NP Nucleus pulposus

NGF Nerve growth facto

PBS Phosphate-buffered saline

SHC Sodium hydrogen carbonate

SF Silk fibroin

TE Tissue engineering

TGF Transforming growth factor

TNF Tumor necrosis factor

UPAL Ultra-purified alginate gel

ACKNOWLEDGEMENTS

This research has been supported by REMIX, funded by the European Union's Horizon 2020 research, and innovation program under the Maria Sklodowska-Curie grant agreement n. 778078, from the Italian Ministry for Education, University and Research (MIUR) through the Departments of Excellence and Regenera Project, and foundation VRT (Fondazione Volarizzazione Ricerca Trentina).

REFERENCES

[1] Zhang L, Zhang W, Hu Y, *et al.* Systematic Review of Silk Scaffolds in Musculoskeletal Tissue Engineering Applications in the Recent Decade. ACS Biomater Sci Eng 2021; 7(3): 817-40.
[http://dx.doi.org/10.1021/acsbiomaterials.0c01716] [PMID: 33595274]

[2] Kandel R, Roberts S, Urban JPG. Tissue engineering and the intervertebral disc: the challenges. Eur Spine J 2008; 17(S4) (Suppl. 4): 480-91.
[http://dx.doi.org/10.1007/s00586-008-0746-2] [PMID: 19005701]

[3] Pattappa G, Li Z, Peroglio M, Wismer N, Alini M, Grad S. Diversity of intervertebral disc cells: phenotype and function. J Anat 2012; 221(6): 480-96.
[http://dx.doi.org/10.1111/j.1469-7580.2012.01521.x] [PMID: 22686699]

[4] Buckley CT, Hoyland JA, Fujii K, Pandit A, Iatridis JC, Grad S. Critical aspects and challenges for intervertebral disc repair and regeneration-Harnessing advances in tissue engineering. JOR Spine 2018; 1(3): e1029.
[http://dx.doi.org/10.1002/jsp2.1029] [PMID: 30895276]

[5] Fearing BV, Hernandez PA, Setton LA, Chahine NO. Mechanotransduction and cell biomechanics of the intervertebral disc. JOR Spine 2018; 1(3): e1026.
[http://dx.doi.org/10.1002/jsp2.1026] [PMID: 30569032]

[6] Nachemson A. Intradiscal measurements of pH in patients with lumbar rhizopathies. Acta Orthop Scand 1969; 40(1): 23-42.
[http://dx.doi.org/10.3109/17453676908989482] [PMID: 4312806]

[7]   Sun Z, Liu B, Luo ZJ. The immune privilege of the intervertebral disc: Implications for intervertebral disc degeneration treatment. Int J Med Sci 2020; 17(5): 685-92.
        [http://dx.doi.org/10.7150/ijms.42238] [PMID: 32210719]

[8]   Teraguchi M, Yoshimura N, Hashizume H, *et al.* Prevalence and distribution of intervertebral disc degeneration over the entire spine in a population-based cohort: the Wakayama Spine Study. Osteoarthritis Cartilage 2014; 22(1): 104-10.
        [http://dx.doi.org/10.1016/j.joca.2013.10.019] [PMID: 24239943]

[9]   Kim HS, Wu PH, Jang IT. Lumbar Degenerative Disease Part 1: Anatomy and Pathophysiology of Intervertebral Discogenic Pain and Radiofrequency Ablation of Basivertebral and Sinuvertebral Nerve Treatment for Chronic Discogenic Back Pain: A Prospective Case Series and Review of Literature. Int J Mol Sci 2020; 21(4): 1483.
        [http://dx.doi.org/10.3390/ijms21041483] [PMID: 32098249]

[10]   Wang D, Chen Y, Cao S, *et al.* Cyclic Mechanical Stretch Ameliorates the Degeneration of Nucleus Pulposus Cells through Promoting the ITGA2/PI3K/AKT Signaling Pathway. Oxid Med Cell Longev 2021; 2021: 1-11.
        [http://dx.doi.org/10.1155/2021/6699326] [PMID: 33815660]

[11]   Guo X, Zhou J, Tian Y, Kang L, Xue Y. Biomechanical effect of different plate-to-disc distance on surgical and adjacent segment in anterior cervical discectomy and fusion - a finite element analysis. BMC Musculoskelet Disord 2021; 22(1): 340.
        [http://dx.doi.org/10.1186/s12891-021-04218-4] [PMID: 33836709]

[12]   Kadow T, Sowa G, Vo N, Kang JD, Fearing BV, Hernandez PA, *et al.* Molecular basis of intervertebral disc degeneration and herniations: what are the important translational questions? Clin Orthop Relat Res 2015; 473(6): 1903-12.
        [http://dx.doi.org/10.1007/s11999-014-3774-8] [PMID: 25024024]

[13]   Teraguchi M, Yoshimura N, Hashizume H, *et al.* Progression, incidence, and risk factors for intervertebral disc degeneration in a longitudinal population-based cohort: the Wakayama Spine Study. Osteoarthritis Cartilage 2017; 25(7): 1122-31.
        [http://dx.doi.org/10.1016/j.joca.2017.01.001] [PMID: 28089899]

[14]   Adams MA, Roughley PJ. What is intervertebral disc degeneration, and what causes it? Spine 2006; 31(18): 2151-61.
        [http://dx.doi.org/10.1097/01.brs.0000231761.73859.2c] [PMID: 16915105]

[15]   van Uden S, Silva-Correia J, Oliveira JM, Reis RL. Current strategies for treatment of intervertebral disc degeneration: substitution and regeneration possibilities. Biomater Res 2017; 21(1): 22.
        [http://dx.doi.org/10.1186/s40824-017-0106-6] [PMID: 29085662]

[16]   Huang YC, Urban JPG, Luk KDK, Luk KDK. Intervertebral disc regeneration: do nutrients lead the way? Nat Rev Rheumatol 2014; 10(9): 561-6.
        [http://dx.doi.org/10.1038/nrrheum.2014.91] [PMID: 24914695]

[17]   Binch ALA, Fitzgerald JC, Growney EA, Barry F. Cell-based strategies for IVD repair: clinical progress and translational obstacles. Nat Rev Rheumatol 2021; 17(3): 158-75.
        [http://dx.doi.org/10.1038/s41584-020-00568-w] [PMID: 33526926]

[18]   Lyu F, Cui H, Pan H, Cheung KMC, Cao X, Iatridis JC. Painful intervertebral disc degeneration and in fl ammation: from laboratory evidence to clinical interventions Bone Res 2021 (9 October 2020); 7

[19]   Tendulkar G, Chen T, Ehnert S, Kaps HP, Nüssler AK. Intervertebral Disc Nucleus Repair: Hype or Hope? Int J Mol Sci 2019; 20(15): 3622.
        [http://dx.doi.org/10.3390/ijms20153622] [PMID: 31344903]

[20]   Shankar H, Scarlett JA, Abram SE. Anatomy and pathophysiology of intervertebral disc disease. Tech Reg Anesth Pain Manage 2009; 13(2): 67-75.
        [http://dx.doi.org/10.1053/j.trap.2009.05.001]

[21]   Kadow T, Sowa G, Vo N, Kang JD. Molecular basis of intervertebral disc degeneration and herniations: what are the important translational questions? Clin Orthop Relat Res 2015; 473(6): 1903-12.
[http://dx.doi.org/10.1007/s11999-014-3774-8] [PMID: 25024024]

[22]   Wu PH, Kim HS, Jang IT. Intervertebral Disc Diseases PART 2: A Review of the Current Diagnostic and Treatment Strategies for Intervertebral Disc Disease. Int J Mol Sci 2020; 21(6): 2135.
[http://dx.doi.org/10.3390/ijms21062135] [PMID: 32244936]

[23]   Mu X, Wei J, A J, Li Z, Ou Y. The short-term efficacy and safety of artificial total disc replacement for selected patients with lumbar degenerative disc disease compared with anterior lumbar interbody fusion: A systematic review and meta-analysis. PLoS One 2018; 13(12): e0209660.
[http://dx.doi.org/10.1371/journal.pone.0209660] [PMID: 30592739]

[24]   Zigler J, Gornet MF, Ferko N, Cameron C, Schranck FW, Patel L. Comparison of Lumbar Total Disc Replacement With Surgical Spinal Fusion for the Treatment of Single-Level Degenerative Disc Disease: A Meta-Analysis of 5-Year Outcomes From Randomized Controlled Trials. Global Spine J 2018; 8(4): 413-23.
[http://dx.doi.org/10.1177/2192568217737317] [PMID: 29977727]

[25]   Dowdell J, Erwin M, Choma T, Vaccaro A, Iatridis J, Cho SK. Intervertebral Disk Degeneration and Repair. Neurosurgery 2017; 80(3S): S46-54.
[http://dx.doi.org/10.1093/neuros/nyw078] [PMID: 28350945]

[26]   Stergar J, Gradisnik L, Velnar T, Maver U. Intervertebral disc tissue engineering : A brief review. (Figure 1) 130-7.

[27]   Tang G, Zhou B, Li F, *et al.* Advances of Naturally Derived and Synthetic Hydrogels for Intervertebral Disk Regeneration. Front Bioeng Biotechnol 2020; 8(June): 745.
[http://dx.doi.org/10.3389/fbioe.2020.00745] [PMID: 32714917]

[28]   Rockwood DN, Preda RC, Yücel T, Wang X, Lovett ML, Kaplan DL. Materials fabrication from Bombyx mori silk fibroin. Nat Protoc 2011; 6(10): 1612-31.
[http://dx.doi.org/10.1038/nprot.2011.379] [PMID: 21959241]

[29]   Agostinacchio F, Kaplan DL, Mu X, Dirè S, Motta A. *In Situ* 3D Printing: Opportunities with Silk Inks. Trends Biotechnol 2020; 1-12.
[PMID: 33279280]

[30]   Floren M, Migliaresi C, Motta A. Processing Techniques and Applications of Silk Hydrogels in Bioengineering. J Funct Biomater 2016; 7(3): 26.
[http://dx.doi.org/10.3390/jfb7030026] [PMID: 27649251]

[31]   Costa JB, Silva-Correia J, Ribeiro VP, da Silva Morais A, Oliveira JM, Reis RL. Engineering patient-specific bioprinted constructs for treatment of degenerated intervertebral disc. Mater Today Commun 2019; 19: 506-12. [Internet].
[http://dx.doi.org/10.1016/j.mtcomm.2018.01.011]

[32]   Park SH, Gil ES, Cho H, *et al.* Intervertebral disk tissue engineering using biphasic silk composite scaffolds. Tissue Eng Part A 2012; 18(5-6): 447-58.
[http://dx.doi.org/10.1089/ten.tea.2011.0195] [PMID: 21919790]

[33]   Chung TW, Chen WP, Tai PW, Lo HY, Wu TY. Roles of Silk Fibroin on Characteristics of Hyaluronic Acid/Silk Fibroin Hydrogels for Tissue Engineering of Nucleus Pulposus. Materials (Basel) 2020; 13(12): 2750.
[http://dx.doi.org/10.3390/ma13122750] [PMID: 32560556]

[34]   Kazezian Z, Joyce K, Pandit A. The Role of Hyaluronic Acid in Intervertebral Disc Regeneration. Appl Sci (Basel) 2020; 10(18): 6257.
[http://dx.doi.org/10.3390/app10186257]

[35]   Choi UY, Joshi HP, Payne S, *et al.* An injectable hyaluronan–methylcellulose (HAMC) hydrogel

combined with wharton's jelly-derived mesenchymal stromal cells (WJ-MSCs) promotes degenerative disc repair. Int J Mol Sci 2020; 21(19): 7391.
[http://dx.doi.org/10.3390/ijms21197391] [PMID: 33036383]

[36]   Russo F, Ambrosio L, Peroglio M, *et al.* A hyaluronan and platelet-rich plasma hydrogel for mesenchymal stem cell delivery in the intervertebral disc: An organ culture study. Int J Mol Sci 2021; 22(6): 2963.
[http://dx.doi.org/10.3390/ijms22062963] [PMID: 33803999]

[37]   Choi Y, Park MH, Lee K. Tissue Engineering Strategies for Intervertebral Disc Treatment Using Functional Polymers. Polymers (Basel) 2019; 11(5): 872.
[http://dx.doi.org/10.3390/polym11050872] [PMID: 31086085]

[38]   Ura K, Yamada K, Tsujimoto T, Ukeba D, Iwasaki N, Sudo H. Ultra-purified alginate gel implantation decreases inflammatory cytokine levels, prevents intervertebral disc degeneration, and reduces acute pain after discectomy. Sci Rep 2021; 11(1): 638.
[http://dx.doi.org/10.1038/s41598-020-79958-9] [PMID: 33436742]

[39]   Tsujimoto T, Sudo H, Todoh M, *et al.* An acellular bioresorbable ultra-purified alginate gel promotes intervertebral disc repair: A preclinical proof-of-concept study. EBioMedicine 2018; 37: 521-34.
[http://dx.doi.org/10.1016/j.ebiom.2018.10.055] [PMID: 30389504]

[40]   Xu P, Guan J, Chen Y, *et al.* Stiffness of photocrosslinkable gelatin hydrogel influences nucleus pulposus cell properties *in vitro*. J Cell Mol Med 2021; 25(2): 880-91.
[http://dx.doi.org/10.1111/jcmm.16141] [PMID: 33289319]

[41]   Borde B, Grunert P, Härtl R, Bonassar LJ. Injectable, high-density collagen gels for annulus fibrosus repair: An *in vitro* rat tail model. J Biomed Mater Res A 2015; 103(8): 2571-81.
[http://dx.doi.org/10.1002/jbm.a.35388] [PMID: 25504661]

[42]   Friedmann A, Baertel A, Schmitt C, *et al.* Intervertebral Disc Regeneration Injection of a Cell-Loaded Collagen Hydrogel in a Sheep Model. Int J Mol Sci 2021; 22(8): 4248.
[http://dx.doi.org/10.3390/ijms22084248] [PMID: 33921913]

[43]   Alinejad Y, Adoungotchodo A, Grant MP, *et al.* Injectable Chitosan Hydrogels with Enhanced Mechanical Properties for Nucleus Pulposus Regeneration. Tissue Eng Part A 2019; 25(5-6): 303-13.
[http://dx.doi.org/10.1089/ten.tea.2018.0170] [PMID: 30251916]

[44]   Moriguchi Y, Mojica-Santiago J, Grunert P, *et al.* Total disc replacement using tissue-engineered intervertebral discs in the canine cervical spine. PLoS One 2017; 12(10): e0185716.
[http://dx.doi.org/10.1371/journal.pone.0185716] [PMID: 29053719]

[45]   Pieri A, Byerley AM, Musumeci CR, Salemizadehparizi F, Vanderhorst MA, Wuertz-Kozak K. Electrospinning and 3D bioprinting for intervertebral disc tissue engineering. JOR Spine 2020; 3(4): e1117.
[http://dx.doi.org/10.1002/jsp2.1117] [PMID: 33392454]

[46]   Sun B, Lian M, Han Y, *et al.* A 3D-Bioprinted dual growth factor-releasing intervertebral disc scaffold induces nucleus pulposus and annulus fibrosus reconstruction. Bioact Mater 2021; 6(1): 179-90.
[http://dx.doi.org/10.1016/j.bioactmat.2020.06.022] [PMID: 32913927]

CHAPTER 14

Rapid Prototyping in Biomedical Applications: Advanced Scopes, Capabilities and Challenges

Akib Jabed[1], **Maliha Rahman**[1] and **Md Enamul Hoque**[2,*]

[1] *Department of Materials Science and Engineering, Rajshahi University of Engineering and Technology (RUET), Rajshahi, Bangladesh*

[2] *Department of Biomedical Engineering, Military Institute of Science and Technology (MIST), Dhaka, Bangladesh*

Abstract: Rapid prototyping (RP) is an advanced technique of fabricating a physical model, or complex assembly where computer-aided design (CAD) plays a significant role. The RP technique offers numerous advantages including providing information such as how a product will look like and/or perform, and in the first stage of the design and manufacturing cycle, allowing switches and improvements to be implemented earlier in the system. It acts quickly and reduces the risk of later/final stage costly errors. RP is considered to be an automated and cost-effective technique as it does not require special tools, involves minimal intervention of the operator, and minimizes material wastage. Different types of RP techniques are now commercially available and serving accordingly in many fields. By using rapid prototyping, engineers can produce and/or upgrade medical instruments that include surgical fasteners, scalpels, retractors, display systems, and so on. Tablets having a sustained drug release capability are also being manufactured by RP. Rehabilitation engineering also uses RP including the fabrication of biomedical implants and prostheses and craniofacial and maxillofacial surgeries. This chapter aims to provide an overview of rapid prototyping technology and various RP machines available commercially. This chapter also includes the applications of the RP technique in biomedical engineering focusing on the advanced scopes, capabilities, and challenges in the upcoming days.

Keywords: Biomedical, Computer-aided design, Manufacturing, Polymer, Rapid prototyping, Rehabilitation.

INTRODUCTION

Rapid prototyping (RP) is one of the cutting-edge manufacturing techniques that can directly fabricate the physical model with the 3D computer-aided design (CAD) data [1]. Rapid prototyping has become an imperative part of the manu:

* **Corresponding author Md Enamul Hoque:** Department of Biomedical Engineering, Military Institute of Science and Technology (MIST), Dhaka, Bangladesh; E-mail: enamul1973@bme.mist.ac.bd

Mohd Fauzi Mh Busra, Daniel Law Jia Xian, Yogeswaran Lokanathan and Ruszymah Haji Idrus (Eds.)

facturing industry providing the flexibility to create more realistic prototypes faster and implement changes instantly.

Rapid prototyping sometimes refers to additive manufacturing (AM), digital fabrication, solid imaging, and laser prototyping [2]. There are six commercially available different rapid prototyping models. Each of the models has a unique strength [3]. The layered manufacturing process is mainly used nowadays in commercial technologies. Rapid prototyping is used in industries, engineering laboratories, medicals, manufacturing facilities, *etc.* because of its low cost [4 - 6].

Also, RP refers to "solid freedom fabrication (SFF)". This is a popular technology and is very easy to fabricate. RP technology is very popular nowadays because of its high customization, fast product development, and reduced time to market [7].

To design any complex shape in the polymer, RP plays a significant role. Due to the unique combination offered by thermoplastic materials in product design nowadays, they are used in all sorts of industries from automobiles to medical and consumer products. The Stereolithography (SLA) machines are based on the polymerization of a photosensitive resin. A wire of thermoplastic polymer is used in fused deposition modeling (FDM). Material selection is an important factor in rapid prototyping. Several polymers including acrylonitrile butadiene styrene (ABS), acrylic, polyphenylsulfone, polycarbonate, and nylon are commonly used in prototyping, which offer outstanding durability, functionality, and strength. These polymer prototypes play a vital role in the biomedical field *e.g.* CT scans, diagnosis, MRI, to find out the tumor and defected tissue, *etc* [8].

RAPID PROTOTYPING PROCESS

All RP technologies consist of five basic steps. Here the basic process steps are discussed below:

  i. Building a CAD model of the desired product.
 ii. Converting the CAD model into the STL format.
iii. Slicing the STL format into thin cross-sectional layers.
 iv. Building the model one layer above another.
  v. Cleaning and finishing the model.

Formation of CAD Model

At first, we will prepare a model of the object using a CAD file. There are lots of software packages available commercially for this purpose. This will give us more accurate 3D models than wireframe modelers like AutoCAD. The designer may use the existing CAD file or can make a file for prototyping. This step is the same for all RP systems.

Conversion from Cad to STL

Different CAD packages have different algorithms to represent solid objects. To set up consistency, the STL (Stereolithography) format has been accepted as the standard for RP technology. The second step is to alter the CAD file into STL format. This format will give us a three-dimensional surface like planar triangles. The file gives the coordinates of the vertices and contains the direction of the outward normal of every triangle. STL format can't give us the curved surface directly or exactly because it uses planer elements. If we increase the number of triangles, it will improve the approximation. As a result, it will produce large-size files. These files require much time to process. So designers must be concerned about the size, accuracy and manageability to create a good and useful STL file. STL format is universal and accepted in all RP systems.

Slice STL Format

Several programs and systems are available for designers to adjust the size, location, and orientation of the model. Orientation creation is important for several reasons.

  i. The design properties of RP are different or vary from one coordinate to another.
 ii. Part orientation partially determines the quantity of time required to create a model.
iii. Placing the shortest dimension in the direction will reduce the number of layers that reduce the build time.

Depending on the build technique, the pre-processing software slices the model from 0.01 mm to 0.7 mm thick [3]. The program also produces an auxiliary structure to support the model. Supports are useful for thin-walled sections, internal cavities, overhangs, *etc*. The prototypes are usually weaker in the z-direction (vertical) than in the x-y direction.

Layer by Layer Formation

This is the actual step of manufacturing the part. Using different types of RP technologies, it creates or builds one layer at a time from a paper, polymer, or powdered metal. Most machines are independent but sometimes need little human intervention.

Clean and Finish

This is a post-processing step. This step removes the prototype from the machine and shifts it from any support. Photosensitive materials are sometimes used. But before using it, it is fully cured. Prototypes require little surface treatment and cleaning. If one wants to increase its durability and appearance, one can paint or seal it [3]. All the steps of the RP process are summarized in (Fig. **1**). as a flowchart.

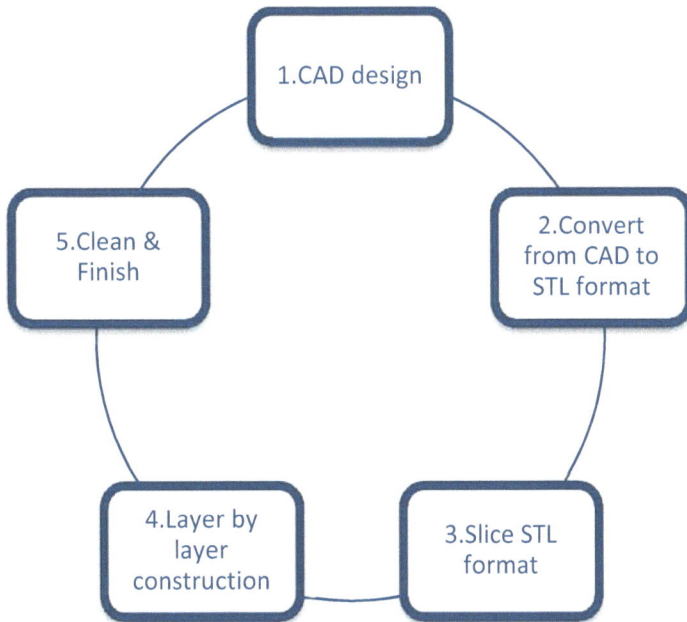

Fig. (1). A flowchart of a rapid prototyping process.

CATEGORIES OF RAPID PROTOTYPING

Rapid prototyping techniques can be categorized based on different features. Based on the precision of the product, there are two types of RP:

  i. High Fidelity
 ii. Low Fidelity

High Fidelity is also referred to as hi-fi or high-fi. It is mainly a computer-based process. The final product in this high fidelity is complete resemblance to the design. The "high" in high fidelity refers to comprehensiveness. High fidelity not only covers the user interface (UI) of the product but also covers the user experience (UX). High fidelity is expensive. It is more time-consuming to switch the design. If we need any visual design of our product we can use it. Again, if we want the transition or animation of any object, we can use hi-fi. The aesthetics of the created prototype give an endemic feeling which is a drawback of hi-fi [9].

Low Fidelity is a low-tech concept and it is simple. It is a quick process. In low fidelity, there is a noticeable difference between the final product and the prototype. These prototypes are distinguished by low technology implantation. This is not as expensive as hi-fi. If we need quick feedback on our concepts, we can use low fidelity. The greatest excellence in this method is its speed [9].

Also based on the state of materials used, Rapid prototyping is mainly of three types [10]. These are:

   i. Liquid-based
  ii. Solid-based
 iii. Powder-based

In the **liquid-based RP,** materials are in the liquid state at the beginning stage of this process. The base material can inhale a polymer. Liquid-based RP technology mainly works based on the 'Photo curing' principle [10]. Parts are built into this system in a vat with the help of laser radiation (UV range) of photo-curable resin. Mainly this resin is solidified by laser radiation and forms a hardened layer. With the help of an elevation system, the layer is lowered and then allowed to form another layer over it. This will continue until the full system is complete. There are lots of variations in this technique. This mainly depends on the type of laser or light, the type of elevation, the type of resin, *etc* [11]. Various liquid-based RP processes are- Multi-Jet Modeling (MJM), Drop on Demand Inkjet (DODI), Poly Jet, Stereolithography (SLA), *etc*.

In the **solid-based RP** system, materials are in the solid state. It can give a shape like laminate, roll, pellets, or wire. Different solid-based RP methods are:

• Joining method or Cutting and Glueing
• Fusion method or Melting and Solidifying

These processes are different from one another and sometimes laser is used to produce prototypes in these methods. Widely used solid-based RP technologies include Fused Deposition Modeling (FDM) and Laminated Object Manufacturing (LOM) [10].

In **Powder-based RP** methods, the starting materials are common in the form of powder of metal, plastic, ceramic or even composites [12]. Powder-based prototyping mainly works based on the binding or joining principle. Laser or binder or glue can be used in this system. It is used to achieve the joining effect. Binder materials are deposited on a layer of powder particles. It happens in a selective area and continues until we get the desired part. Post-processing is important in this system to remove unbonded particles [13]. Representative methods of powder-based RP include ZCorp's 3D Printing (3DP), Selective Laser Sintering (SLS), Selective Laser Melting (SLM), Electron Beam Melting (EBM), and Direct Metal Laser Sintering (DMLS) [10].

PROMINENT POLYMER RAPID PROTOTYPING TECHNIQUES

This section discusses the main rapid prototyping techniques for polymer fabrication briefly. These techniques are:

  i. Selective Laser Sintering (SLS)
 ii. Laminated Object Manufacturing (LOM)
iii. Stereolithography (SLA)
iv. Fused Deposition Modeling (FDM)

Table 1. Prominent Rapid Prototyping Methods and the State of Input Materials [14].

Methods	Building Materials
SLS	Polymer powders
LOM	Special papers or polymer sheets
SLA	Photopolymer
FDM	Thermoplastics

Stereolithography (SLA)

In this technique, the section is produced in a vat. That vat contains a liquid. This liquid is a photo-curable resin acrylate [15]. The SLA machines build 3D parts by scanning this liquid resin through laser light or ultraviolet light, as illustrated in (Fig. **2**). When SLA resin is exposed to certain wavelengths of light, a polymerization reaction starts and the liquid resin is cured into very thin layers. Liquid resin is solidified due to heat radiated from the laser beam [16]. The liquid is replenished and leveled between layers [12].

Selective Laser Sintering (SLS)

In this system, mainly roller is used. Fine polymeric powder such as polystyrene, polyamide, and polycarbonate is spread onto the substrate. The overall fabrication process is shown schematically in Fig. (**3**). Temperature is raised below its melting point before starting CO_2 laser scanning. This is done to minimize thermal distortion and increase fusion to the previous layer. The laser is controlled in such a way that those grains which are attached to the laser beam are affected first. When the laser beam slaves a slice then the bed is lowered. After lowering the bed, a powder feed chamber is raised. This powder will spread the build area with the help of a counter-rotating roller. The support structure is not required in this process. The un-sintered powder acts as support. It is cleaned. After that, it can be recycled when the model is complete [15]. Prototypes are manufactured from a polymer and ceramics in this process. Recently composite materials are widely studied in this process [14]. Calcium phosphates, hydroxyapatite (HAp), polylactides, polyetheretherketone (PEEK), and polycaprolactones are fabricated in the SLS system [18 - 20]. The schematic figure of SLS is given below:

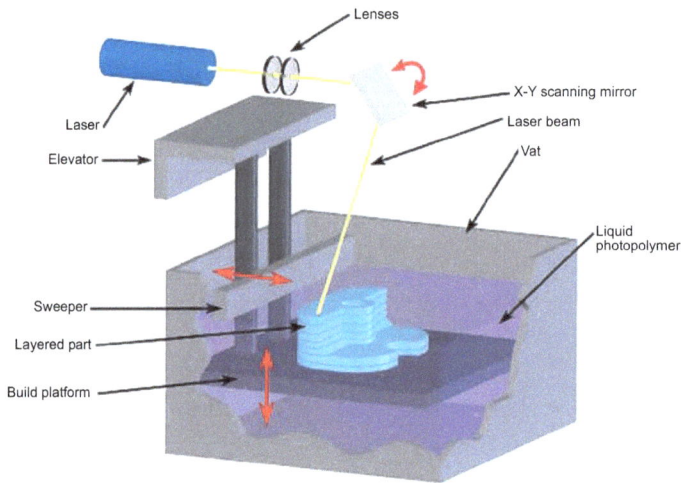

Fig. (2). Stereolithography (SLA) [17].

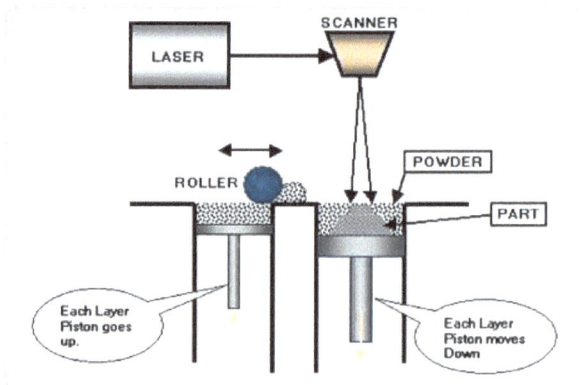

Fig. (3). Selective Laser Sintering (SLS) [21].

Fused Deposition Modeling (FDM)

This is one of the most widely used methods in RP. It uses polymer filament as starting materials to build parts. At first, a thermoplastic filament is extruded from a coil. After that, materials are sent through the extrusion nozzle. This nozzle is heated to the plastic's melting point. The flow of melted plastic is ensured. The nozzle is joined to a mechanical head. This helps to move over the table. This occurs due to slice geometry. It produces a thin bead from that extruded plastic. Then the plastics harden instantly after being extruded and finally bonds to the layer below. After completing a layer, the platform holds a part. The part moves vertically which is shown in Fig. (**4**). to start depositing a new layer above the previous one.

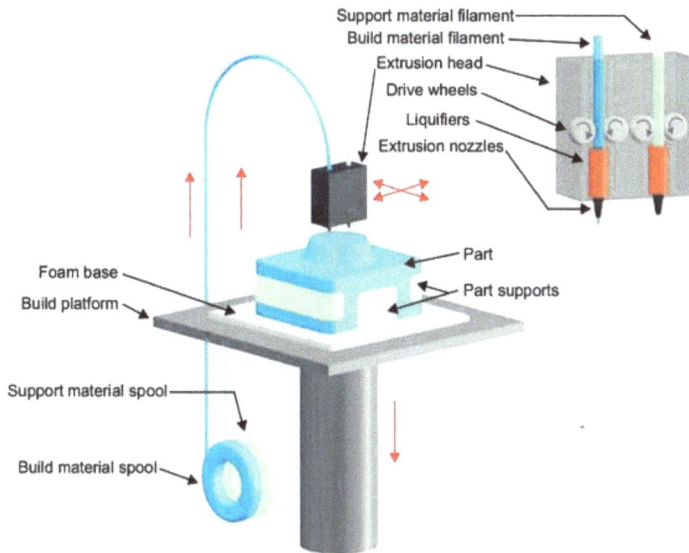

Fig. (4). Fused Deposition Modeling (FDM) [22].

The production system is furnished with another nozzle in the head which is in parallel. With an overhang angle, less than 45° from the horizontal, it helps to support materials from the building prop. The support materials can be broken in the future due to their poor quality. FDM machines can construct parts from pure materials including elastomers, polycarbonate (PC), nylon PA12, ULTEM1010 or mixed materials. In recent times, water-soluble support structures are also used. Due to their internal porous structure, generated by the process, it is possible to diffuse manufactured parts with epoxy resin for sealing parts and make them stronger [23 - 26]. FDM is also used in polymer-ceramics composites [27].

Laminated Object Manufacturing (LOM)

In this method, prefabricated foils are cut by a CO_2 laser beam (25-30 watt). It is similar to the sliced 3D CAD file and it is bonded above the preceding layer. The adjacent layers are joined together with the help of glue, soldering, ultrasonic technique, or diffusion welding. A heated roller is passed over the sheet of the material on the build platform to make an object. Then melting and pressing are also needed to complete it. By using a computer-controlled laser, it is used to cut the object into the desired shape. Sometimes, it is cut into a crosshatch shape. It is easy to remove the object if it is fully printed. No chemical reaction is necessary here, that's why larger parts are made in this method. The process is demonstrated in (Fig. **5**). Mcor Technologies Ltd., Irish companies are to bring LOM into the mainstream. This machine produces an affordable model that's why it is used by artists, architects and product developers. By using this technology, composites can also be fabricated with some extra steps [28, 29].

BENEFITS AND CHALLENGES OF RAPID PROTOTYPING

Table 2. Major Benefits and Challenges of Rapid Prototyping [31, 32].

Benefits	Challenges
1. **Faster new product development** – RP technology allows new product design and development to be completed in a reduced time frame.	1. **Accuracy**- Accuracy and quality are extremely important in manufacturing biomedical prototypes. Quality control is still a downside of the RP process.
2. **Material wastage**-Rapid prototypes are subjected to less wastage of materials. It is one of the most important advantages of the RP technology.	2. **Initial cost & maintenance cost** - This system needs high initial costs. Especially for biomedical prototypes, rapid prototyping equipment and materials are costly. Again extra expense is added for each revision and modification of the product.
3. **Output**-Good throughput capabilities are achieved.	3. **Skilled labor**- Skilled personnel is required to use RP technology properly. Without proper training in this high technology, the fabrication of the prototype is risky. It may cause huge materials wastage and economic failure to the industries. In biomedical engineering without skilled labor, faulty prototypes even can bring disaster to someone's life.
4. **Automated process**- It's a well-automated process involving no or little supervision during the building process. That also eliminates or reduces working risk.	
5. **Concise roadmap**- Little pre-preparation and post-processing steps are required.	4. **Limited range of materials**-There is a limitation on the choice of materials we can use as raw materials.
6. **Exploring new designs**- RP technology provides the freedom to explore a new design. The ability to thoroughly test and refine a concept minimizes costly design flaws, which might not be evident during an early assessment.	5. **Size limitation-** Another drawback of RP technology is that it may not be appropriate for large model production.

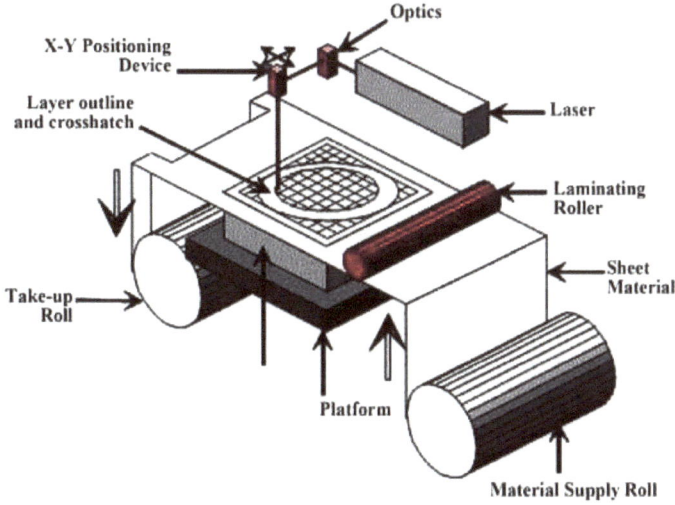

Fig. (5). Laminated Object Manufacturing (LOM) [30].

APPLICATIONS OF RAPID PROTOTYPING TECHNOLOGY

Manufacturing industries are leaning toward RP technology for its key benefit *e.g.* the potential to reduce costs, improve productivity and reduce lead time [14]. RP technologies are successfully used in many industries. Such as:

- Mechanical engineering
- Electrical appliances
- Textile
- Furniture design
- Architectural interior design
- Reverse engineering application
- Rapid tooling
- Arts and crafts
- Footwear designing
- The medical field

Mechanical Engineering

Before the invention of rapid prototyping, mechanical prototypes were machined, which makes the process expensive and slow. For building functional prototypes directly from the CAD program, rapid prototyping technologies are becoming more influential in the mechanical industries. RP gives us the comfort of easy flow analysis. With the help of RP technology, an engineer can determine the point of stress concentration easily. Sometimes it is used as a proof of concept.

Electrical Appliances

With the help of RP technology, household electrical appliances, for example-power socket driver, ambient colored lamp driver, fan control driver, *etc*. are broadly manufactured. To manufacture a special contour in an electrical system, RP technology is very important.

Furniture Designing

Prototype furniture, for example- chair, table, couch, *etc*. are designed with the help of RP technology [33]. The model allows us to determine the effective points of permanent joints and to achieve low weight.

Architectural Interior Design

To design stature, proto-house, the Mobius house, wall mountings, or toys, RP technology plays a significant role [34]. RP technologies give a good surface finish and an aesthetic look in the interior design.

Footwear Designing

Footwear prototypes are manufactured by the RP technique. Because of this technique, this type of footwear is now much stronger and more comfortable. Complicated designs, for example- 3D printed shoes, 3D printer sneakers, *etc*. are manufactured by this technology. The reliability is better than the conventional one.

Aerospace & Automobile Industry

For design, tolerance, visual verification, clearances, inspection, 3D casting, fit, *etc*. RP technologies play an important role in this industry. Crafts, complex components, car parts, *etc*. are produced by RP technology.

Rapid Tooling

Complicated parts & tools are manufactured in RP technologies. The wind tunnel model injection mold plug, ultrasound sensor wedge, *etc*. are manufactured by the RP technology. The RP technology improves its strength and gives a high production rate [35].

RAPID PROTOTYPING IN THE BIOMEDICAL & MEDICAL FIELD

RP technology has developed quickly over the past few decades and showed its technological growth in various domains [36]. Rapid prototyping is used in the medical field to manufacturing complex prototypes *e.g.* to make the model of cranioplasty implants. 3D CAM or CAD is used to develop new products. It helps in research and shortens the implementation time. We can easily convert CT or MRI results into CAD files and evaluate them. After finding out the bone abnormality or anatomical issue, RP technology generates a proper design to manufacture the required model for treatment [37].

RP in Tissue Engineering and Regeneration

The loss of the structure and function of an organ or tissue is a common biomedical fact. Damaged organs or tissue can be replaced by a fabricated scaffold by applying some advanced technologies *e.g.* RP technology. Constructing the same kind of organ or tissue that mimics biomechanical properties is a complex thing to do [38, 39]. The scaffold has a porous structure to facilitate nutrients, oxygen diffusion and waste materials [40]. It permits proliferation, cell adhesion, and separation for surgical implantations. The scaffold has a compatible carrier structure so that it fastens the healing process of injured or damaged tissue or organs. Designing scaffolds, customized for each patient, with the structural intricacies of the tissue being replaced, is practically impossible through traditional manufacturing approaches. Cartilage or bone tissue scaffolds need complex structures to produce strength, structural integrity, and a good microenvironment for the growth of tissues and cells. Hence, several advanced fabricating technologies have been developed to artificially rebuild a scaffold [41]. With the help of RP techniques, the resolution of the scaffolds can be improved without any change in handleability, shape, and strength. This technique will facilitate the control of bone growth, optimization of mechanical properties, investigation of bioactive process materials, and development of hybrid biological materials [11]. RP technology such as fused deposition modeling or multiphase jet solidification or 3D plotting is used to manufacture scaffolds. By using RP technology, we can manufacture complex shapes directly from the computer model of the defect site and maintain their dimensions quite easily and thus it can save lives [42, 43]. A Bioplotter machine such as EnvisionTEC GmbH is used in tissue engineering. Fig. (**6**). represents the fabrication process and the developed scaffolds.

RP for Diagnosis

Diagnosis of an internal organ remains challenging for physicians. A physical model that mimics the internal organ, provides a platform for intelligent diagnosis and helps to take subsequent treatment decisions. Studies have shown that precise bio-models fabricated by advanced RP techniques make the diagnosis tests more realistic, rapid controlled, or cost-effective [45 - 48]. RP technologies are successfully used to produce devices, constructed of polymer or glass or wax for diagnostic purposes [49 - 51]. The thermometer is an important diagnostic, medical device. This is also manufactured by rapid prototyping. Electrocardiographs are also a complex device to determine the electrical activity of the heart. This is also developed by the rapid prototyping process. Stethoscopes and ophthalmoscopes are also designed by rapid prototype techniques.

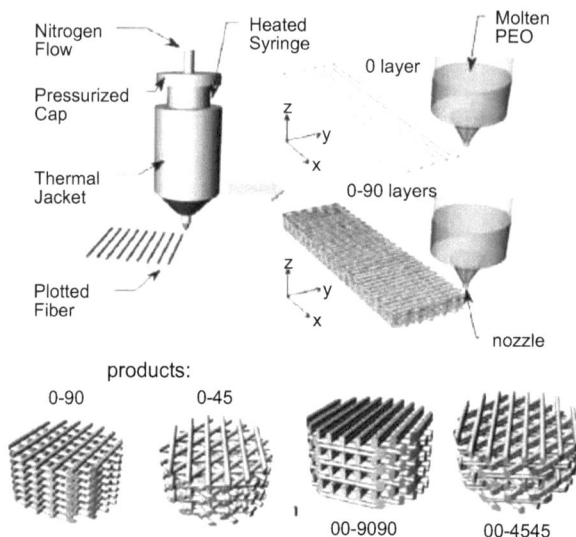

Fig. (6). Building a 3D Scaffold through a Jet or Nozzle in a Layered Fashion by RP Techniques [44].

RP in Dentistry

Dentistry is another prime field of application of rapid prototypes. Due to the aesthetic importance of customized implants, personalized approaches facilitated by rapid prototyping are very common in dentistry. The dental models are used in orthodontic treatment planning. Rapid prototyping could become a new tool for fabricating brackets, maxillofacial prostheses, and other precision accessories for specific needs [52, 53]. Curettes, operative burs, excavators, and probes types of devices are manufactured by rapid prototyping process nowadays.

RP for Medical Devices

Using rapid prototypes in the biomedical sector will help us to upgrade display systems, medical instruments, scalpels, surgical fasteners, *etc*. Rapid prototype technology not only designs medical devices but also manufactures them. Aid devices are also manufactured by RP. Selective laser sintering or stereolithography is used to construct aid devices. Drug dosage forms are also manufactured by RP because it has a complex shape. It is hard to design in any other method than RP. Tablets that preserve drugs are also designed and manufactured by rapid prototyping. It minimizes adverse drug reactions and provides safety.

RP in Prosthesis

RP plays a vital role in implantation and prostheses. Nowadays with the help of RP, prostheses are particularly manufactured for a patient. It doesn't cost much, that's why patients from the third world now can easily afford prostheses, which were once limited to the developed countries. Now doctors can easily customize them and fit prostheses in the patient's body. Artificial limbs and heart valves are also manufactured by using RP technologies. Braces, bone plates, pacemakers, and eyeglasses are also fabricated in RP technologies.

RP in Surgery

RP is a significant tool for surgical planning and simulation. Surgeons can get the real impression of the complex organ before surgical intervention, using the models of complex organs developed by RP technology. These models produced by RP technology increase surgical accuracy [54, 55]. Prototyped models are also used to demonstrate the tumor and foreign growth in bodies. Stereolithography is the most common for this purpose. It has reliable features like development in color resin or transparency [56]. Scalpers, scissors, and saws are the most traditional cutting surgical device. By using RP techniques, it becomes very easy to fabricate more accurate surgical devices. Sutures, cautery is a hemostatic instrument. These types of surgical instruments are made by using RP techniques. A surgical pinzette is a holding surgical instrument. This is also fabricated by using rapid prototyping technologies. Surgical needles, surgical mesh, and surgical blades are also manufactured by using these techniques nowadays.

Materials Used in Biomedical Engineering

The selection of materials is an important thing in biomedical applications. Like hydrogel is used for cell culture. Thermo reversible hydrogel is advanced biomedical material. With the help of RP technologies, cells are directly patterned or printed [57 - 59]. Temporary scaffolds are produced from biodegradable polymers by RP technology within which the bone tissues can be regenerated [60, 61]. Ceramics are used largely in biomedical applications. Ceramics are used as molds for the fabrication of metal clinical implants. Cast metal and 3D-printed ceramic mold are used in a knee prosthesis. RP plays an important role in this system [62]. If there is any possibility of corrosion, fatigue cracking or ion elution, using ceramics will solve this problem [63]. Ceramics have some additional characteristics such as bioactivity (HAp), chemical stability, and bioinertia (alumina/zirconia) [64].

FUTURE DEMANDS

Tissue Engineering to Biofabrication

A lot of developments have occurred in tissue engineering in recent years. The artificial creation of living cells, scaffolds, and extracellular matrices is common now which helps in tissue engineering.

RP is one of the most emergent technologies used in tissue engineering that relate bioprinters to bioplotters. Biological materials are used to directly produce biodevices that are the same as body tissue [65, 66]. Bioplotter machine is systematically tested with different biomaterials such as calcium phosphate, agar, collagen, chitin, gelatin, biopolymers, bioinks, *etc.* The printer head is used to deposit biodegradable polymers together with cells to the intended organs or tissues. But it has two limitations such as multiple cell types and the weak mechanical strength of hydrogel struts [11]. Research is going on to produce soft tissues synthetically by the production of muscle fibers [67], the production of the artificial liver [68], and the reconstruction of the epidermis [69, 70].

Improve Biological Systems

The day when RP technology will be widely used is not very far away from us to allow direct customized implant printing, developing advanced biomaterials that are similar to the human body and manufacturing facilities connected to the operating room in hospitals. Arrays of actuators and sensors would be organized into the artificially produced anatomical elements to produce self-healing capabilities, self-diagnostic abilities possibly by design strategies used in the improvement of self-repairing materials and self-sensitive and structures [71, 72]. It is necessary to enhance the biological system for patients' safety. Some systems or methods can be used to improve the system and research more to do better from now.

Pharmaceuticals and Sustainable Growth

Rapid prototyping has tightened its position within the pharmaceutical area, as it can serve as a platform for prototyping at a low cost [73]. RP technologies have a huge prospective to upgrade the properties of pharmaceutical products and can help to improve the microstructure of drugs to find an alternative way to supply [74].

CONCLUSIONS

Rapid prototyping is a blessed technology in the manufacturing industry. In the past few years, rapid prototyping technologies have gained access to various fields all over the world. But it has brought a significant impact on the biomedical field. Rapid prototypes reduce turnaround time in product development and give dimensionally accurate production [12]. Nowadays there are several commercial RP methods including SLA, SLS, LOM, FDM, *etc*. The selection of an appropriate rapid prototyping process relies on the geometry of the parts to be designed, machine parameters, the application of the parts, and their properties [75]. Further development in the RP technology will enable fast and accurate production. This chapter covers the rapid prototyping process, prominent methods of rapid prototyping for fabricating polymers and their working principles. This review has also described various fields of applications of rapid prototyping focusing on the significance of RP in the biomedical field, the main challenges, and the future demands of rapid prototypes. More innovation in the field of rapid prototyping process can make it more acceptable and reliable in near future for biomedical applications.

LIST OF ABBREVIATIONS

AM   Additive manufacturing

CAD   Computer-aided design

FDM   Fused Deposition Modeling

LOM   Laminated Object Manufacturing

RP   Rapid prototyping

SLS   Selective Laser Sintering

SLA   Stereolithography

REFERENCES

[1]   Maurya NK, Rastogi V, Singh P. An overview of mechanical properties and form error for rapid prototyping. CIRO J Manuf Sci Technol 2020; 29: 53-70.
      [http://dx.doi.org/10.1016/j.cirpj.2020.02.003]

[2]   Chua CK, Leong KF, An J. Introduction to rapid prototyping of biomaterials. Rapid Prototyping of Biomaterials 2020; pp. 1-15.

[3]   Mahindru DV, Priyanka Mahendru SR, Tewari Ganj L. Review of rapid prototyping-technology for the future Global journal of computer science and technology 2013 May 31..

[4]   Hanser Gebhardt A. Rapid Prototyping 2003.

[5]   https://3dprintingindustry.com/news/metalmaker-3d-launches-rapid-prototyping-service-for-3d-printed-metal-parts-142735/

[6]   https://www.rapidmade.com/3d-printing-in-the-medical-industry/

[7]   Hoque ME. 2011.https://www.intechopen.com/books/307

[8]   https://www.gtvinc.com/different-materials-used-rapid-prototyping-services/

[9]   Ibragimova E. High-fidelity prototyping: What, When, Why and How? 2016.   https://blog. prototypr.io/high-fidelity-prototyping-what-when-why-and-how- f5bbde6a7fd4

[10]   Short DB, Sirinterlikci A, Badger P, Artieri B. Environmental, health, and safety issues in rapid prototyping. Rapid Prototyping J 2015; 21(1): 105-10.
[http://dx.doi.org/10.1108/RPJ-11-2012-0111]

[11]   Touri M, Kabirian F, Saadati M, Ramakrishna S, Mozafari M. Additive manufacturing of biomaterials− the evolution of rapid prototyping. Adv Eng Mater 2019; 21(2): 1800511.
[http://dx.doi.org/10.1002/adem.201800511]

[12]   Chang KH. Rapid Prototyping. In: Chang KH, Ed. e-Design. 2015; pp. 743-86.
[http://dx.doi.org/10.1016/B978-0-12-382038-9.00014-4]

[13]   Sachs EM, Haggerty JS, Cima MJ, Williams PA. inventors; Massachusetts Institute of Technology, assignee. Three-dimensional printing techniques. United States patent US 5,340,656 1994 Aug 23..

[14]   hua CK, Leong KF, Lim CS, Eds. Rapid Prototyping: Principles and Applications. 2003.

[15]   Pham DT, Dimov SS. Rapid prototyping processes. Rapid Manufacturing. London: Springer 2001; pp. 19-42.
[http://dx.doi.org/10.1007/978-1-4471-0703-3_2]

[16]   Xu X, Goyanes A, Trenfield SJ, *et al.* Stereolithography (SLA) 3D printing of a bladder device for intravesical drug delivery. Mater Sci Eng C 2021; 120: 111773.
[http://dx.doi.org/10.1016/j.msec.2020.111773] [PMID: 33545904]

[17]   Rapid Prototyping - Stereolithography (SLA) [internet]. [cited 2021 Aug 8]. https://www. custompartnet.com/wu/stereolithography

[18]   Tan KH, Chua CK, Leong KF, *et al.* Scaffold development using selective laser sintering of polyetheretherketone–hydroxyapatite biocomposite blends. Biomaterials 2003; 24(18): 3115-23.
[http://dx.doi.org/10.1016/S0142-9612(03)00131-5] [PMID: 12895584]

[19]   Williams JM, Adewunmi A, Schek RM, *et al.* Bone tissue engineering using polycaprolactone scaffolds fabricated *via* selective laser sintering. Biomaterials 2005; 26(23): 4817-27.
[http://dx.doi.org/10.1016/j.biomaterials.2004.11.057] [PMID: 15763261]

[20]   Bukharova TB, Antonov EN, Popov VK, *et al.* Biocompatibility of tissue engineering constructions from porous polylactide carriers obtained by the method of selective laser sintering and bone marrow-derived multipotent stromal cells. Bull Exp Biol Med 2010; 149(1): 148-53.
[http://dx.doi.org/10.1007/s10517-010-0895-2] [PMID: 21113479]

[21]   SLS- (Selective Laser Sintering) [Internet]. [cited 2021 Aug 8]. Available from: https://www. arptech.com.au/sls.html

[22]   Fused Deposition Modeling (FDM) [Internet]. [cited at 2021 Aug 8]. Available from: https://www. custompartnet.com/wu/fused-deposition-modeling

[23]   Hutmacher DW, Schantz T, Zein I, Ng KW, Teoh SH, Tan KC. Mechanical properties and cell cultural response of polycaprolactone scaffolds designed and fabricated *via* fused deposition modeling. J Biomed Mater Res 2001; 55(2): 203-16.
[http://dx.doi.org/10.1002/1097-4636(200105)55:2<203::AID-JBM1007>3.0.CO;2-7]   [PMID: 11255172]

[24]   Dudek P. FDM 3D printing technology in manufacturing composite elements. Arch Metall Mater 2013; 58(4): 1415-8.
[http://dx.doi.org/10.2478/amm-2013-0186]

[25]   Ning F, Cong W, Qiu J, Wei J, Wang S. Additive manufacturing of carbon fiber reinforced thermoplastic composites using fused deposition modeling. Compos, Part B Eng 2015; 80: 369-78.

[http://dx.doi.org/10.1016/j.compositesb.2015.06.013]

[26]   Garg HK, Singh R. Comparison of wear behavior of ABS and Nylon6—Fe powder composite parts prepared with fused deposition modelling. J Cent South Univ 2015; 22(10): 3705-11.
[http://dx.doi.org/10.1007/s11771-015-2913-z]

[27]   Kalita SJ, Bose S, Hosick HL, Bandyopadhyay A. Development of controlled porosity polymer-ceramic composite scaffolds *via* fused deposition modeling. Mater Sci Eng C 2003; 23(5): 611-20.
[http://dx.doi.org/10.1016/S0928-4931(03)00052-3]

[28]   Klosterman D, Chartoff R, Graves G, Osborne N, Priore B. Interfacial characteristics of composites fabricated by laminated object manufacturing. Compos, Part A Appl Sci Manuf 1998; 29(9-10): 1165-74.
[http://dx.doi.org/10.1016/S1359-835X(98)00088-8]

[29]   Klosterman DA, Chartoff RP, Osborne NR, *et al.* Development of a curved layer LOM process for monolithic ceramics and ceramic matrix composites. Rapid Prototyping J 1999; 5(2): 61-71.
[http://dx.doi.org/10.1108/13552549910267362]

[30]   Suresh G, Narayana KL, Mallik MK. A review on development of medical implants by rapid prototyping technology. Int J Pure Appl Math 2017; 117(21): 257-76.

[31]   What is Rapid Prototyping, protyping techniques, benefits and limitations [Internet]. Available from: https://engineeringproductdesign.com/knowledge-base/rapid-prototyping-techniques/

[32]   Hoque M, Prasad RG. Rapid prototyping technology in bone tissue engineering. J Appl Mech Eng 2013; 2: 124.

[33]   Kieback B, Neubrand A, Riedel H. Processing techniques for functionally graded materials. Mater Sci Eng A 2003; 362(1-2): 81-106.
[http://dx.doi.org/10.1016/S0921-5093(03)00578-1]

[34]   Novakova-Marcincinova L, Novak-Marcincin J. Experimental testing of materials used in fused deposition modeling rapid prototyping technology InAdvanced Materials Research. Trans Tech Publications Ltd. 2013; Vol. 740: pp. 597-602.

[35]   Chuk RN, Thomson VJ. A comparison of rapid prototyping techniques used for wind tunnel model fabrication. Rapid Prototyping J 1998; 4(4): 185-96.
[http://dx.doi.org/10.1108/13552549810239030]

[36]   Lu B, Li D, Tian X. Development trends in additive manufacturing and 3D printing. Engineering (Beijing) 2015; 1(1): 085-9. Epub ahead of print
[http://dx.doi.org/10.15302/J-ENG-2015012]

[37]   Hoque ME, Chuan YL. Desktop robot based rapid prototyping system: an advanced extrusion based processing of biopolymers into 3D tissue engineering scaffolds. Rapid prototyping technology-Principles and functional requirements. 2011 Sep; 26: 105-34.

[38]   Hoque ME, Chuan YL. Desktop robot based rapid prototyping system: an advanced extrusion based processing of biopolymers into 3D tissue engineering scaffolds. Rapid prototyping technology-Principles and functional requirements. 2011 Sep; 26: 105-34.

[39]   Qu H. Additive manufacturing for bone tissue engineering scaffolds. Mater Today Commun 2020; 24: 101024.
[http://dx.doi.org/10.1016/j.mtcomm.2020.101024]

[40]   yadav P, Beniwal G, Saxena KK. A review on pore and porosity in tissue engineering. Mater Today Proc 2021; 44: 2623-8.
[http://dx.doi.org/10.1016/j.matpr.2020.12.661]

[41]   Liu N, Ye X, Yao B, *et al.* Advances in 3D bioprinting technology for cardiac tissue engineering and regeneration. Bioact Mater 2021; 6(5): 1388-401.
[http://dx.doi.org/10.1016/j.bioactmat.2020.10.021] [PMID: 33210031]

[42]   Kalita SJ. Rapid prototyping in biomedical engineering: structural intricacies of biological materials. Bio integration of Medical Implant Materials. Woodhead Publishing 2010; pp. 349-97.
[http://dx.doi.org/10.1533/9781845699802.3.349]

[43]   Hoque ME. Rapid Prototyping Technology - Principles and Functional Requirements; 2011. [Internet]. [cited 2020 Apr 19]. Available from: https://www.intechopen.com/books/rapid-prototyping-technology-principles-and-functional-requirements

[44]   Hoque ME, Chuan YL, Pashby I. Extrusion based rapid prototyping technique: An advanced platform for tissue engineering scaffold fabrication. Biopolymers 2012; 97(2): 83-93.
[http://dx.doi.org/10.1002/bip.21701] [PMID: 21830198]

[45]   Nie W, Zhang J, Wang Z, Wang C, Liu Z. [Rapid-prototyping manufacture of human scoliosis based on laminated object technology]. Sheng Wu I Hsueh Kung Cheng Hsueh Tsa Chih 2008; 25(6): 1260-3.
[PMID: 19166188]

[46]   Court LE, Seco J, Lu XQ, *et al.* Use of a realistic breathing lung phantom to evaluate dose delivery errors a. medical physics. 2010 Nov; 37(11): 5850-7.

[47]   Erdelt KJ, Lamper T. Development of a device to simulate tooth mobility 2010; 55: 273-78.

[48]   Lantada AD, Morgado PL. Rapid prototyping for biomedical engineering: current capabilities and challenges. Annu Rev Biomed Eng 2012; 14(1): 73-96.
[http://dx.doi.org/10.1146/annurev-bioeng-071811-150112] [PMID: 22524389]

[49]   Ke K, Hasselbrink EF Jr, Hunt AJ. Rapidly prototyped three-dimensional nanofluidic channel networks in glass substrates. Anal Chem 2005; 77(16): 5083-8.
[http://dx.doi.org/10.1021/ac0505167] [PMID: 16097742]

[50]   Bhagat AAS, Jothimuthu P, Papautsky I. Photodefinable polydimethylsiloxane (PDMS) for rapid lab-on-a-chip prototyping. Lab Chip 2007; 7(9): 1192-7.
[http://dx.doi.org/10.1039/b704946c] [PMID: 17713619]

[51]   Kaigala GV, Ho S, Penterman R, Backhouse CJ. Rapid prototyping of microfluidic devices with a wax printer. Lab Chip 2007; 7(3): 384-7.
[http://dx.doi.org/10.1039/b617764f] [PMID: 17330171]

[52]   Faber J, Berto PM, Quaresma M. Rapid prototyping as a tool for diagnosis and treatment planning for maxillary canine impaction. Am J Orthod Dentofacial Orthop 2006; 129(4): 583-9.
[http://dx.doi.org/10.1016/j.ajodo.2005.12.015] [PMID: 16627189]

[53]   Quadri S, Kapoor B, Singh G, Tewari R. Rapid prototyping: An innovative technique in dentistry. Journal of Oral Research and Review 2017; 9(2): 96.
[http://dx.doi.org/10.4103/jorr.jorr_9_17]

[54]   Petzold R, Zeilhofer HF, Kalender WA. Rapid prototyping technology in medicine—basics and applications. Comput Med Imaging Graph 1999; 23(5): 277-84.
[http://dx.doi.org/10.1016/S0895-6111(99)00025-7] [PMID: 10638658]

[55]   Deokar ND, Thakur DA. Design development and analysis of femur bone by using rapid prototyping International journal of engineering development and research 2016.

[56]   Medical Applications of Rapid Prototyping [Internet]. [cited 2020 Apr 27]. Available from: https://additive3d.com/medical-applications-rapid-prototyping/

[57]   Awad HA, Quinn Wickham M, Leddy HA, Gimble JM, Guilak F. Chondrogenic differentiation of adipose-derived adult stem cells in agarose, alginate, and gelatin scaffolds. Biomaterials 2004; 25(16): 3211-22.
[http://dx.doi.org/10.1016/j.biomaterials.2003.10.045] [PMID: 14980416]

[58]   Raghunath J, Rollo J, Sales KM, Butler PE, Seifalian AM. Biomaterials and scaffold design: key to tissue-engineering cartilage. Biotechnol Appl Biochem 2007; 46(Pt 2): 73-84.

[PMID: 17227284]

[59]   Ladet S, David L, Domard A. Multi-membrane hydrogels. Nature 2008; 452(7183): 76-9.
[http://dx.doi.org/10.1038/nature06619] [PMID: 18322531]

[60]   Biswas MC, Jony B, Nandy PK, *et al.* Recent Advancement of Biopolymers and Their Potential Biomedical Applications. J Polym Environ 2021; 1-24.

[61]   Anita Lett J, Sagadevan S, Fatimah I, *et al.* Recent advances in natural polymer-based hydroxyapatite scaffolds: Properties and applications. Eur Polym J 2021; 148: 110360.
[http://dx.doi.org/10.1016/j.eurpolymj.2021.110360]

[62]   Curodeau A, Sachs E, Caldarise S. Design and fabrication of cast orthopedic implants with freeform surface textures from 3-D printed ceramic shell. J Biomed Mater Res 2000; 53(5): 525-35.
[http://dx.doi.org/10.1002/1097-4636(200009)53:5<525::AID-JBM12>3.0.CO;2-1]   [PMID: 10984701]

[63]   Clarke IC. Role of ceramic implants. Design and clinical success with total hip prosthetic ceramic-t--ceramic bearings. Clin Orthop Relat Res 1992; 1(282): 19-30.
[PMID: 1516312]

[64]   Bose S, Darsell J, Hosick HL, Yang L, Sarkar DK, Bandyopadhyay A. Processing and characterization of porous alumina scaffolds. J Mater Sci Mater Med 2002; 13(1): 23-8.
[http://dx.doi.org/10.1023/A:1013622216071] [PMID: 15348200]

[65]   Basha RY. TS SK, Doble M. Design of biocomposite materials for bone tissue regeneration. Mater Sci Eng C 2015; 57: 452-63.
[http://dx.doi.org/10.1016/j.msec.2015.07.016]

[66]   Mironov V, Trusk T, Kasyanov V, Little S, Swaja R, Markwald R. Biofabrication: a 21st century manufacturing paradigm. Biofabrication 2009; 1(2): 022001.
[http://dx.doi.org/10.1088/1758-5082/1/2/022001] [PMID: 20811099]

[67]   Bian W, Bursac N. Engineered skeletal muscle tissue networks with controllable architecture. Biomaterials 2009; 30(7): 1401-12.
[http://dx.doi.org/10.1016/j.biomaterials.2008.11.015] [PMID: 19070360]

[68]   Wang X, Yan Y, Zhang R. Rapid prototyping as a tool for manufacturing bioartificial livers. Trends Biotechnol 2007; 25(11): 505-13.
[http://dx.doi.org/10.1016/j.tibtech.2007.08.010] [PMID: 17949840]

[69]   Wang X, Tuomi J, Mäkitie AA, Poloheimo KS, Partanen J, Yliperttula M. The integrations of biomaterials and rapid prototyping techniques for intelligent manufacturing of complex organs. In: Lazinica R, Ed. Advances in Biomaterials Science and Applications in Biomedicine. 2016; pp. 437-63.

[70]   Staudenmaier R, Hoang NT, Mandlik V, *et al.* Customized tissue engineering for ear reconstruction. Adv Otorhinolaryngol 2010; 68: 120-31.
[http://dx.doi.org/10.1159/000314567] [PMID: 20442566]

[71]   Suresh G, Narayana KL, Mallik MK. Laser engineered net shaping process in development of bio-compatible implants: An overview. Journal of Advanced Research in Dynamical and Control Systems 2017; 9: 745-55.

[72]   Ghosh SK, Ed. Self-healing materials: fundamentals, design strategies, and applications. Weinheim: Wiley-vch 2009.

[73]   Svane R, Pedersen T, Hirschberg C, Rantanen J. Rapid prototyping of miniaturized powder mixing geometries. J Pharm Sci 2021; 110(7): 2625-8.
[http://dx.doi.org/10.1016/j.xphs.2021.03.019] [PMID: 33775671]

[74]   Yu DG, Zhu LM, Branford-White CJ, Yang XL. Three-dimensional printing in pharmaceutics: promises and problems. J Pharm Sci 2008; 97(9): 3666-90.
[http://dx.doi.org/10.1002/jps.21284] [PMID: 18257041]

[75]   Hoque ME. Robust formulation for the design of tissue engineering scaffolds: A comprehensive study on structural anisotropy, viscoelasticity and degradation of 3D scaffolds fabricated with customized desktop robot based rapid prototyping (DRBRP) system. Mater Sci Eng C 2017; 72: 433-43.
       [http://dx.doi.org/10.1016/j.msec.2016.11.019] [PMID: 28024607]

CHAPTER 15

Cells in Vascular Tissue Engineering Research

Ubashini Vijakumaran[1], Nur Atiqah Haron[1], Heng J. Wei[1], Mohamad Fikeri Ishak[1] and **Nadiah Sulaiman[1,*]**

[1] Centre for Tissue Engineering and Regenerative Medicine, Faculty of Medicine, Universiti Kebangsaan Malaysia, 56000, Cheras, Kuala Lumpur, Malaysia

Abstract: Fabrication of off-the-shelf small diameter vascular graft as an alternative to current autologous graft in clinical setting *i.e.*, internal mammary artery and saphenous veins has yet to be perfected. With cardiovascular diseases (CVD) topping the list of the causes of death worldwide, alternative vascular graft is especially crucial in patients with a lack of autologous grafts. Successful re-vascularisation could substantially lower the progression of CVD and mortality rate. This chapter delves into cells that are vital in developing a tissue engineered vascular graft (TEVG), ranging from the native tissue on the vascular bed to the potential cells that could be utilized, compounds that possibly could improve the available grafts and stents and future TEVG design.

Keywords: Blood vessel, Cardiovascular diseases, Coronary artery bypass grafting, Tissue-engineered vascular graft, Vascular bed.

CELLS IN VASCULAR TISSUE ENGINEERING RESEARCH

Cardiovascular diseases (CVDs) represent the leading cause of global mortality and morbidity to date, with ischaemic heart diseases accounting for the majority of CVD-related mortalities. The aforementioned manifestation of CVD develops as a result of acute arterial occlusion in the coronary arteries leading to impaired coronary circulation, consequently, causing cardiac tissue damage and myocardial infarction [1, 2]. Therefore, rapid restoration of coronary perfusion is essential to limit ischaemic tissue damage and improve clinical outcomes. Pharmaceutical therapies and lifestyle modifications represent two of the most common non-invasive treatment options for the management of CVD [3], but invasive vascular bypass surgical procedures such as coronary artery bypass grafting (CABG) remain an indispensable treatment option for patients with severe arterial occlusions that require extended revascularisation [4 - 6]. The saphenous vein

---

* **Corresponding author Nadiah Sulaiman:** Centre for Tissue Engineering and Regenerative Medicine, 12th Floor, Clinical Block, Universiti Kebangsaan Malaysia Medical Centre, Jalan Yaacob Latif, Bandar Tun Razak, Cheras, Kuala Lumpur, Malaysia; E-mail: nadiahsulaiman@ukm.edu.my

(SV) and internal thoracic artery (ITA) are autologous vessels that represent the benchmark for small diameter (<6 mm) vascular bypass procedures, but they are limited by the scarce supply present in the body and the need for invasive autograft surgery to harvest them. In addition, harvested vessels are often of poor quality (excessively thick or thin), rendering them unusable [7 - 9]. Furthermore, prior vascular bypass procedures utilizing SVs have shown low long-term patency rates with approximately 50% failure rates and 10 years post-implantation [7, 10]. Therefore, there is a need to improve current treatment to increase available graft patency or provide alternatives to currently available grafts that work better if not at par.

Blood vessels carry oxygen and nutrients to all parts of the body. Therefore, a fundamental understanding of the vascular structure is necessary in order to design and develop suitable grafts for specific clinical applications *i.e.*, in peripheral artery diseases bypass grafting (PABG), coronary artery bypass grafting (CABG), or arteriovenous graft (AVG). Many of the different blood vessel beds (Fig. **1**). have similar main structural characteristics with few particular differences.

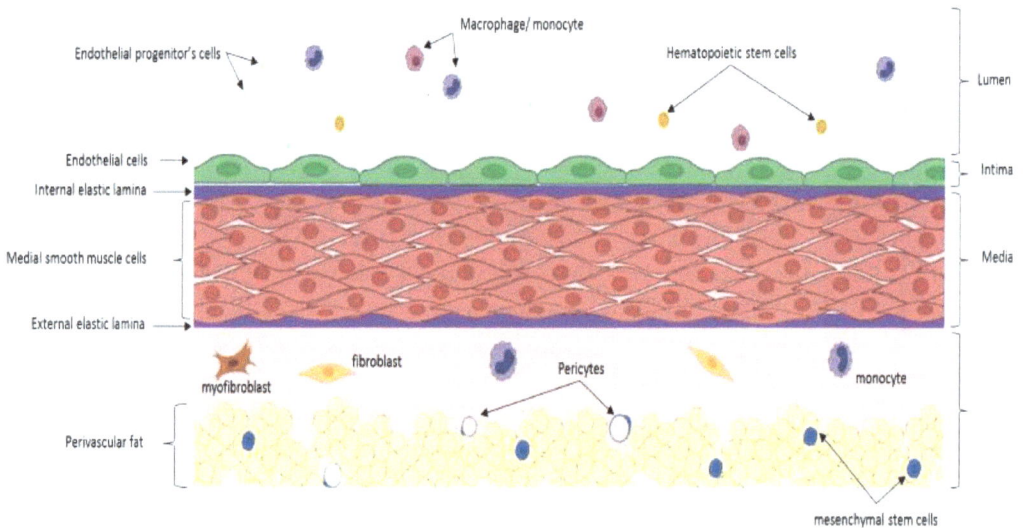

Fig. (1). A schematic illustration of layers of the blood vessel wall. The outermost layer (adventitia), mostly composed of collagen and elastic fibres with pericytes that surround the microvascular and nerve endings are in this layer. As the layer consists of elastic fibres, it enables the vessel to stretch to a certain extent and become flexible. The middle layer (media), mainly consists of densely packed smooth muscle cells and is located in between a layer of elastic laminae which are prominent in the artery and poorly defined in vein structure. The innermost layer is known as intima. This layer is mainly made up of a single layer of endothelial cells. The thickness of each layer may differ between the artery and the vein and also depends on the location of the vessels. Image created with Biorender.com.

Native Cells on Vascular Bed

Endothelial Cells

In general, tunica intima of arteries, veins, and capillaries is made up of endothelial cells (EC), that are attached on a thin sheet-like structure primarily composed of laminin, collagens, fibronectin, proteoglycan, and other macromolecules [11, 12]. These cells and their structural components are critically involved in controlling physiological functions including coagulation, haemostatic balance, permeability, and proliferation, as well as in the transport of immune cells [12].

Endothelial cells are the blood-contacting layer positioned on the lumen of the blood vessel. This cell forms a single layer that lines all blood vessels and regulates connections between the bloodstream and surrounding tissues. The luminal membrane of EC is directly in contact with blood elements and circulating cells, while a glycoprotein plasma membrane splits the basolateral surface from the neighbouring tissues which are secreted and tied by the EC itself to its cell membrane. The EC's shape varies but has a commonly elongated thin morphology between 30- 50 μm length, 10-30 μm wide and 0.1-10 μm thick [13]. ECs are positioned along the axis of the vessel in the wall of vascular, a structural property that minimizes the shear stress applied by the flowing blood [14].

Smooth Muscle Cells

Intima is positioned under the plasma membrane which separates ECs from the internal elastic laminae (IEL) formed by several layers of contractile vascular smooth muscle cells (SMC) which interweave with collagen-rich ECM and elastic fibres. Tunica media, on the other hand, consists of SMC, collagen, elastin, and proteoglycans that provide vessel strength and serve as a vascular tone receptor [12]. Underneath the basement membrane, normal vessels have media without intima beginning at the IEL, followed by concentric lamellar units made up of elastic fibres and SMCs separated by interlaminar matrix collagens, proteoglycans, glycoproteins, microfibrils, and ground matter [15].

Fibroblasts

In vascular anatomy and physiology, the fibroblast is found in the adventitial or the outermost layer of blood vessels. These cells are responsible for the vascular remodelling and the pathophysiology of neointimal formation. Morphologically, fibroblasts are flat, spindle-shaped cells that have high affinity to tissue culture plastic [16]. Fibroblasts are of mesenchymal origin with the ability to secrete extracellular matrix proteins. The matrix protein expression is reliant on the level of cellular activation and it can also be synthesized by other cell types such as smooth muscle cells, *etc* [17].

Pericytes

Eberth first identified pericytes in the late 19th century and the cells were later isolated by Rouget from the capillary wall [18, 19]. Pericytes were found embedded within the basement membrane. Pericytes control the EC cell cycle at the capillary level and contribute to the development of the basement membrane to stabilise the vascular wall [20]. The localization of pericytes is often confused with smooth muscle cells (SMCs), macrophages, fibroblasts, and even epithelial cells.

Overall, endothelial cells, smooth muscle cells, fibroblasts, and pericytes collectively work together to ensure normal vessel physiology and maintain vessel structural integrity.

Potential Cells for TEVG Fabrication

Cells for vascular tissue engineering are derived from the different adult stem cells and progenitor cells. These cells are isolated from diverse sources such as peripheral blood, umbilical cord, placenta, bone marrow, and white adipose tissue to improve the fabrication of a vascular graft [21]. Multipotent and pluripotent stem cells have great potential for vascular tissue engineering. Mesenchymal stem cells (MSC) are autologous adult multipotent stem cells that showed rapid differentiation potential towards vascular lineages, thus a beneficial trait in balancing the inflammatory response and encouraging healing [22 - 24].

Mesenchymal stem cells are adult stromal non-hematopoietic cells isolated from bone marrow. MSC is well known for its multi-potency which is the ability to differentiate into osteoblasts, chondrocytes, ECs, SMCs, and osteocytes [25]. However, several factors such as soluble growth factors, the interaction between similar and different types of cells, mechanical stimulus, and extracellular matrix proteins influence the differentiation of MSCs [26]. These cells are spindle-like in shape and can adhere to polymeric surfaces like plastic [27]. Antiplatelet adhesion property plays a significant role in the patency of the TEVGs after grafting. Based on platelet adhesion assay, MSCs, and ECs have similar antiplatelet adhesion properties [28].

The common precursors of immune cells and all blood lineages are hematopoietic stem cells (HSCs), which can differentiate into specific blood cells that monitor immune function, the balance of homeostasis, and response to microorganisms and inflammation [29, 30]. Till and McCulloch were the first to propose the idea of HSCs. The pioneering findings showed that single BM cells can regenerate and thus create the origin of multi-potential HSCs. It is only the cells in the hematopoietic system that have the ability for both multipotency and auto-renewal [29]. To repopulate decellularised canine carotid arteries, SMCs, and ECs were isolated from canine HSCs. The fabricated TEVGs had a suture strength that is equivalent to innate carotid arteries and the grafts remained patent for 8 weeks post-surgery in a canine model [31].

The successful reprogramming of human pluripotent stem cells (iPSCs) shows impressive self-renewability and differentiability into virtually any type of somatic cells, including vascular smooth muscle cells and endothelial cells [29, 32]. Human iPSCs could be a possible cell source for large-scale production of TEVGs, with comparable abilities and immune compatibility to the host [32]. The discovery of iPSCs has provided us with unique access to early human blood production as well as an endless supply of clinically relevant cells that could be used in immunotherapies [30]. Autologous iPSCs can be directly derived from a patient's somatic cells and applied to TEVG fabrication to avoid future immunogenic issues. However, due to the time-consuming iPSCs production, the application of autologous iPSCs for TEVG generation is still impractical in clinical use [32].

Endothelial progenitor cells (EPCs) population can be successfully isolated from peripheral blood-derived mononuclear cells from healthy subjects, utilizing magnetic bead, positive selection of two cell surface antigens which are CD34 and CD309 [33]. Amongst phenotypically diverse progeny of EPCs, a rarely isolated sub-population, which is around 1 to 4 cells/ml is termed blood outgrowth endothelial cells (BOECs), or endothelial colony forming cells that are particularly attractive in vascular tissue engineering applications [34, 35]. Attractive BOECs features, making it a favorable TEVG design, include a high proliferation rate, robust expansion potential, and simple sourcing *via* venepuncture. Venepunctures are far less risky than isolating ECs from the surplus tissue [34]. A few colonies reach confluency in minimal time from its higher proliferation rate and expansion potential. Thus BOECs seem like a quintessential cell candidate for vascular tissue engineering applications.

Strategies in Vascular Graft Improvement

Naturally-derived materials are well-suited for vascular graft development due to their biodegradable properties and good compatibility with the human mechanism rather than synthetic materials. Graft fabricated or incorporated with natural ingredients could easily integrate with the native vessel [36]. Plant-derived molecules are enriched with antioxidant, anti-inflammatory, and antiatherogenic properties. Their vascular protective nature makes them a suitable candidate to be incorporated in tissue-engineered vascular grafts (TEVGs).

Plant-base Compounds

Polyphenols are abundantly distributed in green plants, tea leaves, olives, and fruits. Recent studies had uncovered their potential as antioxidant, anti-inflammatory, and vascular protection properties [37]. For instance, Hydroxytyrosol (HT) a major polyphenol present in olive oil is extensively being studied for its cardioprotection ability. HT was proven to improve endothelial dysfunction and haemostatic profiles in vitro [38]. Hydroxytyrosol was also reported to positively regulate the antioxidant defence system in vascular endothelial cells (Fig. **2**). (ECs) [39]. Hydroxytyrosol promotes endothelial wound repair, increases cell proliferation and protects cells against H_2O_2 cytotoxicity through the activation of Akt and ERK1/2 [40, 41]. Interestingly, HT was also involved in the inhibition of platelet aggregation *via* a reduction of thromboxane synthesis and an increase in the production of nitric oxide [42].

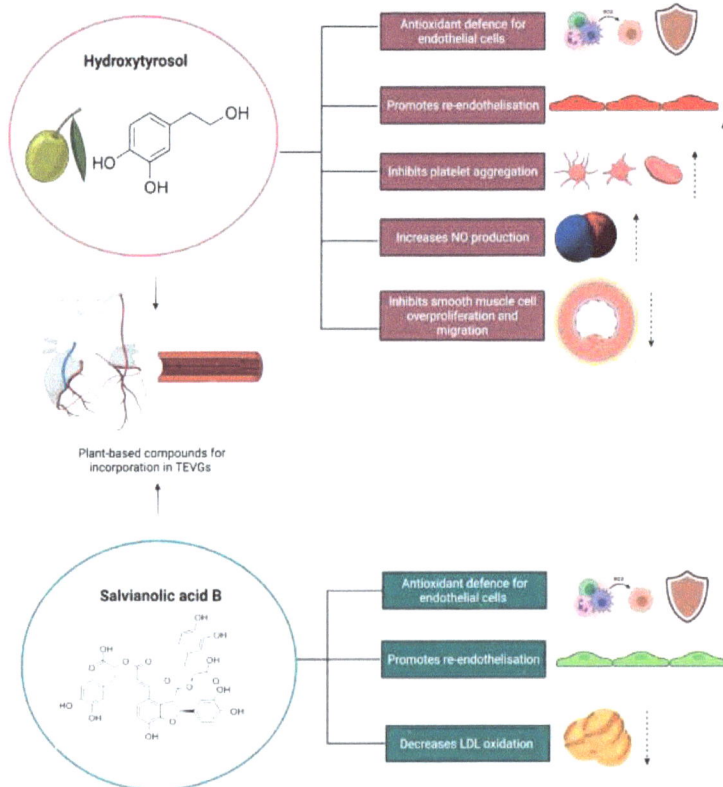

Fig. (2). Summary of plant-based compounds' properties for incorporation in TEVGs.

Neointimal hyperplasia is one of the reasons for TEVGs failures, where smooth muscle cells (SMCs) tend to migrate to the intimal region, a response triggered by ECs injury. Hydroxytyrosol was elucidated to inhibit the migration of SMCs [43]. Therefore, the incorporation of HT to the vascular graft could possibly reduce post grafting complications. Moreover, salvianolic acid B from the *Salvia miltiorrhiza* plant was also noted to prevent neointimal hyperplasia with apoptosis induction in over-proliferating cells by upregulating p53 expression levels [44]. In another study by Wang, salvianolic acid B performs reendothelisation with the help of EC in intimal hyperplasia by suppressing LDL oxidation through the reduction of ROS [45].

Drugs and Growth Factors

Growth factors for vascular graft have been studied over decades [34, 46, 47]. Usually, growth factors are incorporated as a coating on the luminal surface of the graft or in the production of the graft scaffold. Vascular endothelial growth factor VEGF is a crucial factor that is involved in angiogenesis [48, 49]. VEGF increased reendothelization, however, it also enhanced intimal hyperplasia in the rat model [48]. In contrast, recent research by Smith reported that VEGF enhanced ECs proliferation without any drawbacks. They elaborated that VEGF could capture flowing ECs from the blood and promote reendothelisation and subsequently increase the patency of acellular tissue-engineered vessels (A-TEVs) positioned into the arterial system of an ovine animal model [50].

Alongside this, Heparin, an anticoagulant was also utilized in TEVG fabrication to overcome complications such as thrombosis and restenosis. Researchers have developed a vascular graft by incorporating heparin into the lumen of ePTFE to increase the interaction with blood and cells. The graft successfully decreased platelet adhesion (Fig. **3**). whilst increasing EC and BOEC adhesion and proliferation, NO production, and expression of endothelial-specific markers [48]. Paclitaxel and Sirolimus are other antiproliferative agents that have also been reported to improve TEVG. Paclitaxel coated in the luminal part of the vascular graft effectively prevented the progression of neointimal hyperplasia while inhibiting a tiny amount of myofibroblast infiltration within the graft wall [51]. In the same manner, sirolimus-loaded hybrid tissue-engineered vascular graft (RM-HTEV) was fabricated by Yang *et al*. The drug-integrated nanofibrous layer shows greater mechanical strength and possesses slow drug releasing property which efficiently increases ECs proliferation, and migration with long-term patency [52].

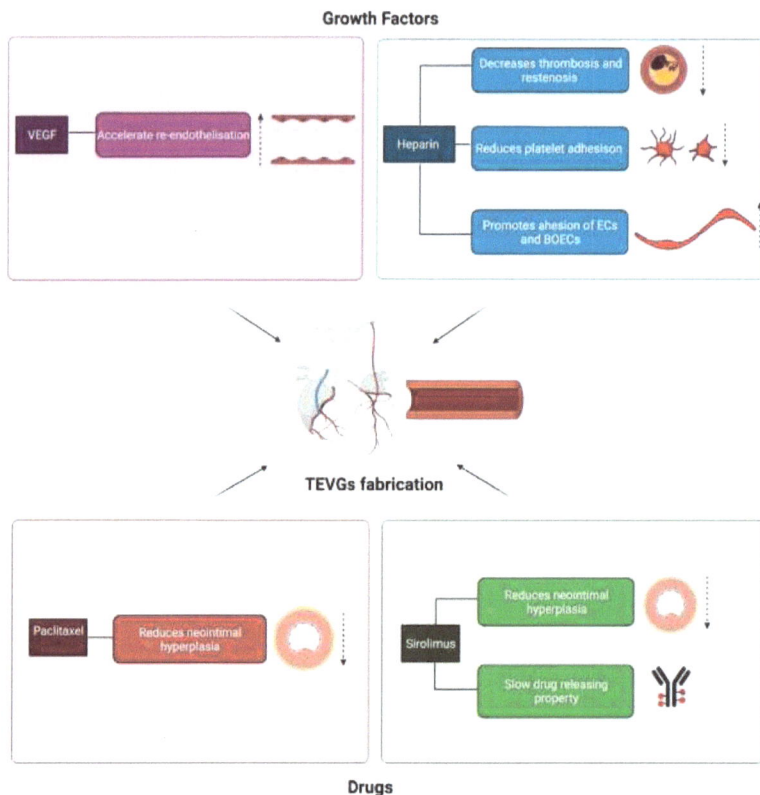

Fig. (3). A schematic illustration of growth factors and drugs properties for TEVGs fabrication.

CONCLUSION

The development of tissue-engineered vascular graft (TEVG) is a promising alternative to the current autologous graft. This chapter summarized cells, plant-base and growth factor-based approaches for the enhancement of TEVGs. Native cells such as Ecs, plant-based antioxidants and growth factors are among potential candidates to aid the revascularization of TEVGs while inhibiting thrombosis, platelet adhesion, and intimal hyperplasia formation. Hence, this approach could possibly ameliorate graft patency as well.

ACKNOWLEDGEMENT

All the authors would like to express our gratitude to the Faculty of Medicine, UKM, for guidance and resources to complete this review.

REFERENCES

[1]   Lozano R, Naghavi M, Foreman K, *et al.* Global and regional mortality from 235 causes of death for 20 age groups in 1990 and 2010: a systematic analysis for the Global Burden of Disease Study 2010.

Lancet 2012; 380(9859): 2095-128.
[http://dx.doi.org/10.1016/S0140-6736(12)61728-0] [PMID: 23245604]

[2]   Virani SS, Alonso A, Benjamin EJ, *et al.* Heart Disease and Stroke Statistics—2020 Update: A Report From the American Heart Association. Circulation 2020; 141(9): e139-596.
[http://dx.doi.org/10.1161/CIR.0000000000000757] [PMID: 31992061]

[3]   Abdulhannan P, Russell DA, Homer-Vanniasinkam S. Peripheral arterial disease: a literature review. Br Med Bull 2012; 104(1): 21-39.
[http://dx.doi.org/10.1093/bmb/lds027] [PMID: 23080419]

[4]   Mohr FW, Morice MC, Kappetein AP, *et al.* Coronary artery bypass graft surgery versus percutaneous coronary intervention in patients with three-vessel disease and left main coronary disease: 5-year follow-up of the randomised, clinical SYNTAX trial. Lancet 2013; 381(9867): 629-38.
[http://dx.doi.org/10.1016/S0140-6736(13)60141-5] [PMID: 23439102]

[5]   Weintraub WS, Grau-Sepulveda MV, Weiss JM, *et al.* Comparative effectiveness of revascularization strategies. N Engl J Med 2012; 366(16): 1467-76.
[http://dx.doi.org/10.1056/NEJMoa1110717] [PMID: 22452338]

[6]   Spadaccio C, Benedetto U. Coronary artery bypass grafting (CABG) *vs.* percutaneous coronary intervention (PCI) in the treatment of multivessel coronary disease: quo vadis? —a review of the evidences on coronary artery disease. Ann Cardiothorac Surg 2018; 7(4): 506-15.
[http://dx.doi.org/10.21037/acs.2018.05.17] [PMID: 30094215]

[7]   Harskamp RE, Lopes RD, Baisden CE, de Winter RJ, Alexander JH. Saphenous vein graft failure after coronary artery bypass surgery: pathophysiology, management, and future directions. Ann Surg 2013; 257(5): 824-33.
[http://dx.doi.org/10.1097/SLA.0b013e318288c38d] [PMID: 23574989]

[8]   Pashneh-Tala S, MacNeil S, Claeyssens F. The Tissue-Engineered Vascular Graft—Past, Present, and Future. Tissue Eng Part B Rev 2016; 22(1): 68-100.
[http://dx.doi.org/10.1089/ten.teb.2015.0100] [PMID: 26447530]

[9]   Conte MS. Critical appraisal of surgical revascularization for critical limb ischemia. J Vasc Surg 2013; 57(2) (Suppl.): 8S-13S.
[http://dx.doi.org/10.1016/j.jvs.2012.05.114] [PMID: 23336860]

[10]   Klinkert P, Post PN, Breslau PJ, van Bockel JH. Saphenous vein versus PTFE for above-knee femoropopliteal bypass. A review of the literature. Eur J Vasc Endovasc Surg 2004; 27(4): 357-62.
[http://dx.doi.org/10.1016/j.ejvs.2003.12.027] [PMID: 15015183]

[11]   Chelladurai P, Seeger W, Pullamsetti SS. Matrix metalloproteinases and their inhibitors in pulmonary hypertension. Eur Respir J 2012; 40(3): 766-82.
[http://dx.doi.org/10.1183/09031936.00209911] [PMID: 22523364]

[12]   Eble J, Niland S. The extracellular matrix of blood vessels. Curr Pharm Des 2009; 15(12): 1385-400.
[http://dx.doi.org/10.2174/138161209787846757] [PMID: 19355976]

[13]   Krüger-Genge A, Blocki A, Franke RP, Jung F. Vascular Endothelial Cell Biology: An Update. Int J Mol Sci 2019; 20(18): 4411.
[http://dx.doi.org/10.3390/ijms20184411] [PMID: 31500313]

[14]   Lu D, Kassab GS. Role of shear stress and stretch in vascular mechanobiology. J R Soc Interface 2011; 8(63): 1379-85.
[http://dx.doi.org/10.1098/rsif.2011.0177] [PMID: 21733876]

[15]   Bacakova L, Travnickova M, Filova E, Matějka R, Stepanovska J, Musilkova J, *et al.* The Role of Vascular Smooth Muscle Cells in the Physiology and Pathophysiology of Blood Vessels. Muscle Cell and Tissue - Current Status of Research Field 2018.
[http://dx.doi.org/10.5772/intechopen.77115]

[16]   Wang HD, Rätsep MT, Chapman A, Boyd R. Adventitial fibroblasts in vascular structure and

function: the role of oxidative stress and beyondThis review is one of a selection of papers published in a Special Issue on Oxidative Stress in Health and Disease. Can J Physiol Pharmacol 2010; 88(3): 177-86.
[http://dx.doi.org/10.1139/Y10-015] [PMID: 20393583]

[17] Chlupáč J, Filová E, Bačáková L. Blood vessel replacement: 50 years of development and tissue engineering paradigms in vascular surgery. Physiol Res 2009; 58 (Suppl. 2): S119-40.
[http://dx.doi.org/10.33549/physiolres.931918] [PMID: 20131930]

[18] Attwell D, Mishra A, Hall CN, O'Farrell FM, Dalkara T. What is a pericyte? J Cereb Blood Flow Metab 2016; 36(2): 451-5.
[http://dx.doi.org/10.1177/0271678X15610340] [PMID: 26661200]

[19] Brown LS, Foster CG, Courtney JM, King NE, Howells DW, Sutherland BA. Pericytes and Neurovascular Function in the Healthy and Diseased Brain. Front Cell Neurosci 2019; 13: 282.
[http://dx.doi.org/10.3389/fncel.2019.00282] [PMID: 31316352]

[20] Armulik A, Genové G, Betsholtz C. Pericytes: developmental, physiological, and pathological perspectives, problems, and promises. Dev Cell 2011; 21(2): 193-215.
[http://dx.doi.org/10.1016/j.devcel.2011.07.001] [PMID: 21839917]

[21] Wang Y, Yin P, Bian GL, *et al.* The combination of stem cells and tissue engineering: an advanced strategy for blood vessels regeneration and vascular disease treatment. Stem Cell Res Ther 2017; 8(1): 194.
[http://dx.doi.org/10.1186/s13287-017-0642-y] [PMID: 28915929]

[22] Jaganathan SK, Supriyanto E, Murugesan S, Balaji A, Asokan MK. Biomaterials in cardiovascular research: applications and clinical implications. BioMed Res Int 2014; 2014: 1-11.
[http://dx.doi.org/10.1155/2014/459465] [PMID: 24895577]

[23] Huang NF, Li S. Mesenchymal stem cells for vascular regeneration. Regen Med 2008; 3(6): 877-92.
[http://dx.doi.org/10.2217/17460751.3.6.877] [PMID: 18947310]

[24] Bajpai VK, Andreadis ST. Stem cell sources for vascular tissue engineering and regeneration. Tissue Eng Part B Rev 2012; 18(5): 405-25.
[http://dx.doi.org/10.1089/ten.teb.2011.0264] [PMID: 22571595]

[25] Rohban R, Pieber TR. Mesenchymal Stem and Progenitor Cells in Regeneration: Tissue Specificity and Regenerative Potential. Stem Cells Int 2017; 2017: 1-16.
[http://dx.doi.org/10.1155/2017/5173732] [PMID: 28286525]

[26] Leal BBJ, Wakabayashi N, Oyama K, Kamiya H, Braghirolli DI, Pranke P. Vascular Tissue Engineering: Polymers and Methodologies for Small Caliber Vascular Grafts. Front Cardiovasc Med 2021; 7: 592361.
[http://dx.doi.org/10.3389/fcvm.2020.592361] [PMID: 33585576]

[27] Homann M, Haehnel JC, Mendler N, *et al.* Reconstruction of the RVOT with valved biological conduits: 25 years experience with allografts and xenografts□. Eur J Cardiothorac Surg 2000; 17(6): 624-30.
[http://dx.doi.org/10.1016/S1010-7940(00)00414-0] [PMID: 10856850]

[28] Drews JD, Miyachi H, Shinoka T. Tissue-engineered vascular grafts for congenital cardiac disease: Clinical experience and current status. Trends Cardiovasc Med 2017; 27(8): 521-31.
[http://dx.doi.org/10.1016/j.tcm.2017.06.013] [PMID: 28754230]

[29] Hadinata IE, Hayward PAR, Hare DL, *et al.* Choice of conduit for the right coronary system: 8-year analysis of Radial Artery Patency and Clinical Outcomes trial. Ann Thorac Surg 2009; 88(5): 1404-9.
[http://dx.doi.org/10.1016/j.athoracsur.2009.06.010] [PMID: 19853082]

[30] Shah PJ, Bui K, Blackmore S, *et al.* Has the in situ right internal thoracic artery been overlooked? An angiographic study of the radial artery, internal thoracic arteries and saphenous vein graft patencies in symptomatic patients. Eur J Cardiothorac Surg 2005; 27(5): 870-5.

[http://dx.doi.org/10.1016/j.ejcts.2005.01.027] [PMID: 15848328]

[31]   Giannico S, Hammad F, Amodeo A, *et al.* Clinical outcome of 193 extracardiac Fontan patients: the first 15 years. J Am Coll Cardiol 2006; 47(10): 2065-73.
[http://dx.doi.org/10.1016/j.jacc.2005.12.065] [PMID: 16697327]

[32]   Chard RB, Johnson DC, Nunn GR, Cartmill TB. Aorta-coronary bypass grafting with polytetrafluoroethylene conduits. J Thorac Cardiovasc Surg 1987; 94(1): 132-4.
[http://dx.doi.org/10.1016/S0022-5223(19)36328-7] [PMID: 3496497]

[33]   PMC E. Europe PMC [Internet]. Europepmc.org. 2022 [cited 18 February 2022]. Available from: https://europepmc.org/article/MED/6336584

[34]   Braghirolli DI, Helfer VE, Chagastelles PC, Dalberto TP, Gamba D, Pranke P. Electrospun scaffolds functionalized with heparin and vascular endothelial growth factor increase the proliferation of endothelial progenitor cells. Biomed Mater 2017; 12(2): 025003.
[http://dx.doi.org/10.1088/1748-605X/aa5bbc] [PMID: 28140340]

[35]   Sarkar S, Sales KM, Hamilton G, Seifalian AM. Addressing thrombogenicity in vascular graft construction. J Biomed Mater Res B Appl Biomater 2007; 82B(1): 100-8.
[http://dx.doi.org/10.1002/jbm.b.30710] [PMID: 17078085]

[36]   Naito Y, Shinoka T, Duncan D, *et al.* Vascular tissue engineering: Towards the next generation vascular grafts. Adv Drug Deliv Rev 2011; 63(4-5): 312-23.
[http://dx.doi.org/10.1016/j.addr.2011.03.001] [PMID: 21421015]

[37]   Bazal P, Gea A, Martínez-González MA, *et al.* Mediterranean alcohol-drinking pattern, low to moderate alcohol intake and risk of atrial fibrillation in the PREDIMED study. Nutr Metab Cardiovasc Dis 2019; 29(7): 676-83.
[http://dx.doi.org/10.1016/j.numecd.2019.03.007] [PMID: 31078364]

[38]   Tejada S, Pinya S, Del Mar Bibiloni M, Tur JA, Pons A, Sureda A. Cardioprotective Effects of the Polyphenol Hydroxytyrosol from Olive Oil. Curr Drug Targets 2017; 18(13): 1477-86.
[PMID: 27719659]

[39]   Storniolo CE, Sacanella I, Mitjavila MT, Lamuela-Raventos RM, Moreno JJ. Bioactive Compounds of Cooked Tomato Sauce Modulate Oxidative Stress and Arachidonic Acid Cascade Induced by Oxidized LDL in Macrophage Cultures. Nutrients 2019; 11(8): 1880.
[http://dx.doi.org/10.3390/nu11081880] [PMID: 31412595]

[40]   Cheng Y, Qu Z, Fu X, Jiang Q, Fei J. Hydroxytyrosol contributes to cell proliferation and inhibits apoptosis in pulsed electromagnetic fields treated human umbilical vein endothelial cells in vitro. Mol Med Rep 2017; 16(6): 8826-32.
[http://dx.doi.org/10.3892/mmr.2017.7701] [PMID: 28990042]

[41]   Pereira-Caro G, Mateos R, Sarria B, Cert R, Goya L, Bravo L. Hydroxytyrosyl acetate contributes to the protective effects against oxidative stress of virgin olive oil. Food Chem 2012; 131(3): 869-78.
[http://dx.doi.org/10.1016/j.foodchem.2011.09.068]

[42]   de Roos B, Zhang X, Rodriguez Gutierrez G, *et al.* Anti-platelet effects of olive oil extract: in vitro functional and proteomic studies. Eur J Nutr 2011; 50(7): 553-62.
[http://dx.doi.org/10.1007/s00394-010-0162-3] [PMID: 21197537]

[43]   Zrelli H, Matsuka M, Araki M, Zarrouk M, Miyazaki H. Hydroxytyrosol induces vascular smooth muscle cells apoptosis through NO production and PP2A activation with subsequent inactivation of Akt. Planta Med 2011; 77(15): 1680-6.
[http://dx.doi.org/10.1055/s-0030-1271073] [PMID: 21590650]

[44]   Huang J, Qin Y, Liu B, Li G, Ouyang L, Wang J. In silicoanalysis and experimental validation of molecular mechanisms of salvianolic acid A-inhibited LPS-stimulated inflammation, in RAW264.7 macrophages. Cell Proliferation. 2013. :n/a-n/a.

[45]   Yang M, You F, Wang Z, Liu X, Wang Y. Salvianolic acid B improves the disruption of high glucose-

mediated brain microvascular endothelial cells *via* the ROS/HIF-1α/VEGF and miR-200b/VEGF signaling pathways. Neurosci Lett 2016; 630: 233-40.
[http://dx.doi.org/10.1016/j.neulet.2016.08.005] [PMID: 27497919]

[46] Nishibe T, Okuda Y, Kumada T, Tanabe T, Yasuda K. Enhanced graft healing of high-porosity expanded polytetrafluoroethylene grafts by covalent bonding of fibronectin. Surg Today 2000; 30(5): 426-31.
[http://dx.doi.org/10.1007/s005950050616] [PMID: 10819478]

[47] Iijima M, Aubin H, Steinbrink M, *et al.* Bioactive coating of decellularized vascular grafts with a temperature-sensitive VEGF-conjugated hydrogel accelerates autologous endothelialization *in vivo*. J Tissue Eng Regen Med 2018; 12(1): e513-22.
[http://dx.doi.org/10.1002/term.2321] [PMID: 27689942]

[48] Kliche S, Waltenberger J. VEGF Receptor Signaling and Endothelial Function IUBMB Life (International Union of Biochemistry and Molecular Biology: Life) 2001; 52(1): 61-6.

[49] Burlacu A, Grigorescu G, Rosca AM, Preda MB, Simionescu M. Factors secreted by mesenchymal stem cells and endothelial progenitor cells have complementary effects on angiogenesis in vitro. Stem Cells Dev 2013; 22(4): 643-53.
[http://dx.doi.org/10.1089/scd.2012.0273] [PMID: 22947186]

[50] Smith RJ Jr, Yi T, Nasiri B, Breuer CK, Andreadis ST. Implantation of VEGF□functionalized cell-free vascular grafts: regenerative and immunological response. FASEB J 2019; 33(4): 5089-100.
[http://dx.doi.org/10.1096/fj.201801856R] [PMID: 30629890]

[51] Baek I, Hwang J, Park J, Kim H, Park JS, Kim DJ. Paclitaxel coating on the terminal portion of hemodialysis grafts effectively suppresses neointimal hyperplasia in a porcine model. J Vasc Surg 2015; 61(6): 1575-1582.e1.
[http://dx.doi.org/10.1016/j.jvs.2014.01.033] [PMID: 24581482]

[52] Yang Y, Lei D, Zou H, *et al.* Hybrid electrospun rapamycin-loaded small-diameter decellularized vascular grafts effectively inhibit intimal hyperplasia. Acta Biomater 2019; 97: 321-32.
[http://dx.doi.org/10.1016/j.actbio.2019.06.037] [PMID: 31523025]

SUBJECT INDEX

A

Acid(s) 4, 19, 58, 77, 80, 82, 84, 92, 99, 100, 104, 105, 122, 123, 125, 126, 145, 165, 177, 178, 179, 199, 216, 218, 224, 239, 240, 244, 245, 279
  acetic 82
  alginic 100
  aminolauric 4
  formic 77
  hyaluronic 84, 99, 104, 105, 177, 178, 224, 239, 240, 244
  lactic 92, 123, 178
  lactide 218
  nucleic 80
  polyglycolic (PGA) 92, 122, 123, 145, 179, 216
  polylactic 19, 84, 122, 123, 145, 165, 224
  salvianolic 279
  sebacic 125, 126
Activation 26, 129, 193, 276
  cellular 26, 276
  immune 129
  osteoclast 193
Adhesion 36, 37, 38, 102, 105, 107, 124, 125, 127, 128, 129, 143, 161, 164
  connective tissue 143
  protein 38
Aging population 141
Alginate, calcium 164
Anaerobic glycolysis 234
Analysis, thermogravimetric 224
Angiogenesis 40, 42, 173, 192, 195, 202, 204, 205, 279
Angiopoietin 194
Anti-inflammatory 27, 198, 223
  agents 27, 223
  cytokine 198
  response 27
Antibacterial 97, 98, 149, 176
  activity 98, 149
  agent 97

efficiency 176
Antimicrobial agents 149
Antioxidant 181, 277, 278
Antiplatelet adhesion properties 276
Apicoectomy 93
Apoptosis 27, 158, 161
Applications 92, 98, 165, 176
  arthroplasty 176
  dental 92
  endodontic 98
  ocular 165
Atherosclerosis 130, 131
Atom transfer radical polymerisation (ATRP) 36
Atomic force microscopy (AFM) 219

B

Bacterial nanocellulose 99
Balance, haemostatic 275
Bare-metal stents (BMS) 17
Biochemical signaling 120
Biodegradable 215, 277
  polymeric 215
  properties 277
Blood 236, 277
  nucleus barrier (BNB) 236
  outgrowth endothelial cells (BOECs) 277
Bone 8, 95, 141, 172, 173, 175, 178, 182, 183, 191, 192, 193, 195, 202, 203, 204, 263
  craniofacial 8
  defective 173
  defects 141, 172, 175, 182, 195, 202
  deficiencies 95
  formation, peroxide-induced 202
  fracture 172, 191, 193
  growth 193, 195, 203, 263
  lacunae formation 204
  loss, periodontitis-induced 95
  marrow stromal cells 178
  mineralisation 192

www.ingramcontent.com/pod-product-compliance
Lightning Source LLC
Chambersburg PA
CBHW050811220326
41598CB00006B/179